Diamond-based materials for biomedical applications

Related titles:

Surface modification of biomaterials: Methods analysis and applications
(ISBN 978-1-84569-640-5)

Coatings for biomedical applications
(ISBN 978-1-84569-568-2)

Biointegration of medical implant materials: Science and design
(ISBN 978-1-84569-509-5)

Details of these books and a complete list of titles from Woodhead Publishing can be obtained by:

- visiting our web site at www.woodheadpublishing.com
- contacting Customer Services (e-mail: sales@woodheadpublishing.com; fax: +44 (0) 1223 832819; tel.: +44 (0) 1223 499140 ext. 130; address: Woodhead Publishing Limited, 80 High Street, Sawston, Cambridge CB22 3HJ, UK)
- contacting our US office (e-mail: usmarketing@woodheadpublishing.com; tel.: (215) 928 9112; address: Woodhead Publishing, 1518 Walnut Street, Suite 1100, Philadelphia, PA 19102-3406, USA)

If you would like e-versions of our content, please visit our online platform: www.woodheadpublishingonline.com. Please recommend it to your librarian so that everyone in your institution can benefit from the wealth of content on the site.

We are always happy to receive suggestions for new books from potential editors. To enquire about contributing to our Biomaterials series, please send your name, contact address and details of the topic/s you are interested in to laura.overend@woodheadpublishing.com. We look forward to hearing from you.

The Woodhead team responsible for publishing this book:
Commissioning Editor: Laura Overend
Publications Coordinator: Adam Davies
Project Editor: Cathryn Freear
Editorial and Production Manager: Mary Campbell
Production Editor: Adam Hooper
Freelance Project Manager: Annette Wiseman
Copyeditor: Eilidh McGregor
Proofreader: Simon Webber
Cover Designer: Terry Callanan

Woodhead Publishing Series in Biomaterials: Number 55

Diamond-based materials for biomedical applications

Edited by

R. Narayan

WOODHEAD PUBLISHING

Oxford Cambridge Philadelphia New Delhi

Published by Woodhead Publishing Limited,
80 High Street, Sawston, Cambridge CB22 3HJ, UK
www.woodheadpublishing.com
www.woodheadpublishingonline.com

Woodhead Publishing, 1518 Walnut Street, Suite 1100, Philadelphia,
PA 19102-3406, USA

Woodhead Publishing India Private Limited, G-2, Vardaan House,
7/28 Ansari Road, Daryaganj, New Delhi – 110002, India
www.woodheadpublishingindia.com

First published 2013, Woodhead Publishing Limited

British Library Cataloguing in Publication Data
A catalogue record for this book is available from the British Library.

Library of Congress Control Number: 2012955384

ISBN 978-0-85709-340-0 (print)
ISBN 978-0-85709-351-6 (online)
ISSN 2049-9485 Woodhead Publishing Series in Biomaterials (print)
ISSN 2049-9493 Woodhead Publishing Series in Biomaterials (online)

The publisher's policy is to use permanent paper from mills that operate a sustainable forestry policy, and which has been manufactured from pulp which is processed using acid-free and elemental chlorine-free practices. Furthermore, the publisher ensures that the text paper and cover board used have met acceptable environmental accreditation standards.

Typeset by RefineCatch Limited, Bungay, Suffolk
Printed by MPG Printgroup, UK

Contents

Contributor contact details

(* = main contact)

Editor

Roger J. Narayan
Joint Department of Biomedical Engineering
University of North Carolina and North Carolina State University
Raleigh, NC
USA

E-mail: roger_narayan@unc.edu

Chapter 1

Roger J. Narayan* and Ryan D. Boehm
Joint Department of Biomedical Engineering
University of North Carolina and North Carolina State University
Raleigh, NC
USA

E-mail: roger_narayan@unc.edu

Anirudha V. Sumant
Center for Nanoscale Materials
Argonne National Laboratory
Argonne, IL
USA

E-mail: sumant@anl.gov

Chapter 2

Sabine Szunerits* and Rabah Boukherroub
Institut de Recherche Interdisciplinaire (IRI, USR 3078)
Université Lille1, Parc de la Haute Borne
50 Avenue de Halley – BP 70478
59658 Villeneuve d'Ascq
France

E-mail: Sabine.Szunerits@iri.univ-lille1.fr

Chapter 3

Margarida Amaral
Department of Material and Ceramics Engineering
University of Aveiro
3810-193 Aveiro
Portugal

E-mail: margarida.amaral@ua.pt

Chapter 4

Mariangela Fedel
Department of Industrial Engineering and BIOtech Research Centre on Biomedical Technologies
University of Trento, Italy
Via delle Regole 101
38123-I Mattarello
Trento
Italy

E-mail: mariangela.fedel@ing.unitn.it

Chapter 5

Shane A. Catledge*, Vinoy Thomas and Yogesh K. Vohra
University of Alabama at Birmingham
Center for Nanoscale Materials and Biointegration (CNMB)
Dept. of Physics
1300 University Blvd
310 Campbell Hall
Birmingham AL
35294-1170
USA

E-mail: catledge@uab.edu

Chapter 6

Orlando Auciello*
Materials Science Division
Argonne National Laboratory
9700 South Cass Av., Lemont
Illinois, 60439
USA

E-mail: auciello@anl.gov

and

University of Texas –Dallas
Department of Materials Science and Engineering and Department of Bioengineering
Box 830688 EC-32
Richardson
TX 75083-0688
USA

E-mail: orlando50@aol.com

Pablo Gurman
Materials Science Division
Argonne National Laboratory
9700 South Cass Av., Lemont
Illinois, 60439
USA

Alejandro Berra
Universidad Nacional de Buenos Aires
Facultad de Medicina
Uribury 950
Buenos Aires C1121ABG
Argentina

Mario Saravia
Hospital Austral
Av. Juan de Garay 125
Ciudad Autónoma de Buenos Aires, (C1063ABB) –
Pilar
Buenos Aires
Argentina

Roberto Zysler
Centro Atómico Bariloche
Av. Bustillos 9500
Bariloche, Rio Negro 8400
Argentina

Chapter 7

Ying-Chieh Chen*
Department of Applied Science
National Hsinchu University of Education
Hsin-Chu 300
Taiwan

E-mail: yingchiehchen@gmail.com

and

Department of Medicine
Center for Biomedical Engineering
Brigham and Women's Hospital
Harvard Medical School
Boston
MA 02115
USA

Don-Ching Lee
Institute of Cellular and System Medicine
National Health Research Institutes
Miaoli 350
Taiwan

Nyan-Hwa Tai
Department of Materials Science and Engineering
National Tsing-Hua University
Hsin-Chu 300
Taiwan

Ing-Ming Chiu
Institute of Cellular and System Medicine
National Health Research Institutes
Miaoli 350
Taiwan

and

Department of Life Sciences
National Chung Hsing University
Tai-Chung 420
Taiwan

and

Department of Internal Medicine
The Ohio State University
Columbus
OH 43210
USA

Chapter 8

Abebe E. Mengesha
College of Pharmacy & Health Sciences
Drake University
2507 University Avenue
Des Moines
IA 50311-4505
USA

Bi-Botti C. Youan*
Laboratory of Future Nanomedicines and Theoretical Chronopharmaceutics
University of Missouri-Kansas City
Kansas City
MO 64108
USA

E-mail: youanb@umkc.edu

Chapter 9

Alexander Kromka*, Oleg Babchenko, Tibor Izak, Stepan Potocky, Marian Varga, Bohuslav Rezek, Alexej Sveshnikov and Pavel Demo
Institute of Physics
Academy of Sciences of the Czech Republic, v.v.i.
Cukrovarnická 10
Praha 6,162 00
Czech Republic

E-mail: kromka@fzu.cz

Chapter 10

Dr Anna Karczemska
Technical University of Lodz
Institute of Turbomachinery
Poland

E-mail: anna.karczemska@p.lodz.pl

Woodhead Publishing Series in Biomaterials

1 **Sterilisation of tissues using ionising radiations**
Edited by J. F. Kennedy, G. O. Phillips and P. A. Williams

2 **Surfaces and interfaces for biomaterials**
Edited by P. Vadgama

3 **Molecular interfacial phenomena of polymers and biopolymers**
Edited by C. Chen

4 **Biomaterials, artificial organs and tissue engineering**
Edited by L. Hench and J. Jones

5 **Medical modelling**
R. Bibb

6 **Artificial cells, cell engineering and therapy**
Edited by S. Prakash

7 **Biomedical polymers**
Edited by M. Jenkins

8 **Tissue engineering using ceramics and polymers**
Edited by A. R. Boccaccini and J. Gough

9 **Bioceramics and their clinical applications**
Edited by T. Kokubo

10 **Dental biomaterials**
Edited by R. V. Curtis and T. F. Watson

11 **Joint replacement technology**
Edited by P. A. Revell

12 **Natural-based polymers for biomedical applications**
Edited by R. L. Reiss et al

13 **Degradation rate of bioresorbable materials**
Edited by F. J. Buchanan

14 **Orthopaedic bone cements**
Edited by S. Deb

15 **Shape memory alloys for biomedical applications**
Edited by T. Yoneyama and S. Miyazaki

16 **Cellular response to biomaterials**
Edited by L. Di Silvio

17 **Biomaterials for treating skin loss**
Edited by D. P. Orgill and C. Blanco

18 **Biomaterials and tissue engineering in urology**
Edited by J. Denstedt and A. Atala

19 **Materials science for dentistry**
B. W. Darvell

20 **Bone repair biomaterials**
Edited by J. A. Planell, S. M. Best, D. Lacroix and A. Merolli
21 **Biomedical composites**
Edited by L. Ambrosio
22 **Drug-device combination products**
Edited by A. Lewis
23 **Biomaterials and regenerative medicine in ophthalmology**
Edited by T. V. Chirila
24 **Regenerative medicine and biomaterials for the repair of connective tissues**
Edited by C. Archer and J. Ralphs
25 **Metals for biomedical devices**
Edited by M. Ninomi
26 **Biointegration of medical implant materials: science and design**
Edited by C. P. Sharma
27 **Biomaterials and devices for the circulatory system**
Edited by T. Gourlay and R. Black
28 **Surface modification of biomaterials: methods analysis and applications**
Edited by R. Williams
29 **Biomaterials for artificial organs**
Edited by M. Lysaght and T. Webster
30 **Injectable biomaterials: science and applications**
Edited by B. Vernon
31 **Biomedical hydrogels: biochemistry, manufacture and medical applications**
Edited by S. Rimmer
32 **Preprosthetic and maxillofacial surgery: biomaterials, bone grafting and tissue engineering**
Edited by J. Ferri and E. Hunziker
33 **Bioactive materials in medicine: design and applications**
Edited by X. Zhao, J. M. Courtney and H. Qian
34 **Advanced wound repair therapies**
Edited by D. Farrar
35 **Electrospinning for tissue regeneration**
Edited by L. Bosworth and S. Downes
36 **Bioactive glasses: materials, properties and applications**
Edited by H. O. Ylänen
37 **Coatings for biomedical applications**
Edited by M. Driver
38 **Progenitor and stem cell technologies and therapies**
Edited by A. Atala
39 **Biomaterials for spinal surgery**
Edited by L. Ambrosio and E. Tanner
40 **Minimized cardiopulmonary bypass techniques and technologies**
Edited by T. Gourlay and S. Gunaydin
41 **Wear of orthopaedic implants and artificial joints**
Edited by S. Affatato
42 **Biomaterials in plastic surgery: breast implants**
Edited by W. Peters, H. Brandon, K. L. Jerina, C. Wolf and V. L. Young
43 **MEMS for biomedical applications**
Edited by S. Bhansali and A. Vasudev

44 **Durability and reliability of medical polymers**
Edited by M. Jenkins and A. Stamboulis
45 **Biosensors for medical applications**
Edited by S. Higson
46 **Sterilisation of biomaterials and medical devices**
Edited by S. Lerouge and A. Simmons
47 **The hip resurfacing handbook: a practical guide to the use and management of modern hip resurfacings**
Edited by K. De Smet, P. Campbell and C. Van Der Straeten
48 **Developments in tissue engineered and regenerative medicine products**
J. Basu and J. W. Ludlow
49 **Nanomedicine: technologies and applications**
Edited by T. J. Webster
50 **Biocompatibility and performance of medical devices**
Edited by J-P. Boutrand
51 **Medical robotics: minimally invasive surgery**
Edited by P. Gomes
52 **Implantable sensor systems for medical applications**
Edited by A. Inmann and D. Hodgins
53 **Non-metallic biomaterials for tooth repair and replacement**
Edited by P. Vallittu
54 **Joining and assembly of medical materials and devices**
Edited by Y. Norman Zhou and M. D. Breyen
55 **Diamond-based materials for biomedical applications**
Edited by R. Narayan
56 **Nanomaterials in tissue engineering: fabrication and applications**
Edited by A. K. Gaharwar, S. Sant, M. J. Hancock and S. A. Hacking
57 **Biomimetic biomaterials: structure and applications**
Edited by A. Ruys
58 **Standardisation in cell and tissue engineering: methods and protocols**
Edited by V. Salih
59 **Inhaler devices: fundamentals, design and drug delivery**
Edited by P. Prokopovich
60 **Bio-tribocorrosion in biomaterials and medical implants**
Edited by Yu Yan
61 **Microfluidics for biomedical applications**
Edited by X-J. James Li and Y. Zhou
62 **Decontamination in hospitals and healthcare**
Edited by J. T. Walker
63 **Biomedical imaging: applications and advances**
Edited by P. Morris
64 **Characterization of biomaterials**
Edited by M. Jaffe, W. Hammond, P. Tolias and T. Arinzeh

Part I

Introduction to diamond-based materials for medical applications

1

Introduction to medical applications of diamond particles and surfaces*

R. J. NARAYAN and R. D. BOEHM, University of North Carolina and North Carolina State University, USA
and A. V. SUMANT, Argonne National Laboratory, USA

DOI: 10.1533/9780857093516.1.3

Abstract: Diamond has been considered for use in several medical applications due to its unique mechanical, chemical, optical, and biological properties. In this chapter, methods for preparing synthetic diamond surfaces and particles are described. In addition, recent developments involving the use of diamond in prostheses, sensing, imaging, and drug delivery applications are reviewed. These developments suggest that diamond-containing structures will provide significant improvements in the diagnosis and treatment of medical conditions over the coming years.

Key words: microcrystalline diamond, nanocrystalline diamond, nanodiamond, biocompatibility, medical applications.

1.1 Introduction

Diamond is an allotrope of carbon that is being considered for use in several medical applications.[1] Ramachandran determined that the crystal structure of diamond consists of two close packed interpenetrating face centered cubic lattices; one lattice is shifted with respect to the other along the elemental cube space diagonal by one-quarter of its length.[2] If one approximates carbon atoms as equal diameter rigid spheres, the filling of this construction is 34%.[3] Due to the carbon–carbon distance (1.54 A), diamond crystal exhibits the highest atomic density (1.76×10^{23} cm^{-3}) of any solid. The very high bond energy between two carbon atoms (83 kcal/mol) and the directionality of tetrahedral bonds are the main reasons for the high strength of diamond. Diamond demonstrates the highest Vickers hardness value of all materials (10 000 kg/mm^2). The tribological properties of diamond are also impressive; the coefficient of friction of polished diamond is 0.07 in argon and 0.05 in humid air. Diamond is resistant to corrosion except in an oxygen atmosphere at temperatures over 800°C. In addition, type IIa diamond exhibits the highest thermal conductivity of all materials (20 W cm^{-1} K^{-1} at room temperature).

* Please note that this chapter was originally published in *Materials Today*, 14(4), Narayan, R. J., Boehm, R. D. and Sumant, A. V., 'Medical applications of diamond particles and surfaces', 154–163, Copyright (2011), and is reused here with permission from Elsevier.

1.2 Growth of synthetic diamond

The graphite-diamond transformation at thermodynamic equilibrium necessitates the use of very high temperatures and pressures. Bundy *et al.* at General Electric developed a high pressure–high temperature approach for creating diamond from graphite in the 1950s.[4] This technique creates small diamond crystals that are commonly utilized for polishing, cutting, and grinding. Growth of diamond coatings at low pressure using hydrocarbon pyrolysis was first reported by Eversole *et al.* at Union Carbide in 1962.[5] In the late 1960s and early 1970s, Derjaguin *et al.* and Angus *et al.* introduced the concept of activating a mixture containing hydrogen and a hydrocarbon gas for low-pressure chemical vapor deposition of diamond coatings.[6,7] For example, Angus *et al.* demonstrated deposition of diamond layers on natural diamond powder by thermal decomposition of methane at a temperature of 1050°C and a pressure of 0.3 Torr.[7] In these methods, diamond coatings are grown from an activated gas phase; this phase contains hydrogen (~99%) as well as methane or other carbon-containing gases. Activation of the gas commonly involves the use of a hot filament, combustion flame, plasma, or a combination of these approaches. Diamond coatings are formed by the decomposition of activated hydrocarbon species into excited carbon atoms. Diamond coatings are commonly deposited on metallic substrates for minimizing wear, corrosion, and metal release; for example, a diamond-coated metallic implant will behave mechanically as the metallic substrate and chemically as the diamond coating.

Several parameters must be considered in deposition of microcrystalline diamond coatings. Hydrogen serves several roles, including termination of carbon dangling bonds, stabilization of diamond clusters, removal of sp^2-hybridized carbon from the surface, and abstraction of hydrogen from carbon–hydrogen bonds on the surface.[8] The chemical properties of the substrate regulate the structure of the diamond coating.[9] Diamond coating growth on cobalt, ferrous alloys, and nickel alloys is challenging because nucleation of diamond is hindered by high carbon diffusion rates within these materials.[10] Formation of graphite is commonly observed on copper and other elements that contain partially filled electron shells.

Growth of microcrystalline diamond on non-diamond surfaces involves scratching of the substrate to promote diamond nucleation and/or use of an interlayer between the diamond coating and the non-diamond substrate. Ultrasonic seeding of the substrate with ultradispersed detonation diamond has also been used to increase nucleation of diamond.[11,12] It should be noted that scratching may alter the surface in a poorly defined manner; non-uniform features may limit use of the coated material in medical applications. In addition, heterogeneous films containing diamond and graphitic carbon may be created on substrates that are scratched with diamond paste.[13]

An interlayer material (e.g. titanium nitride, aluminum nitride, and tungsten carbide) can promote diamond nucleation and facilitate coating adhesion through relief of interfacial stresses.[14] Properties of the interlayer material include: a similar thermal expansion coefficient value to that of diamond for reducing thermal stresses; low diffusivity of carbon for increasing diamond nucleation; and small lattice mismatch with diamond as well as with the bulk material. Silicon nitride is frequently utilized as a bulk material due to the fact that it exhibits a low coefficient of thermal expansion. In addition, silicon nitride exhibits high fracture toughness and high hardness values.[15,16] Furthermore, silicon nitride is compatible with diamond CVD deposition temperatures (650–1000°C).

Significant academic and industrial research activities are under way to create nanocrystalline diamond coatings. The term nanocrystalline diamond is utilized for describing materials that contain grain sizes below 100 nm, usually 10–100 nm (Fig. 1.1).[17] The mechanism for nanocrystalline diamond growth, which involves a hydrogen-rich growth chemistry, is similar to that for microcrystalline diamond or polycrystalline diamond growth. Competitive crystal growth results in a columnar texture that is oriented in the growth direction and coarsening grain sizes with film thickness (van der Drift growth). By controlling the initial nucleation density and the growth parameters, one can limit re-nucleation density and maintain grain sizes from 10 nm to 100 nm for nanocrystalline diamond films up to a few micrometers in thickness. When film thickness exceeds a few micrometers, nanocrystalline diamond becomes conventional microcrystalline diamond; in this situation, roughness increases with film thickness.

Nanocrystalline diamond coatings exhibit small crystallite sizes; these materials are considered to be appropriate for tribological applications due to their relatively smooth surfaces. Amaral *et al.* examined the wear behavior of nanocrystalline

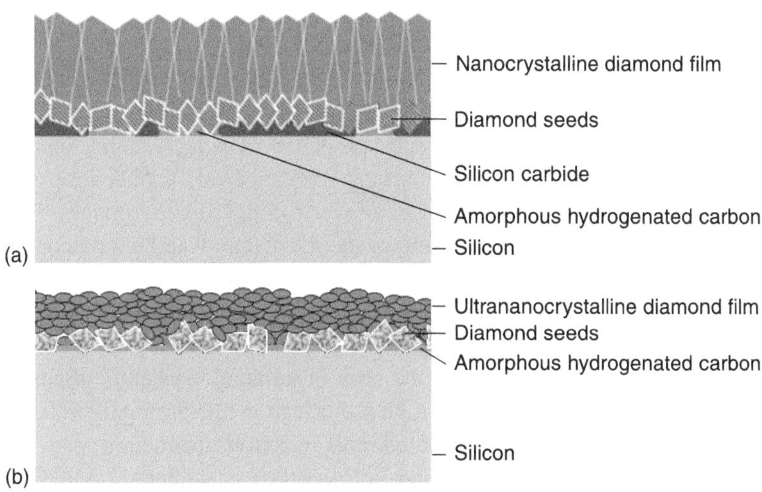

1.1 Schematic explaining the possible nucleation mechanisms of (a) nanocrystalline diamond and (b) ultrananocrystalline diamond. Reprinted from Butler and Sumant[17] with permission of the author.

diamond; steady-state friction coefficients of 0.01–0.05 in unlubricated environments and water-lubricated environments were observed.[18] The wear rate under water lubrication was $1.9 \times 10^{-10} mm^3 N^{-1} m^{-1}$; testing in Hank's balanced salt solution revealed similar friction (0.06) and wear data. Testing in dilute fetal bovine serum revealed a higher coefficient of friction (0.10); this finding was associated with protein attachment. Wear behavior in Ringer's solution and synthetic serum was impressive; final wear rates of $\sim 10^{-10} mm^3 N^{-1} m^{-1}$ were obtained.

The term ultrananocrystalline diamond was coined by researchers at Argonne National Laboratory to distinguish their form of diamond from other forms of diamond on the basis of grain size. Ultrananocrystalline diamond contains grains with sizes below 10 nm, usually between 2 nm and 5 nm. Ninety-five to ninety-eight percent of the material, in the form of sp^3-hybridized carbon, is found in these grains; the remaining material, in the form of sp^2-hybridized carbon, resides at atomically abrupt grain boundaries.[19,20] Ultrananocrystalline diamond films are produced in an argon-rich, hydrogen-deficient environment using microwave plasma-enhanced chemical vapor deposition. Films grown from plasmas containing ~99% argon and ~1% methane are able to grow directly on SiO_2 as carbon dimers (C_2) form a silicon carbide nucleation layer. Work by Sumant *et al.* and Naguib *et al.* has indicated that a tungsten interlayer reduces the incubation time for diamond nucleation due to the low diffusion coefficient of carbon in tungsten; as a result, ultrananocrystalline diamond coatings may be grown with lower surface roughness values (4–6 nm), lower thickness values, and an absence of interfacial voids.[21,22] High re-nucleation ($\sim 10^{11} cm^{-2} s^{-1}$) and minimal re-gasification of small grains occur due to a limited amount of hydrogen in the plasma.[19,20] In addition, ultrananocrystalline diamond can be deposited at temperatures as low as 400°C, facilitating use of this material in complementary metal-oxide-semiconductor (CMOS)-compatible microelectromechanical systems (MEMS) or nanoelectromechanical systems (NEMS).[23]

The exceptional chemical and physical properties of nanocrystalline diamond and ultrananocrystalline diamond determine the medical applications of these materials.[19,20] The chemical and physical properties of nanocrystalline diamond and ultrananocrystalline diamond determine the medical applications of these materials.[19,20] Figure 1.2 shows scanning electron microscopy images that depict typical surface morphologies of nanocrystalline diamond and ultrananocrystalline diamond films, respectively.[23,24] There is a distinct difference in surface morphologies of nanocrystalline diamond and ultrananocrystalline diamond films. Nanocrystalline diamond shows some grain faceting along with some secondary nucleation. On the other hand, no grain faceting can be seen in ultrananocrystalline diamond; this morphology is attributed to a very high re-nucleation rate during film growth.

Figure 1.3(a) contains a selected area electron diffraction pattern for a nanocrystalline diamond coating on a silicon (100) substrate; (111), (022), (113), (222), (004), and (133) reflections of cubic diamond were observed.[25] The bright ring was assigned to diamond-like carbon and/or amorphous glassy carbon within the coating. No significant scattering attributable to graphite crystallites was

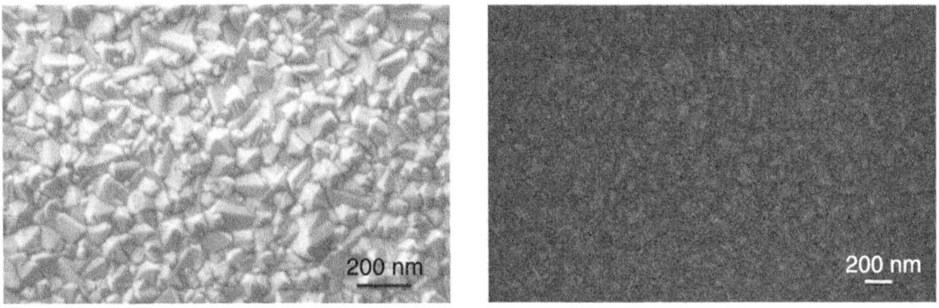

(a) (b)

1.2 Scanning electron micrograph images depicting typical surface morphologies of (a) nanocrystalline diamond and (b) ultrananocrystalline diamond films. Reprinted from Sumant *et al.* (2010, 2007)[23,24] with permission of the author.

noted. Grain boundaries of ~1 nm and 2–4 nm rectangular crystallites were noted in the transmission electron micrograph (Fig. 1.3(b)).

Nanodiamond particles may be produced using a variety of methods. Detonation nanodiamond was originally produced in the Soviet Union.[26] Nanodiamond particles are commonly prepared by detonating carbon-containing explosives under a rapid

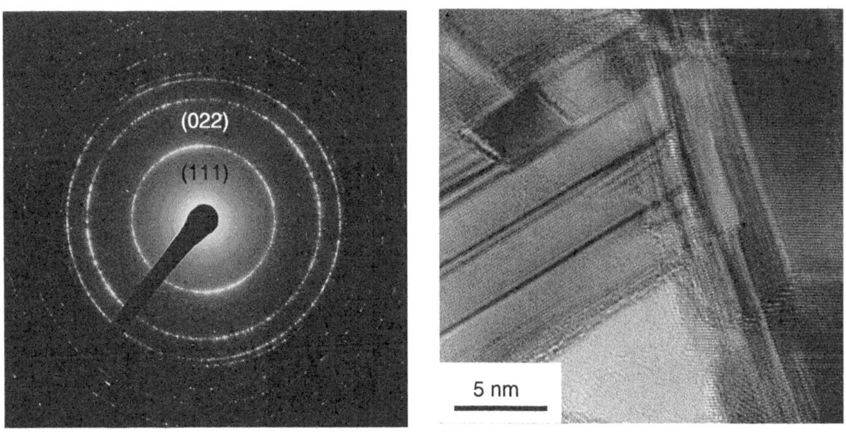

(a) (b)

1.3 (a) Selected area electron diffraction pattern of the nanocrystalline diamond coating. In this image, sharp Bragg reflections from the first two planes are indicated. The rings were indexed as (111), (022), (113), (222), (004), and (133) from the diamond cubic structure. The bright ring around the center represents the amorphous glassy carbon or diamond-like carbon material. (b) High-resolution transmission electron micrograph of the nanocrystalline diamond coating. Rectangular crystallites were observed (with a size of 2–4 nm). Reprinted from Narayan, *et al.*[25] with permission from Elsevier.

cooling rate (≥3000 K/min); the resulting polyhedral structures exhibit a narrow particle size distribution and a small particle size (3.5–6 nm).[27,28] A cooling gas (e.g. carbon dioxide or an inert gas) is used to prevent the formation of graphite and other non-diamond materials.[29] After synthesis, removal of non-diamond non-carbon impurities by means of acid washing, ball milling, and/or batch ultrasonication is performed.[30] For example, Adadurov *et al.* described preparation of nanodiamond particles using either an X-ray-amorphous form of carbon (e.g. carbon black) or graphite; explosives (e.g. PETN and hexogen) were used to create temperatures of 2000–6000°C and dynamic pressures of 3–60 GPa.[26] Figure 1.4 shows transmission

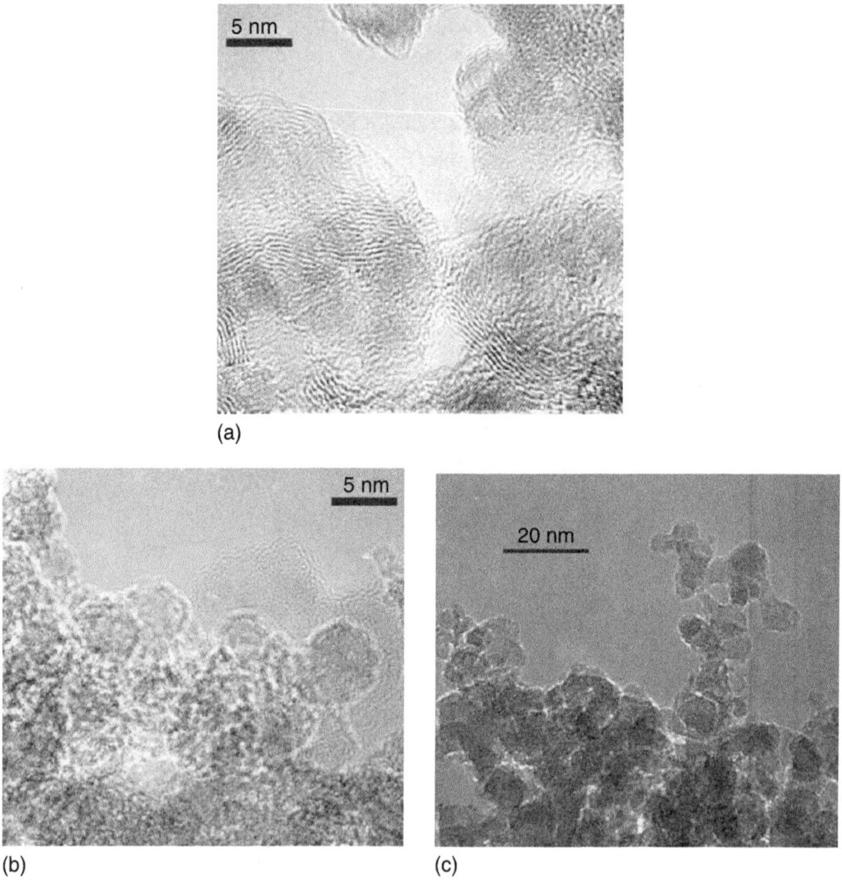

1.4 Transmission electron microscopy photographs (200 keV) of nanodiamond aggregate (NDA): (a) pristine material (sample N2 in the source manuscript) (soot), (b) pristine material (N4 in the source manuscript) after washing with hot nitric acid, (c) a recent commercial product (B2 in the source manuscript). Reprinted from Krueger *et al.*[28] with permission from Elsevier.

electron micrographs of nanodiamond aggregates, including (a) pristine raw soot, (b) pristine soot after washing with hot nitric acid, and (c) a commercially available product. Krueger *et al.* described the use of stirred-media milling with ceramic beads (with a diameter of 0.1 mm) in order to obtain four to five nanodiamond particles.[28] High temperature–high pressure growth combined with ball milling may also be used to prepare ≥4 nm nanodiamond particles.[31]

1.3 Diamond-based medical devices

Diamond coatings have been applied to a number of medical devices in recent years, including temporomandibular joint prostheses, heart valves, and microelectromechanical systems, for the purpose of extending implant lifetime. Fries *et al.* performed microwave plasma chemical vapor deposition of 3 μm-thick nanostructured diamond films on objects that were similar in shape to components of temporomandibular joint prostheses.[32] Raman spectroscopy was used to demonstrate the uniform chemical composition of the nanostructured diamond coating on the surface of the titanium–aluminum–vanadium alloy condyle component. Nanoindentation hardness measurements showed that coating hardness was 60 ± 5 GPa. Papo *et al.* deposited single layer nanocrystalline diamond films and multilayer nanocrystalline/microcrystalline/nanocrystalline diamond films on Ti-6Al-4V components, which were similar in shape to the fossa and condyle components of a temporomandibular joint prosthesis.[33] Wear testing in a mandibular movement simulator corresponding to two years of clinical use was performed; micro-Raman scans of the wear-tested components revealed no film loss and some film damage. The multilayer nanocrystalline/microcrystalline/nanocrystalline diamond film showed better wear resistance than the single layer nanocrystalline diamond film.

Jozwik *et al.* deposited nanocrystalline diamond on an artificial heart valve ring using plasma-assisted chemical vapor deposition.[34] Good coverage of the nanocrystalline diamond coating on the surface of the titanium ring was noted. Raman spectroscopy and scanning electron microscopy of the nanocrystalline diamond-coated ring after mechanical fatigue testing indicated that the coating was in good condition. The nanocrystalline diamond coating remained on the entire surface after fatigue testing. Amaral *et al.* deposited nanocrystalline diamond coatings on Si_3N_4–bioglass substrates using hot filament chemical vapor deposition.[35] Pin-on-flat wear studies in Hanks' balanced salt solution and dilute fetal bovine serum provided coefficient of friction values of 0.01–0.02 and 0.06–0.09, respectively; the higher wear rate obtained with fetal bovine serum was attributed to attachment of proteins. Wear rates in Hanks' balanced salt solution and dilute fetal bovine serum were $k \sim 10^{-10}\,mm^3N^{-1}m^{-1}$ and $k \sim 10^{-9} - 10^{-8}\,mm^3N^{-1}m^{-1}$, respectively.

Pecheva *et al.* described processing of a composite material containing apatite and 4–6 nm nanodiamond on AISI 316L stainless steel by means of potentiostatic deposition; this coating exhibited no residual stress or cracks.[36] The composite coating exhibited better adhesion, ductility, and Vickers hardness than pure apatite. The apatite–nanodiamond coating also demonstrated biological activity; formation of a hydroxyapatite layer in simulated body fluid was observed. This material may be used to prevent release of metal ions, inhibit fibrous tissue growth, and prevent blood coagulation in medical devices. Huang *et al.* created single-layer and multilayer nanofilms containing 2–8 nm nanodiamond particles by means of a layer-by-layer deposition approach.[37] *In vitro* studies involving RAW 264.7 murine macrophages showed that the dexamethasone–nanodiamond composite nanofilms attenuated inflammatory cytokine levels. Use of these materials as anti-inflammatory implant coatings and drug delivery devices has been considered.[30,37]

Conventional MEMS are commonly fabricated using silicon; however, silicon demonstrates undesirable mechanical and tribological properties, including poor brittle fracture strength and a tendency to adhere to surfaces (stiction). Sumant *et al.* and Carpick *et al.* utilized atomic force microscopy to examine the nanoscale adhesion and friction behavior of ultrananocrystalline diamond surfaces; Sumant *et al.* showed that hydrogen-terminated ultrananocrystalline diamond exhibited a work of adhesion value of $10.2 \pm 0.4\,mJ/m^2$, which is lower than work of adhesion values associated with saturated hydrocarbon interfaces.[24,38] This work of adhesion value was entirely attributed to van der Waals forces. Tribological studies involving self-mated ultrananocrystalline diamond surfaces have demonstrated friction coefficients as low as $\mu < 0.007$ under test conditions with sufficient humidity.[39] It should also be noted that ultrananocrystalline diamond exhibits hardness and Young's modulus values of ~98 GPa and ~980 GPa, respectively. Several methods for preparing diamond-based MEMS, including conformal coating, selective deposition, and lithographic patterning, have been described.[40,41] Diamond film can be deposited as a thin, conformal coating using chemical vapor deposition. For example, high aspect ratio and low aspect ratio silicon tips were coated with ultrananocrystalline diamond films.[40] The selective deposition process involves growth of ultrananocrystalline diamond on only part of the substrate. Growth of ultrananocrystalline diamond requires a nucleation layer; in selective deposition, a portion of the substrate is seeded. It should be noted that the feature resolution obtained using this method is limited by the grain size. Figure 1.5 shows freestanding 1-μm-thick diamond propellers, which are supported by 100 μm tall silicon platforms.[40] The long arms in these structures are flat, which indicates that the ultrananocrystalline diamond films are nearly stress-free. Lithographic patterning may also be used to prepare multilayer structures; in this method, a thin diamond film is deposited on a sacrificial release layer (e.g. SiO_2). For example, lithographic patterning of a diamond-based MEMS may involve the following steps: deposition of an ultrananocrystalline diamond coating on a thermal SiO_2 layer, deposition of a SiO_2 layer, patterning of SiO_2 with a photoresist using reactive ion etching, etching of ultrananocrystalline diamond using oxygen

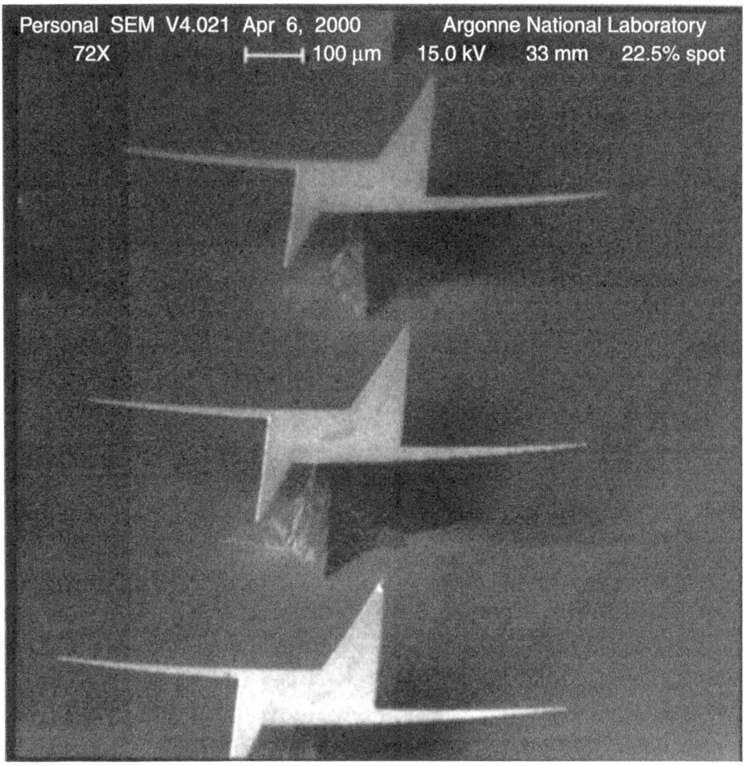

1.5 Scanning electron micrograph of freestanding ultrananocrystalline diamond propellers, which were grown by selective deposition followed by potassium hydroxide etching on silicon posts. Reprinted from Krauss *et al.*[40] with permission from Elsevier.

plasma, and removal of SiO_2 using a hydrofluoric acid wet etch and/or a gas etch. Krauss *et al.* demonstrated processing of multilevel structures, including a captive rotor, using a combination of selective deposition and lithographic etching.[40]

Khanna *et al.* developed lab-on-a-chip structures containing hydrogen-terminated nanocrystalline diamond.[42] In their work, nanocrystalline diamond exhibited the least binding of DNA. In addition, nanocrystalline diamond was shown to exhibit less non-specific attachment than glass, polydimethylsiloxane, polymethylmethacrylate, silicon dioxide, silicon, or SU-8. These results suggest that nanocrystalline diamond may be used to provide high sensitivity and high throughput in lab-on-chip devices. In subsequent work, Khanna *et al.* created microspikes using nanocrystalline diamond.[43] They incorporated the spikes in a microfluidic chamber, which may be placed within a lab-on-chip system. The microspikes increased the mechanical lysis efficiency for B16-F10 (ATCC

CRL-6475) murine melanoma cells compared with non-textured glass. An increase in fluorescence of ~400% was observed. It is interesting to note that performance of the microspikes did not diminish after multiple ultrasonic vibration/wash cycles.

Bijnens *et al.* developed an immunosensor containing nanocrystalline diamond; in this sensor, anti-C reactive protein antibodies were physically adsorbed to the surface of hydrogen-terminated nanocrystalline diamond.[44] Real-time monitoring of C-reactive proteins was demonstrated; for example, 1 μM C-reactive protein was detected with a 30 minute reaction time. Diamond nanowire-based nucleic acid sensors have recently been developed. Nebel *et al.* described fabrication of diamond nanowires through use of an electrochemical phenyl-linker molecule attachment and functionalized thiol-modified DNA.[45] Sensitivity to hybridization of complementary DNA sequences with a concentration of 2 pM over a 3 mm^2 sensor area was demonstrated. No degradation in DNA bonding was noted over 30 hybridization/denaturation cycles.

Diamond is also an attractive material for use in cell-based biosensors. Ariano *et al.* demonstrated adhesion, growth, and viability of GT1-7 neuronal cells (neuronal line of hypothalamic origin) on diamond surfaces.[46] Cells plated on H^- or O^- terminated nanocrystalline diamond samples were shown to adhere, proliferate, and exhibit somatic Ca^{2+} activity. Their work suggested that hydrogen-terminated nanocrystalline diamond is a transparent, biocompatible, and conductive material for cell-based biosensors. Due to its optical transparency, stable electrical conductivity, and mechanical robustness, Ariano *et al.* examined the use of diamond in the fabrication of multielectrode arrays.[47] They demonstrated fabrication of electrodes out of conductive H-terminated diamond for recording electrical signals from excitable cells. Multiparametrical recordings of electrical activity from cultured neuronal networks were demonstrated.

In addition, diamond is being considered for use in neural prostheses. Arrays of solution-gate field-effect transistors were fabricated by Dankerl *et al.* using hydrogen-terminated single-crystalline diamond substrates.[48] Adhesion of cardiomyocyte-like (HL-1) and human embryonic kidney (HEK293) cells was demonstrated. In addition, potassium currents of HEK293 cells were activated with the patch-clamp technique and observed with field-effect transistors. Furthermore, stability of the device in phosphate buffered saline electrolyte solutions for at least 7 days was noted.

Xiao *et al.* discussed the development of retinal prostheses in which ultrananocrystalline diamond served as an inert coating.[49] Electrochemical inactivity and very low leakage currents were demonstrated using cyclic voltammetry. Ultrananocrystalline diamond implanted in rabbit eyes was not associated with intraocular inflammation; however, acute tissue reactions and silicon degradation were observed with incomplete ultrananocrystalline diamond coatings. Their work suggested that intact nanocrystalline diamond coatings are appropriate hermetic coatings for retinal implants. Bonnauron *et al.* utilized detonation nanodiamond seeding and bias enhanced nucleation in order to create diamond-containing microelectrode arrays on three-dimensional glass substrates; such devices may find use in retinal implants.[50]

Rezek *et al.* recently evaluated the effects of cell growth and protein adsorption on solution-gated field-effect transistors containing hydrogen-terminated nanocrystalline diamond films.[51] Interaction with fetal bovine serum proteins was shown to decrease diamond conductivity; this result was attributed to formation of a 2–4 nm thick protein film on the diamond surface. Incubation of osteoblastic SAOS-2 cells on the diamond field-effect transistor surface was also associated with a decrease in conductivity. It is thought that proteins lower the diamond–electrolyte electronic barrier, enabling alternate mechanisms for the transfer of charge across the diamond–electrolyte interface.

1.4 Functionalization of nanodiamond and nanocrystalline diamond

The functionalization of nanodiamond with biological molecules has attracted significant research activity in recent years. In 2002, Yang *et al.* demonstrated covalent attachment of DNA oligonucleotides to nanocrystalline diamond.[52] In the initial step, an amine-terminated hydrocarbon chain protected with a trifluoroacetamide functional group was attached to nanocrystalline diamond. The diamond surface was illuminated with UV light; this process led to activation of the diamond surface. Next, an electrophilic attack to the cross-linking double bond was carried out. The protected amine was subsequently deprotected, resulting in a primary amine. The amine was then reacted with a cross-linker molecule. The material was finally reacted with thiol-modified DNA. Hybridization reactions with fluorescently tagged oligonucleotides showed no detectable non-specific adsorption. In addition, DNA-modified ultrananocrystalline diamond surfaces showed no measurable decrease in signal intensity after 30 cycles. It is believed that DNA-modified diamond surfaces are more resistant to oxidation than Si–O or thiol–gold interactions. More recently, Popov *et al.* showed ribonucleic acid molecule attachment to a nanocrystalline diamond/amorphous carbon composite; in this study, 1-amino-3-cyclopentene hydrochloride was attached to nanocrystalline diamond using UV irradiation.[53] Haertl *et al.* attached proteins, including catalase and green fluorescent protein, to nanocrystalline diamond using a covalent mechanism.[54] In the initial step, an amine-containing molecule was immobilized on hydrogen-terminated nanocrystalline diamond using a photochemical process; proteins were attached to the surface using peptide bonds. Catalase-modified nanocrystalline diamond electrodes were demonstrated for use as hydrogen peroxide sensors.

Rubio-Retama *et al.* demonstrated immobilization of an enzyme on nanocrystalline diamond.[55] In the initial step, TFA (2,2,2-trifluorine-N-9'-decenil acetamide) was attached to nanocrystalline diamond using a photochemical process. Enzyme attachment involved TFA attachment, TFA deprotection, insertion of a carboxyl group, and immobilization of the enzyme (horseradish peroxidase). The proximity of the horseradish peroxidase heme groups to the nanocrystalline diamond enabled direct electron transfer. This electrode was used to detect hydrogen peroxide in the 0.1–45 mM range; enzymatic activity for the biosensor was constant over 15 days at room temperature. This system may be used in amperometric biosensors or enzyme-linked immunosorbent assays.

In addition, Zhou *et al.* have described covalent immobilization of cytochrome c on boron-doped nanocrystalline diamond.[56] A photochemical reaction was used to chemically modify hydrogen-terminated nanocrystalline diamond surfaces with an undecylenic acid methyl ester. The ester was hydrolyzed under basic conditions to create a monolayer of carboxylic groups; cytochrome c was covalently immobilized on the carboxyl-terminated electrode by means of a carbodiimide coupling reaction. Direct electron transfer between cytochrome c and the electrode was observed. Response to a H_2O_2 concentration between 1 μM and 450 μM was observed; excellent electrocatalytic performance (e.g. low detection limit, rapid response, and high stability) was also noted.

Modification of diamond powders has been demonstrated. For example, Nguyen *et al.* described modification of diamond through a physical adsorption process.[57] Diamond powders (with a size of 100 nm) underwent treatment in oxidative acid solution (concentrated H_2SO_4 and HNO_3 mixture) at elevated temperatures. Non-covalent immobilization of the hen egg white lysozyme enzyme, an antimicrobial protein, was subsequently performed. The enzyme retained significant activity after physical adsorption to the crystallite surface. Co-adsorption of cytochrome c, a heme protein involved with electron transfer within the mitochondrial electron transport chain, on the crystallite surface served to block empty sites, enhance surface crowding, and increase enzyme activity.

Binding of biotin, a B-complex vitamin commonly utilized in *in vitro* biochemical assays, to diamond has also been demonstrated. Neugart *et al.* utilized a surfactant (sodium dodecyl sulfate) to improve stability of nanodiamond solutions and reduce nanodiamond aggregation.[58] After incubation, nanodiamond particles entered the cells within a few minutes. The 50 nm nanodiamond particles were shown to enter the cell via the endosomal pathway. Binding of streptavidin to biotinylated nanodiamond aggregates was also shown. As each streptavidin molecule can bind four biotin molecules, large aggregates were formed.

The Fenton reaction has been used to create functionalized nanodiamond particles. Martin *et al.* exposed raw nanodiamond particles (of particle size 7 nm) to the Fenton reaction in order to remove amorphous soot, increase surface-OH groups, and enable covalent functionalization.[59] They functionalized nanodiamond with thionine; these nanoparticles were shown to enter HeLa cell nuclei. Ninety-seven percent of HeLa cells survived after incubation with nanodiamond–thionine, indicating good biocompatibility.

In recent work, Sreenívasan *et al.* demonstrated salt-solution stable bioconjugation of luminescent nanodiamond particles with barstar:barnase, a high-affinity protein pair.[31] The covalent nature of the luminescent nanodiamond particle–barstar bonding was demonstrated using X-ray photoelectron spectroscopy. Luminescent nanodiamond–barstar conjugates in buffer solutions were noted to be stable over several months. Imaging of luminescent nanodiamond–barstar:barnase-enhanced green fluorescent protein particles within Chinese Hamster Ovary cells was also demonstrated.

1.5 Drug delivery using nanodiamond

Immobilization of chemotherapeutic agents on nanodiamond has been described. Huang *et al.* functionalized 2–8 nm nanodiamond particles with doxorubicin hydrochloride (DOX); DOX is a pharmacologic agent that is used to induce apoptosis (controlled cell death).[60] A detonation technique was used to produce nanodiamond material, which contained hydrophilic functional groups such as -COOH and -OH. Biocompatibility of nanodiamond was demonstrated using a real-time polymerase chain reaction. Genes associated with expression of interleukin-6, tumor necrosis factor α, and inducible nitric oxide synthase were not significantly up-regulated in cells exposed to nanocrystalline diamond, indicating the absence of inflammation.

Sodium chloride was shown to promote the adsorption of doxorubicin hydrochloride onto nanodiamond; 2–10 nm coatings were observed on the nanodiamond particles using transmission electron microscopy. Release of DOX was obtained by removal of sodium chloride. Their work showed that doxorubicin–nanodiamond composites induced cell death in murine macrophage and HT-29 colorectal cancer cells. Furthermore, MTT assays and DNA fragmentation assays revealed that doxorubicin–nanodiamond composites were associated with apoptotic cell death.

Covalent immobilization of paclitaxel on nanodiamond was demonstrated by Liu *et al.*[61] Nanodiamond–paclitaxel (of concentration 0.1–50 μg mL^{-1}) inhibited mitosis and induced apoptosis in A549 human lung cells. Confocal microscopy indicated that the 3–5 nm nanodiamond particles were localized in the cytoplasm and in the microtubules. Nanodiamond–paclitaxel particles were shown to block tumor growth and lung cancer cell formation in xenograft SCID mice. In this study, nanodiamond particles and paclitaxel were joined by an ester bond, which can be broken by esterase enzymes. Nanodiamond particles alone induced neither apoptosis nor mitotic arrest. In addition, delivery of water-insoluble pharmacologic agents has been demonstrated. Chen *et al.* used an acid treatment to remove impurities and form carboxyl groups on the surfaces of nanodiamond particles.[62] The carboxyl groups enabled the nanodiamond suspension to be stable in water. The carboxyl groups were also capable of complexing with poorly water-soluble drugs; for example, attachment of three drugs, purvalanol A (a drug for liver cancer), 4-hydroxytamoxifen (a drug for estrogen receptor-positive breast cancer), and dexamethasone (an anti-inflammatory agent), was demonstrated.

Zhang *et al.* demonstrated plasmid DNA delivery using nanodiamond.[63] They immobilized 800 Da polyethyleneimine, a polycation used for transfection, on the surface of nanodiamond. This material demonstrated high transfection efficiency in a HeLa cell model, which was similar to that of high molecular weight polyethyleneimine (25K). Eighty percent of cells survived in the medium containing polyethyleneimine 800-nanodiamond at concentrations as high as 90 μg/mL. A combination of 800 Da polyethyleneimine and nanodiamond was noted to provide the high transfection efficiency of high molecular weight polyethyleneimine and the low cytotoxicity of low molecular weight polyethyleneimine. The combination of 800 Da polyethyleneimine and nanodiamond may also include other medically relevant agents, such as chemotherapeutic agents and cell-specific targeting molecules.

Chow *et al.* recently utilized a complex containing nanodiamond and doxorubicin for treatment of mammary carcinoma and hepatoblastoma (liver tumor) in a murine model.[64] *In vivo* studies showed that intravenous delivery of nanodiamond–doxorubicin complexes provided increased retention within tumor cells and greater inhibition of tumor growth than intravenous delivery of doxorubicin; no increases in systemic immune response (as indicated by serum interleukin-6), liver toxicity (as indicated by serum alanine transferase), or myelosuppression were associated with nanocrystalline diamond treatment. Although retention of nanodiamond–doxorubicin complexes was enhanced in both tumor tissues and healthy tissues, clearance of the small nanodiamond–doxorubicin complexes from slowly dividing healthy tissue cells prevented systemic apoptosis (programmed cell death) in healthy tissues. Their work suggests that nanodiamond-based chemotherapeutic agents may be useful for treatment of tumors that are resistant to conventional chemotherapeutic agents.

1.6 Imaging with nanodiamond

Several studies have demonstrated imaging of nanodiamond particles within cells and tissues.[65] As noted by Barnard, the fluorescent properties of diamond are associated with point defects, including nitrogen-vacancy and silicon-vacancy defects.[29] Nitrogen-vacancy defects are of particular interest for imaging applications because they exhibit strong absorbance at 560 nm and fluorescence at approximately 700 nm.[65] For example, Yu *et al.* created point defects in diamond, specifically negatively charged nitrogen-vacancy center (N-V)-defects, by means of a two-step process that involved (a) irradiation-induced damage using a 3 MeV proton beam and (b) thermal annealing at 800°C for two hours under vacuum.[66] Synthetic type Ib diamond powders with a nominal size of 100 nm were prepared by irradiation-annealing; these particles exhibited a 10^2-fold enhancement in fluorescence intensity compared with annealed materials. The fluorescent nanodiamond materials were shown to be suitable for epifluorescent imaging. Entry of fluorescent nanodiamond particles to the cell and localization within the cytoplasm was demonstrated. In addition, an MTT assay involving 293T human kidney cells revealed an absence of toxicity.

Chang *et al.* prepared magnetic nanodiamond particles from a mixture of annealed nanodiamond powder and ferrocene powder by means of microwave irradiation-induced arcing; nanodiamond particles with a coercivity field of 155 G and a saturation magnetization of ~10 emu/g were obtained using this approach.[67] Magnetic nanodiamond particles with fluorescent properties were created by grafting fluorescein o-methacrylate onto magnetic nanodiamond particles using microwave irradiation. Ingestion of fluorescent magnetic nanodiamond particles into the cytoplasms of HeLa cells via non-receptor-mediated endocytosis was demonstrated.

Fu *et al.* described bright fluorescence from diamonds at 550–800 nm.[68] Fluorescence of a single 35 nm diamond was noted to be significantly brighter than that of a single Alexa Fluor 546 dye molecule under the same excitation conditions. The nanodiamond particles showed no sign of photobleaching even after 5 minutes of continuous excitation by 532 nm light at a power density of 8×10^3 W/cm^2. Fluorescent 35 nm nanocrystalline diamond particles were incubated with HeLa cells. Vertical cross-section images demonstrated translocation of the fluorescent nanocrystalline diamond particles through the cell membrane. Many fluorescent nanocrystalline diamond particles formed aggregates in the cell. The particles exhibited photostability after continuous excitation for 20 minutes (with a laser power of 100 W/cm^2). Neither photobleaching nor blinking of fluorescence was noted. In addition, tracking of a 35 nm single fluorescent nanocrystalline diamond particle in the cytoplasm of a live HeLa cell was demonstrated.

Nanodiamond has recently been considered for use as a biomarker. For example, Chang *et al.* created bright fluorescent nanodiamonds in large quantities through formation of point defects in synthetic diamond nanocrystallites by means of 40 keV He^+ helium ion irradiation from a radio-frequency ion source.[69] Excellent photostability was observed in the modified 25 nm nanoparticles. Imaging and three-dimensional tracking of fluorescent nanodiamond in a HeLa cell using two-photon excitation microscopy was demonstrated. Biodistribution of nanodiamond has been examined by means of radiolabeling. For example, Yuan *et al.* used radiolabeling, Raman spectrometry, transmission electron microscopy, and UV-visible light spectroscopy to examine biodistribution of iodine 215-labeled ~50 nm nanoparticles in a male ICR murine model.[70] Figure 1.6 shows high-resolution transmission electron microscopy images of digested solutions containing murine liver, lung, and spleen tissues 28 days after nanodiamond particle injection. Sixty percent of nanodiamond particles were observed in the liver at 30 minutes. It is believed that nanocrystalline diamond particles are rapidly captured by opsonization; the nanoparticles are bound by opsonins in the plasma and are subsequently recognized by phagocytes in the reticuloendothelial system.

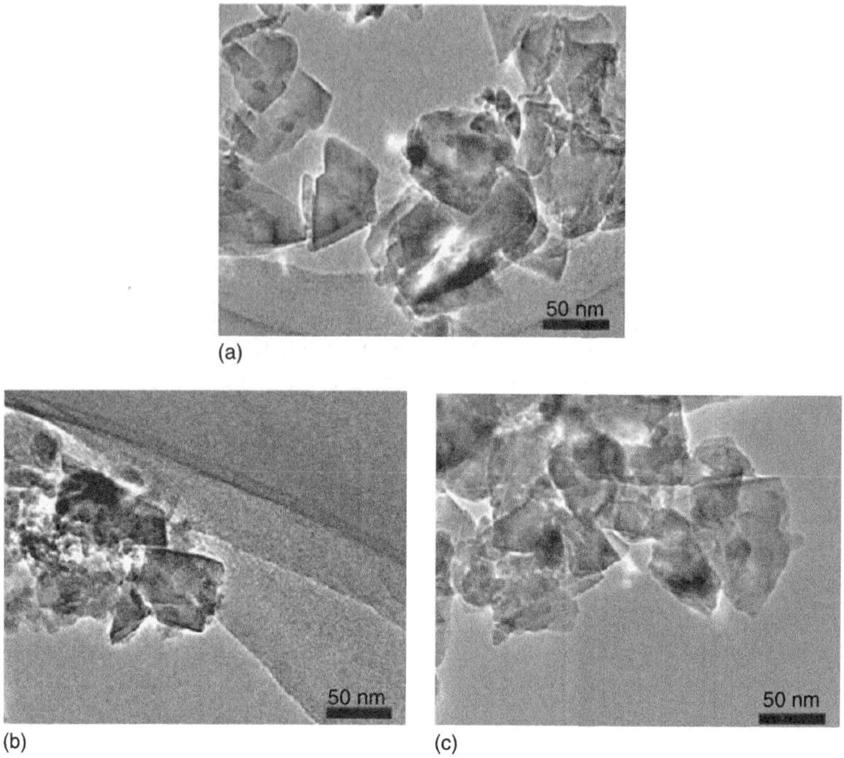

1.6 High-resolution transmission electron microscopy images of digested solution of different mouse tissues at 28 days after intravenous injection of 80 mg/kg body weight nanodiamonds. (a) Liver, (b) spleen, and (c) lung. Reprinted from Yuan *et al.*[70] with permission from Elsevier.

Zhang *et al.* prepared radiolabeled nanodiamond particles and examined the biodistribution of these particles after intratracheal instillation in a Kun Ming mouse model.[71] They showed that a majority of the intratracheally administered ^{188}Re-nanodiamond particles remained in the lungs; however, some particles crossed the blood–air barrier and entered the bone, heart, liver, and spleen. They also observed dose-dependent systemic toxicity involving several tissues; for example, dose-dependent adverse effects on kidney and lung function were observed. Faklaris *et al.* examined the use of a photoluminescent nanodiamond (of size 50 nm) as a biomarker in diagnostic and therapeutic applications.[72] They attributed emission in the red and near-infrared spectral region (575–750 nm) to nitrogen vacancy color centers. In addition, they noted that photoluminescent nanodiamond materials did not exhibit photobleaching or photoblinking. Photoluminescent nanodiamond was shown to enter cells by means of endocytosis; it is believed that this process is mediated by clathrin. Once in the cells, nanodiamond particles were segregated in endosomal and lysosomal vesicles; some of these materials were released into the cytoplasm. *In vitro* studies involving HeLa cells demonstrated an absence of cytotoxicity. These photoluminescent nanodiamond materials may be used for imaging transport and labeling intracellular structures.

The use of labeled nanodiamond has clinical applications; for example, nanodiamond particles containing gadolinium (III) have been considered for use in magnetic resonance imaging (MRI). Manus *et al.* described the use of gadolinium (III)-nanodiamond particles in MRI.[73] An amine-functionalized Gd(III) complex with a six carbon linker was reacted with carboxylic acid groups on the surface of nanodiamond. The hydrodynamic size of gadolinium (III)-nanodiamond decreased from ~128 to ~55 nm after dilution and ultrasonication; the pre-conjugation size of the nanodiamond was ~21 nm. Gadolinium (III)-nanodiamond did not significantly decrease cell viability compared to doxorubicin. In addition, gadolinium (III)-nanodiamond had no significant effect on cytotoxicity in comparison with unmodified nanodiamonds in HeLa cells or unmodified nanodiamonds in NIH/3T3 cells below a concentration of 0.5 mg mL^{-1}. They demonstrated improved performance, including ten-fold greater relaxivity values as well as significantly higher contrast levels, with gadolinium-modified nanodiamond in comparison with conventional Gd(III) complex.

As discussed by Barnard, coherent interfacial Coulombic interactions result in agglomeration of as-prepared nanodiamond particles.[29] Recent work has indicated that functionalization with polyethylene glycol may be used to prevent nanodiamond aggregation. For example, Takimoto *et al.* recently incorporated polyethylene glycol and fluorescein on the surface of diamond.[74] In the initial step, ω-aminododecanoic acid was immobilized on the surface of nanodiamond particles. These fluorescent nanoparticles remained in dispersion within a phosphate-buffered saline physiological solution. In addition, use of the functionalized nanodiamond particles for cellular imaging in HeLa cells was demonstrated.

It should also be noted that Raman spectroscopy may be utilized as a non-invasive contrasting approach with nanodiamond particles.[30] The Raman spectra of materials containing sp^3-hybridized carbon bonds show a strong intensity signal at 1332 cm^{-1}, which is associated with a triply degenerate zone center optical phonon exhibiting F_{2g} symmetry.[75,76] For example, Cheng *et al.* utilized confocal Raman mapping to perform *in vitro* monitoring of interactions between carboxylated nanodiamond-growth hormone complexes and growth hormone receptors in A549 human epithelial cells.[77]

1.7 Conclusion

The results of recent studies have demonstrated the use of diamond in a variety of medical applications, including drug delivery devices, microelectromechanical devices, and cardiovascular devices. However, several challenges for diamond-based materials and devices must be overcome. Reproducible, scalable processes must be developed to facilitate the translation of diamond coatings to clinical use. The short-term toxicity, long-term toxicity, and fate of diamond, impurities, and breakdown products must be carefully considered using medical application-specific parameters.[27,78] Additional work is also necessary to optimize the properties of diamond for particular medical applications. Efforts are under way to increase the density of nitrogen-vacancy point defects in small (<5 nm) nanodiamond particles; for example, Smith *et al.* prepared nanodiamond particles containing nitrogen-vacancy point defects by means of high-energy (2.5 MeV) proton irradiation and thermal annealing.[29,79] The relationships between biological functionality, surface functionalization, purity, and physical properties (e.g. aspect ratio) must also be carefully considered.[30] Furthermore, improved methods for conjugating pharmacologic agents and biological molecules to diamond must be developed.[30] If these hurdles are overcome, diamond-based materials and devices may be translated to use in medical devices, drug delivery, and medical diagnostic applications over the next few decades.

1.8 Acknowledgments

One of the authors (AVS) would like to acknowledge use of the Center for Nanoscale Materials, which is supported by the U. S. Department of Energy, Office of Science, Office of Basic Energy Sciences, under Contract No. DE-AC02-06CH11357.

1.9 References

1. Narayan, R. J., and Boehm, R., Hard as diamonds. *Medical Device Developments* (2010) 2.
2. Ramachandran, G. N., Crystal structure of diamond. *Nature* (1945) 156, 83.
3. Pierson, H., *Handbook of carbon, graphite, and fullerenes: properties, processing, and applications*, Noyes Publications, Park Ridge, NJ (1993).
4. Bundy F. P., Hall H. T., Strong H. M. and Wentorf R. H., Man-Made Diamonds. *Nature* (1955) 176, 51.
5. Eversole, E. G., *Synthesis of Diamond.* Patent number 3,030,187, 1962.
6. Derjaguin, B. V., and Fedoseev, D. B., The synthesis of diamond at low pressure. *Scientific American* (1975) 233, 102.
7. Angus, J.C., Will, H.A. and Stanko, W.S., Growth of diamond seed crystals by vapor deposition. *Journal of Applied Physics* (1968) 39, 2915.
8. Zhou, D., Gruen, D.M., Qin, L.C., *et al.* Control of diamond film microstructure by Ar additions to CH4/H2 microwave plasmas. *Journal of Applied Physics* (1998) 84, 1981.
9. Anthony, T. R., Metastable synthesis of diamond. *Vacuum* (1990) 41, 1356.
10. Kumar, A., Determination of zinc and manganese by differential pulse polarographic technique. *Thin Solid Films* (1997) 308, 209.

11. Williams, O.A., Douhéret, O., Daenen, M., *et al.* Enhanced diamond nucleation on monodispersed nanocrystalline diamond. *Chemical Physics Letters* (2007) 445, 255.
12. Kromka, A., Rezek, B., Remes, Z., *et al.* Formation of continuous nanocrystalline diamond layers on glass and silicon at low temperatures. *Chemical Vapor Deposition* (2008) 14, 181.
13. Kumar, A., *et al.*, Evaluation of buffer layers for hot filament chemical vapor deposition diamond films on silicon substrates. *Thin Solid Films* (1997) 308, 209.
14. Godbole, V.P., Narayan, R., Xu, Z., *et al.* Diamond films and composites on cobalt-chromium alloys. *Materials Science and Engineering B* (1999) 58, 251.
15. Belmonte, M., Fernandes, A.J.S., Costa, F.M., *et al.* Adhesion behaviour assessment on diamond coated silicon nitride by acoustic emission. *Diamond and Related Materials* (2003) 12, 733.
16. Mallika, K., and Komanduri, R., Low pressure microwave plasma assisted chemical vapor deposition (MPCVD) of diamond coatings on silicon nitride cutting tools. *Thin Solid Films* (2001) 396, 146.
17. Butler, J. E., and Sumant, A. V., The CVD of nanodiamond materials. *Chemical Vapor Deposition* (2008) 14, 145.
18. Amaral, M., Abreu, C.S., Fernandes, A.J.S., *et al.* Nanodiamond-based tribosystems. *Surface and Coatings Technology* (2010) 204, 1962.
19. Gruen, D. M., Ultrananocrystalline diamond in the laboratory and the cosmos. *MRS Bulletin* (2001) 26, 771.
20. Jiao, S., Sumant, A., Kirk, M.A., *et al.* Microstructure of ultrananocrystalline diamond films grown by microwave Ar-CH4 plasma chemical vapor deposition with or without added H2. *Journal of Applied Physics* (2001) 90, 118.
21. Sumant, A. V., *et al.*, Large-area low-temperature ultrananocrystalline diamond (UNCD) films and integration with CMOS devices for monolithically integrated diamond MEMS/NEMS-CMOS systems. *SPIE Proceedings: Micro- and Nanotechnology Sensors, Systems, and Applications* (2009) 7318, 71817.
22. Naguib, N.N., Elam, J.W., Birrell, J., *et al.* Enhanced nucleation, smoothness and conformality of ultrananocrystalline diamond (UNCD) ultrathin films via tungsten interlayers. *Chem Phys Lett* (2006) 430, 345.
23. Sumant, A.V., Auciello, O., Carpick, R.W., *et al.* Ultrananocrystalline and nanocrystalline diamond thin films for MEMS/NEMS applications. *MRS Bulletin* (2010) 35, 281.
24. Sumant, A. V., *et al.*, Surface chemistry and bonding configuration of ultrananocrystalline diamond surfaces and their effects on nanotribological properties. *Physical Review B* (2007) 76, 235429.
25. Narayan, R.J., Wei, W., Jin, C., *et al.* Microstructural and biological properties of nanocrystalline diamond coatings. *Diamond and Related Materials* (2006) 15, 1935.
26. Adadurov, G. A., *et al., Methods of producing diamond and/or diamond-like modifications of boron nitride.* United States Patent 4,483,836, 1984.
27. Schrand, A.M., Hens, S.A.C., and Shenderova, O.A., Nanodiamond particles: Properties and perspectives for bioapplications. *Critical Reviews in Solid State and Materials Sciences* (2009) 34, 18.
28. Krueger, A., Valuation of water quality and consumer choice and recognition of beach eco-certification in Tampa Bay area beaches. *Carbon* (2005) 43, 1722.
29. Barnard, A. S., Diamond standard in diagnostics: Nanodiamond biolabels make their mark. *Analyst* (2009) 134, 1751.

30. Lam, R., and Ho, D., Nanodiamonds as vehicles for systemic and localized drug delivery. *Expert Opinion on Drug Delivery* (2009) 6, 883.
31. Sreenivasan, V. K., *et al.*, Barstar: barnase – a versatile platform for colloidal diamond bioconjugation. *Journal of Materials Chemistry* (2001) 21, 65.
32. Fries, M. D., and Vohra, Y.K., Nanostructured diamond film deposition on curved surfaces of metallic temporomandibular joint implant. *Journal of Physics D-Applied Physics* (2002) 35, L105.
33. Papo, M.J., Catledge, S.A., Vohra, Y.K., and Machado, C., Mechanical wear behavior of nanocrystalline and multilayer diamond coatings on temporomandibular joint implants. *Journal of Materials Science: Materials in Medicine* (2004) 15, 773.
34. Jozwik, K., and Karczemska, A., The new generation Ti6Al4V artificial heart valve with nanocrystalline diamond coating on the ring and with Derlin disc after long-term mechanical fatigue examination. *Diamond and Related Materials* (2007) 16, 1004.
35. Amaral, M., Abreu, C.S., Oliveira, F.J., *et al.* Biotribological performance of NCD coated Si3N4-bioglass composites. *Diamond and Related Materials* (2007) 16, 790.
36. Pecheva, E., Pramatarova, L., Hikov, T., *et al.* Apatite-nanodiamond composite as a functional coating of stainless steel (Conference Paper). *Surface and Interface Analysis* (2010) 42, 475.
37. Huang, H., Pierstorff, E., Osawa, E., and Ho, D., Protein-mediated assembly of nanodiamond hydrogels into a biocompatible and biofunctional multilayer nanofilm. *ACS Nano* (2008) 2, 203.
38. Sumant, A.V., Grierson, D.S., Gerbi, J.E., *et al.* Toward the ultimate tribological interface: Surface chemistry and nanotribology of ultrananocrystalline diamond. *Advanced Materials* (2005) 17, 1039.
39. Hamilton, M. A., *et al.*, Environmental Performance Limits of Ultrananocrystalline Diamond Films. *Proceedings of the STLE/ASME International Joint Tribology Conference* (2008) IJTC2008-71198.
40. Krauss, A.R., Auciello, O., Gruen, D.M., *et al.* Ultrananocrystalline diamond thin films for MEMS and moving mechanical assembly devices. *Diamond and Related Materials* (2001) 10, 1952.
41. Auciello, O., Birrell, J., Carlisle, J.A., *et al.* Materials science and fabrication processes for a new MEMS technology based on ultrananocrystalline diamond thin films (Review). *Journal of Physics-Condensed Matter* (2004) 16, R539.
42. Khanna, P., Villagra, A., Kim, S., *et al.* Use of nanocrystalline diamond for microfluidic lab-on-a-chip. *Diamond and Related Materials* (2006) 15, 2073.
43. Khanna, P., Ramachandran, N., Yang, J., *et al.* Nanocrystalline diamond microspikes increase the efficiency of ultrasonic cell lysis in a microfluidic lab-on-a-chip. *Diamond and Related Materials* (2009) 18, 606.
44. Bijnens, N., *et al.*, Synthetic diamond films as a platform material for label-free protein sensors. *Physica Status Solidi A* (2008) 205, 520.
45. Nebel, C.E., Yang, N., Uetsuka, H., *et al.* Diamond nano-wires, a new approach towards next generation electrochemical gene sensor platforms. *Diamond and Related Materials* (2009) 18, 910.
46. Ariano, P., Budnyk, O., Dalmazzo, S., *et al.* On diamond surface properties and interactions with neurons. *European Journal of Physics E* (2009) 30, 149.
47. Ariano, P, Lo Giudice, A, Marcantoni, A, *et al.* diamond-based biosensor for the recording of neuronal activity. *Biosensors and Bioelectronics* (2009) 24, 2046.
48. Dankerl, M., Eick, S., Hofmann, B., *et al.* Diamond transistor array for extracellular recording from electrogenic cells. *Advanced Functional Materials* (2009) 19, 2915.

49. Xiao, X., Wang, J., Liu, C., *et al.* In vitro and in vivo evaluation of ultrananocrystalline diamond for coating of implantable retinal microchips. *Journal of Biomedical Materials Research* (2006) 77B, 273.
50. Bonnauron, M., Saada, S., Mer, C., *et al.* Transparent diamond-on-glass micro-electrode arrays for ex-vivo neuronal study (Conference Paper). *Phys Stat Sol A* (2008) 9, 2126.
51. Rezek, B., Krátká, M., Kromka, A., and Kalbacova, M., Effects of protein inter-layers on cell-diamond FET characteristics. *Biosensors and Bioelectronics* (2010) 26, 1307.
52. Yang, W., Auciello, O., Butler, J.E., *et al.* DNA-modified nanocrystalline diamond thin-films as stable, biologically active substrates. *Nature Materials* (2002) 1, 253.
53. Popov, C., Bliznakov, S., Boycheva, S., *et al.* Nanocrystalline diamond/amorphous carbon composite coatings for biomedical applications. *Diamond and Related Materials* (2008) 17, 882.
54. Härtl A., Schmich E., Garrido J.A., *et al.* Protein-modified nanocrystalline diamond thin films for biosensor applications. *Nature Materials* (2004) 3, 736–742.
55. Rubio-Retama, J., Hernando, J., López-Ruiz, B., *et al.* Synthetic nanocrystalline diamond as a third-generation biosensor support. *Langmuir* (2006) 22, 5837.
56. Zhou, Y., Zhi, J., Zou, Y., *et al.* Direct electrochemistry and electrocatalytic activity of cytochrome c covalently immobilized on a boron-doped nanocrystalline diamond electrode. *Analytical Chemistry* (2008) 80, 4141.
57. Nguyen, T.-T.-B., Chang, H.-C., and Wu, V.W.-K., Adsorption and hydrolytic activity of lysozyme on diamond nanocrystallites. *Diamond and Related Materials* (2007) 16, 872.
58. Neugart, F., Zappe, A., Jelezko, F., *et al.* Dynamics of diamond nanoparticles in solution and cells. *Nano Letters* (2007) 7, 3588.
59. Martín, R., Álvaro, M., Herance, J.R., and García, H., Fenton-treated functionalized diamond nanoparticles as gene delivery system. *ACS Nano* (2010) 4, 65.
60. Huang, H., Pierstorff, E., Osawa, E., and Ho, D., Active nanodiamond hydrogels for chemotherapeutic delivery. *Nano Letters* (2007) 7, 3305.
61. Liu, K.K., Zheng, W.W., Wang, C.C., *et al.* Covalent linkage of nanodiamond-paclitaxel for drug delivery and cancer therapy. *Nanotechnology* (2010) 21, 315106.
62. Chen, M., Pierstorff, E.D., Lam, R., *et al.* Nanodiamond-mediated delivery of water-insoluble therapeutics. *ACS Nano* (2009) 3, 2016.
63. Zhang, X.-Q., Chen, M., Lam, R., *et al.* Polymer-functionalized nanodiamond platforms as vehicles for gene delivery. *ACS Nano* (2009) 3, 2609.
64. Chow, E.K., Zhang, X.-Q., Chen, M., *et al.* Nanodiamond therapeutic delivery agents mediate enhanced chemoresistant tumor treatment. *Science Translational Medicine* (2011) 3, 73ra21.
65. Hui, Y., Cravens, T.E., Ozak, N., and Schultz, D.R., What can be learned from the absence of auroral X-ray emission from Saturn? *Journal of Physics D* (2010) 43, 374021.
66. Yu, S.-J., Kang, M.-W., Chang, H.-C., *et al.* Bright fluorescent nanodiamonds: No photobleaching and low cytotoxicity. *Journal of the American Chemical Society* (2005) 127, 17604.
67. Chang, I.P., Hwang, K.C., and Chiang, C.S., Preparation of fluorescent magnetic nanodiamonds and cellular imaging. *Journal of the American Chemical Society* (2008) 130, 15476–81.
68. Fu C.C., Lee H.Y., Chen K., *et al.* Characterization and application of single fluorescent nanodiamonds as cellular biomarkers. *Proceedings of the National Academy of Sciences USA* (2008) 104, 727.

69. Chang, Y.-R., Lee, H.-Y., Chen, K., *et al.* Mass production and dynamic imaging of fluorescent nanodiamonds. *Nature Nanotechnology* (2008) 3, 284.
70. Yuan, Y., Chen, Y., Liu, J.-H., *et al.* Biodistribution and fate of nanodiamonds in vivo. *Diamond and Related Materials* (2009) 18, 95.
71. Zhang, X.-B., and Peng, J.-Y., Re-ranking algorithm using clustering and relevance feedback for image retrieval (Conference Paper). *Toxicology Letters* (2010) 198, 237.
72. Faklaris, O., Joshi, V., Irinopoulou, T., *et al.* Photoluminescent diamond nanoparticles for cell labeling: Study of the uptake mechanism in mammalian cells. *ACS Nano* (2009) 3, 3955.
73. Manus L.M., Mastarone D.J., Waters E.A., *et al.* Gd(III)-nanodiamond conjugates for MRI contrast enhancement. *Nano Letters* (2009) 10, 484.
74. Takimoto, T., Chano, T., Shimizu, S., *et al.* Preparation of fluorescent diamond nanoparticles stably dispersed under a physiological environment through multistep organic transformations. *Chemistry of Materials* (2010) 22, 3462.
75. Schiferl, D., Nicol, M., Zaug, J.M., *et al.* The diamond 13C/12C isotope Raman pressure sensor system for high-temperature/pressure diamond-anvil cells with reactive samples. *Journal of Applied Physics* (1997) 82, 3256.
76. Levenson, M.D., Flytzanis, C., and Bloembergen, N., Interference of resonant and nonresonant three-wave mixing in diamond. *Physical Review B* (1972) 6, 3962.
77. Cheng, C.-C., Chien, C.-H., Luo, G.-L., *et al.* Ultrathin Si capping layer suppresses charge trapping in HfO xNy/Ge metal-insulator-semiconductor capacitors. *Applied Physics Letters* (2007) 90, 163903.
78. Krueger, A., New carbon materials: biological applications of functionalized nanodiamond materials. *Chemistry: A European Journal* (2008) 14, 1382.
79. Smith B.R., Inglis D.W., Sandnes B., *et al.* Five-nanometer diamond with luminescent nitrogen-vacancy defect centers. *Small* (2009) 5, 1649.

2
Functionalization of diamond surfaces for medical applications

S. SZUNERITS and R. BOUKHERROUB,
Université Lille 1, France.

DOI: 10.1533/9780857093516.1.25

Abstract: Recent advances made in the controlled deposition of diamond thin films with varying morphologies have pushed researchers to consider diamond as an alternative carbon-based material. Surface functionalization is believed to be an effective approach to tune the physical, chemical and electrochemical properties of diamond. Understanding and controlling the functionalization process of diamond surfaces thus holds considerable promise for both fundamental and applied research aspects. This chapter summarizes the state of the art of chemical, photochemical and electrochemical strategies for the grafting of different organic moieties onto diamond.

Key words: surface functionalization, aryldiazonium salt, photochemical modification, amine-termination, oxygen-termination, click chemistry, thiol-yne.

2.1 Introduction

Active attention is currently being paid to the chemical modification of solid substrate surfaces due to their utility as model systems for understanding electron transfer, but also for their potential applications in various fields, including molecular electronics, bioelectronics and sensors.

Diamond, a well-known gemstone, displays outstanding physico-chemical properties that have attracted much attention of the scientific community. The development of controllable methods for the fabrication of high-quality diamond thin films has made diamond interfaces more accessible. Potentially the panel of applications for this material is extremely wide (Nebel and Ristein, 2003; Nebel *et al.*, 2008; Luong *et al.*, 2009). As a wide band gap semiconductor, diamond combines ultimate electronic properties (highest hole mobility, saturation velocity and breakdown voltage among all semiconductors) with exceptional physico-chemical properties. Diamond is, for instance, exceptionally bio-inert giving a high compatibility with living tissues in many biological applications. It has, in addition, one of the largest potential windows for electrochemistry in aqueous solutions (Fortin *et al.*, 2004), a thermal conductivity above that of copper, a remarkable mechanical hardness and an unbeatable transparency from ultraviolet to infrared. Despite the high chemical stability of diamond even in harsh environmental conditions, a myriad of strategies for controllable surface functionalization have been developed. In particular, hydrogen, oxygen, halogen, and amine terminations have been achieved and studied on diamond surfaces. The functionalities on diamond surfaces have been further extended for covalent grafting of organic and biological molecules. Among the chemical modification methods of diamond surfaces, photochemical functionalization with alkenes and electrochemical modification via reduction of aryldiazonium salts are the most widely used strategies. The functionalization of diamond by electrochemical reduction of aryldiazonium salts was first reported by Kuo *et al.*, (Kuo *et al.*, 1999) and much interest was generated subsequently (Wang *et al.*, 2004; Shin *et al.*, 2006a; Uetsuka *et al.*, 2007; Zhong *et al.*, 2009), especially in connection with the biofunctionalization of diamond (Shin *et al.*, 2006b; Wang and Carlisle, 2006; Zhou and Zhi, 2006). The photochemical grafting of alkene-based molecules onto hydrogen-terminated diamond was reported first by Hamers *et al.*, (Hamers *et al.*, 2005; Nichols *et al.*, 2005) some years later. This method is restricted mainly to alkyl compounds, as the presence of aromaticity in the target adsorbates will open up non-selective pathways of attachment to the surface in the presence of UV activation (Zhong *et al.*, 2008a). After a brief discussion of diamond surface modification using electrochemical reduction of aryldiazonium salts and photochemical grafting of alkene compounds, the chapter will focus on methods leading to the formation of amine and oxygen-terminated diamond surfaces, as these functions offer a rich diversity of interfacial reactions with different organic molecules.

2.2 Electrochemical reduction of aryldiazonium salts

The electrochemical reduction of aryldiazonium salts is a very convenient way for the derivatization of a diamond surface with simple aryl molecules (Kuo *et al.*, 1999; Jian *et al.*, 2004; Lud *et al.*, 2006; Shin *et al.*, 2006a, 2006b; Wang and Carlisle, 2006; Zhou and Zhi, 2006; Rezek *et al.*, 2007; Uetsuka *et al.*, 2007). The unique characteristics of aryldiazonium cations are the very strong electron-withdrawing effect of the diazonium moiety and the high stability of dinitrogen as a leaving group. Both factors account for the relative ease of reducing aryldiazonium salts. The electroreduction of aryldiazonium salts proceeds through a concerted mechanism, in which electron transfer and dinitrogen loss are concomitant (Fig. 2.1(a)) (Andrieux and Pinson, 2003). As aryldiazonium cations are reduced at relatively high potentials, the subsequent reduction of the aryl radical generated at the electrode surface does not occur. This approach to link organic thin films onto diamond has been carried out on a range of different diamond interfaces: ultrananocrystalline diamond films (Wang *et al.*, 2004), boron-doped diamond disks (Sarapuu *et al.*, 2005), single-crystalline diamond films with atomically flat surfaces (Shin *et al.*, 2006b; Rezek *et al.*, 2007; Uetsuka *et al.*, 2007) and undoped nanocrystalline diamond (Zhong *et al.*, 2008a). It was

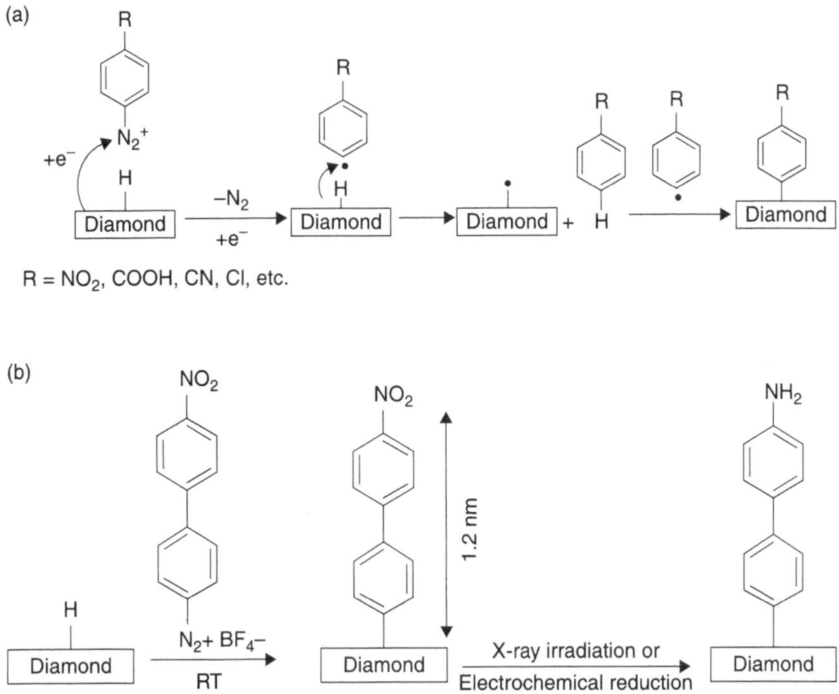

2.1 (a) Electrochemical linking of organic layers through reduction of aryl diazonium salts. (b) Chemical grafting of 4-nitro-l,1-biphenyl-4-diazonium tetrafluoroborate and reduction of the nitro group to amine group by X-ray or electrochemical reduction.

also confirmed that electrochemical diazonium salt reduction takes place on oxidized diamond interfaces; however, to a lesser extent and at ~250 mV more cathodic potentials (Uetsuka *et al.*, 2007).

Although the electrochemical aryldiazonium reduction method is a convenient way for the derivatization of diamond surface, precise control of the density of grafted molecules is not a straightforward task. Phenyl radical species, formed next to nitrogen during the grafting process, react directly with the diamond surface, but also with the phenyl ring grafted onto the surface to form multilayers. A comprehensive review by Pinson and Podvorica discusses monolayer formation achieved by the careful control of grafting parameters such as the amount of charge supplied during the electrochemical grafting and the concentration of the aryldiazonium salts (Pinson and Podvorica, 2005). In addition, the chemical reduction potential of the different aryldiazonium salts with respect to the Fermi level of diamond controls the extent of the reaction (Zhong *et al.*, 2008a). One approach to overcome the problems of multilayer formation using the electrochemical grafting process is the use of chemical grafting processes. In this case, the electrons necessary for the reduction of the diazonium salt are most likely provided by the diamond itself. The advantage of the chemical grafting step is its simplicity and that it can be applied to intrinsic undoped hydrogenated diamond. Ultrananocrystalline diamond was chemically linked to 4-nitro-1,1-biphenyl-4-diazonium tetrafluoroborate by immersing the interface into an acetonitrile solution of the salt under stirring for 72 hours (Lud *et al.*, 2006) (Fig. 2.1(b)). In order to verify the formation of a monolayer of 4-nitro-1,1-biphenyl on the diamond surface, the modified polycrystalline diamond substrate was subjected to an atomic force microscopy (AFM) scratch experiment. From this a layer thickness of 1.2 nm was determined, being in good agreement with the theoretical height of a monolayer (1.208 nm) with a perpendicular orientation of the biphenyl molecules with respect to the surface plane. The electrochemical or X-ray irradiation-induced conversion of the terminal nitro function of a nitrophenyl-terminated diamond surface to the corresponding amine was demonstrated. The radiation-based transformation offers the possibility of X-ray lithography analogous to the chemical lithography using electron irradiation. The electrochemical conversion allows *in situ* coupling of proteins to the electrode surface in a physiological environment.

The use of sodium dodecyl sulfate (SDS) (Yang *et al.*, 2005; Shul *et al.*, 2007), hydrochloric acid (0.1 M) (Zhong *et al.*, 2008a) or ionic liquids (1-butyl-3-methylimidazolium hexafluorophosphate or 1-butyl-3-methylimidazolium methyl sulphate) (Shul, Actis *et al.* 2007) to initiate the reduction of diazonium salts are other means for the chemical grafting of different aromatic molecules onto the diamond surface.

More recently, the advantage of electrochemical grafting via *in situ* generated aryldiazonium salts has been shown (Zhong *et al.*, 2008a, 2008b, 2009). Arylboronic acid ester functionalized BDD was formed in this way by diazotization of the aniline group with $NaNO_2$ (Fig. 2.2). The advantage of this approach

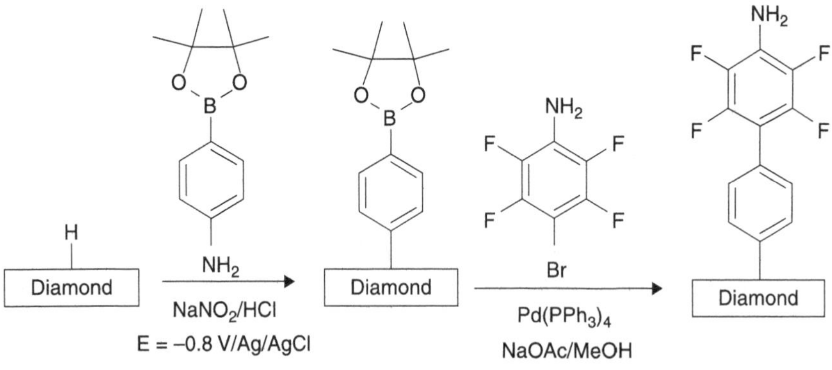

2.2 In situ electrochemical formation of aryldiazonium salts by diazotization of the aniline function with $NaNO_2$ followed by Suzuki coupling.

includes the ease of working with stable aniline precursors and compatibility with lithographic patterning. Furthermore, a Suzuki coupling reaction of the boronic acid ester function with aryl halides such as 4-bromotetrafluoroaniline or 2-(dicyanovinyl)-5-iodobithiophene was demonstrated on such diamond interfaces (Fig. 2.2) (Zhong *et al.* 2008b).

2.3 Photochemical modification

Photochemical initiated chlorination/amination/carboxylation processes of the initially hydrogenated (H-terminated) diamond surface were first introduced (Miller and Brown 1995, 1996; Ando *et al.*, 1996; Takahashi *et al.*, 2003). Based on this concept, ultraviolet irradiation (λ=254 nm) of H-terminated diamond covered with liquid films of an appropriate alkene (e.g. 10-aminodec-1-ene protected with a trifluoroacetamide functional group, vinylferrocene, 1-undecen-11-ol, etc.) (Strother *et al.*, 2002; Yang *et al.*, 2002; Knickerbocker *et al.*, 2003; Hartl *et al.*, 2004; Nakamura *et al.*, 2004; Nichols *et al.*, 2005; Tse *et al.*, 2005; Colavita *et al.*, 2006; Nebel *et al.*, 2006; Nichols *et al.*, 2006; Chong *et al.*, 2007; Rezek *et al.*, 2007; Sun *et al.*, 2007; Wang *et al.*, 2007; Yang *et al.*, 2007; Zhong *et al.*, 2007; Kondo *et al.*, 2008; Ruther *et al.*, 2011) produced organic layers covalently attached to the diamond surface through C-C bonds (Fig. 2.3). Deprotection of the protected amine results in terminal primary amine groups on the diamond surface, which can be used for further covalent attachment of DNA, enzymes, proteins and other molecules.

Although the chemical stability of the resulting monolayer has been confirmed (Yang *et al.*, 2002; Hartl *et al.*, 2004; Lu *et al.*, 2004), questions concerning the structure of the organic films and how the reaction proceeds mechanistically have been only recently clarified (Nichols *et al.*, 2005, 2006; Yang *et al.*, 2007; Zhuang *et al.*, 2010). Figure 2.3 illustrates the proposed mechanism. Illumination of H-terminated diamond, which possesses a negative electron affinity (up to −1.3 eV) results in photoemission of an electron from diamond to a molecular acceptor state in the alkene solution. The excess positive charge in the diamond then mediates nucleophilic attack at surface hydrogen sites by the alkene double bond. No analogous reaction can occur on O-terminated diamond as the positive electron affinity (up to +1.7 eV) prevents such an internal photoemission process.

Recently, Hoeb *et al.* (Hoeb *et al.*, 2010) reported an approach for thermally rather than photochemically activated formation of alkene-derived monolayers on oxygen-terminated diamond surfaces. It was revealed that heating oxidized diamond interface in 1-octadecene selectively attached the alkene to the oxygen-terminated sites via covalent C-O-C bonds. This approach is complementary to the UV initiated reaction of alkenes with diamond, which exhibits the opposite reactivity contrast.

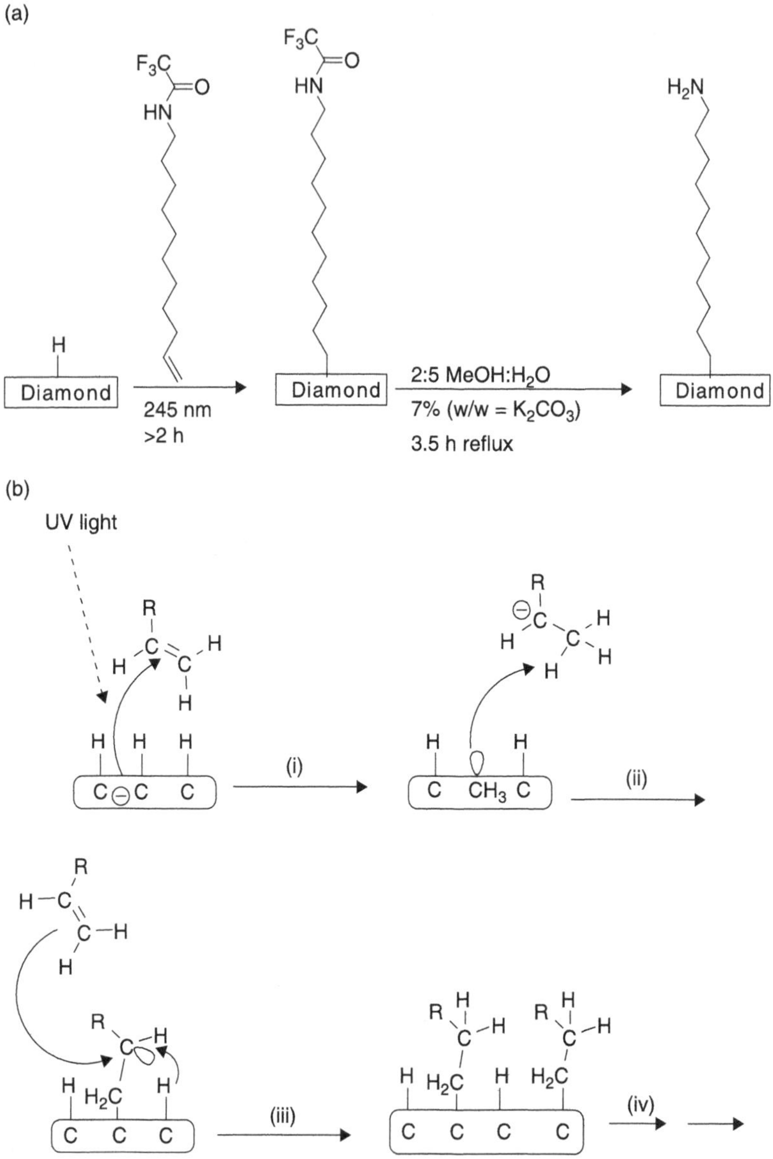

2.3 (a) Photochemical functionalization of diamond with 10-aminodec-1-ene protected with a trifluoroacetamide group. (b) Grafting mechanism of alkenes: (i) electron transfer from diamond to the olefin with hydrogen abstraction resulting in a surface carbon dangling bond, (ii) the dangling bond reacts with an olefin molecule to form diamond–carbon bond, (iii) the olefin abstracts a hydrogen atom of the diamond surface, which becomes a new site for olefin addition, (iv) the H-abstraction results in a chain reaction.

2.4 Preparation of amine-terminated diamond surfaces

The first report on the possibility of forming C-N bonds dates back to 1996 (Miller and Brown 1996; Míguez *et al.*, 2000). It has been shown that amine functions can be directly incorporated onto diamond by reaction of chlorinated diamond with ammonia or methylamine gas under UV irradiation (Fig. 2.4(a)). Along the lines of these results, the group of Kawarada reported on the possibility for direct amination of hydrogen-terminated diamond surface by first partially oxidizing the diamond by UV irradiation at 184.9 nm under oxygen gas, followed by amination for 1 hour at room temperature under UV irradiation at λ = 254 nm in an ammonia gas environment (Yan *et al.*, 2006; Zhang *et al.*, 2006; Kuga *et al.*, 2008) (Fig. 2.4(b)). Furthermore, the authors have used photolithography to pattern the surface to locally immobilize DNA molecules.

More recently, plasma rather than gas phase amination processes have been the focus of attention (Fig. 2.4(c)). We have demonstrated that the use of a cold NH_3 plasma treatment of hydrogenated diamond substrate generates surface terminal amino groups (Szunerits *et al.*, 2007). Such diamond surfaces showed their ability to bind gold nanoparticles (Szunerits *et al.*, 2006, 2007), which favoured electrochemical reduction of oxygen in basic medium. Moreover, the aminated-diamond surface was successfully used for the formation of a peptide array (Coffinier *et al.*, 2007a,b). More recently, a linear-antenna microwave plasma CVD process (Wang *et al.*, 2012) was used to form amine-terminated undoped nanocrystalline diamond thin films. The atomic concentration of nitrogen reached

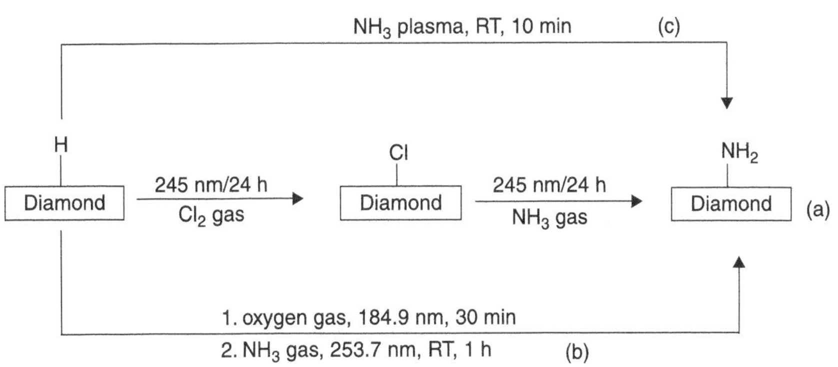

2.4 Preparation of amine-terminated diamond surfaces: (a) two-step procedure based on photochemical irradiation of a hydrogenated surface in the presence of chlorine gas forming Cl-terminated diamond, which reacts further with ammonia gas to form an amine-terminated interface; (b,c) a one-step processes using either NH_3 gas (b) or NH_3 plasma (c).

4.5% with a limited oxidization during the amination process (Fig. 2.5(a)). From the high-resolution N 1s XPS spectrum (Fig. 2.5(b)), a dominated primary amine contribution at 399.4 eV (-NH_2) together with imide and/or secondary amine contribution at 398.4 eV (C=N, C-N-C), and other contribution(s) at 400.8 eV were observed. Based on the diamond structure, it is expected that the sp^3 C-H

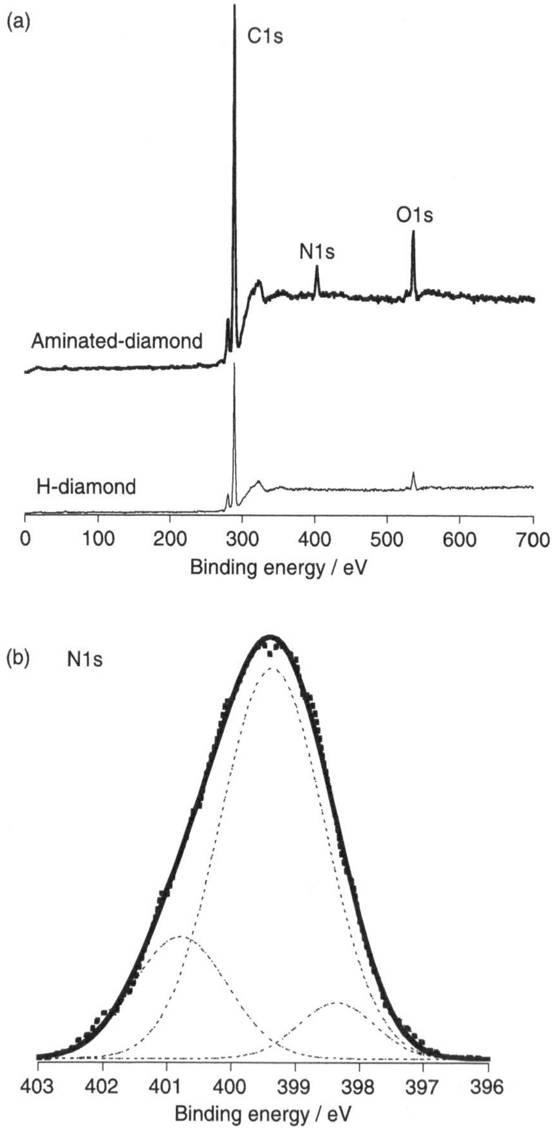

2.5 (a) Wide-range XPS survey spectrum of H-terminated and plasma aminated-diamond surfaces. (b) High resolution N1s XPS spectrum of aminated-diamond.

bonds on the (111) facets will be terminated with -NH_2 groups, whereas the CH_2 bonds on the (100) facets will be transformed to imine (C=N) and/or (C-N-C) functional groups (Szunerits *et al.*, 2006). The aminated-diamond surface was further decorated with horseradish peroxidase (HRP) enzyme using carbodiimide coupling chemistry to form an optical sensor for the detection of hydrogen peroxide (Wang *et al.*, 2012) with a high sensitivity.

2.5 Preparation of oxygen-terminated diamond surfaces

The hydrogen plasma used to deposit diamond thin films by CVD automatically results in an H-terminated surface (Goodwin, 1993; Barjon *et al.*, 2011). To achieve hydrogen termination after growth, the carbon source, mainly methane gas, is switched off and the diamond is exposed to pure hydrogen plasma for a few minutes. In spite of the high stability of H-terminated diamond, oxidation is relatively easy to perform (Boukherroub *et al.*, 2005). The resulting oxidized surface is so stable that it can be recovered only by hydrogen plasma treatment at elevated temperatures. Diverse procedures have been reported for the oxidation of H-terminated surfaces, including thermal (Ando *et al.*, 1993; Pehrsson and Mercer, 2000; John *et al.*, 2003), plasma (Notsu *et al.*, 1999; Yagi *et al.*, 1999) and electrochemical techniques (Popa *et al.*, 1999; Goeting *et al.*, 2000; Notsu *et al.*, 2000; Delabouglise *et al.*, 2003), the use of singlet oxygen (Delabouglise *et al.*, 2003), irradiation with vacuum ultraviolet light (VUV, $\lambda = 172$ nm, $t = 3$ h in the presence of O_2 and H_2O) (Ohta *et al.*, 2004) and ozone treatment (Kanazawa *et al.*, 2003; Riedel *et al.*, 2004; Boukherroub *et al.*, 2005). As oxygen atoms are divalent, they can simultaneously saturate two surface dangling bonds. Consequently, all oxidation techniques result in a combination of surface oxygen moieties including hydroxyl (-OH), ketone (C=O) and ether (C-O-C) groups (Fig. 2.6(a)). The detailed surface composition following oxidation depends sensitively on the specific processing conditions, surface orientation and surface morphology. Characterization of these oxidized diamond surfaces remains a subject of active research (Klausner *et al.*, 2009; Wang *et al.*, 2009; Ghodbane *et al.*, 2010; Mezian *et al.*, 2012). For example, it has been concluded that high concentrations of C-O functions can be obtained on nanocrystalline diamond when oxidized by radio frequency (rf) oxygen plasma, whereas the highest C=O/C-O ratio can be achieved by electrochemical oxidation. Indeed, the diamond surface oxidized by rf plasma was totally free of C=O functions (Ghodbane *et al.* 2010).

X-ray photoelectron spectroscopy (XPS) is mainly used to identify the presence of the different functional groups on the diamond surface. Figure 2.6(b) shows the high-resolution C 1s XPS spectral region of an anodically oxidized diamond surface. It displays next to the bulk diamond component at 285.0 eV (C_2), C-O bonds (i.e. –C–OH or –C–O–C–) at around 286.3 eV (C_3), while further oxidation to –C=O is observed at around 287 eV. Sp^2 impurities are seen at lower energy of about 284.3 eV (C_1).

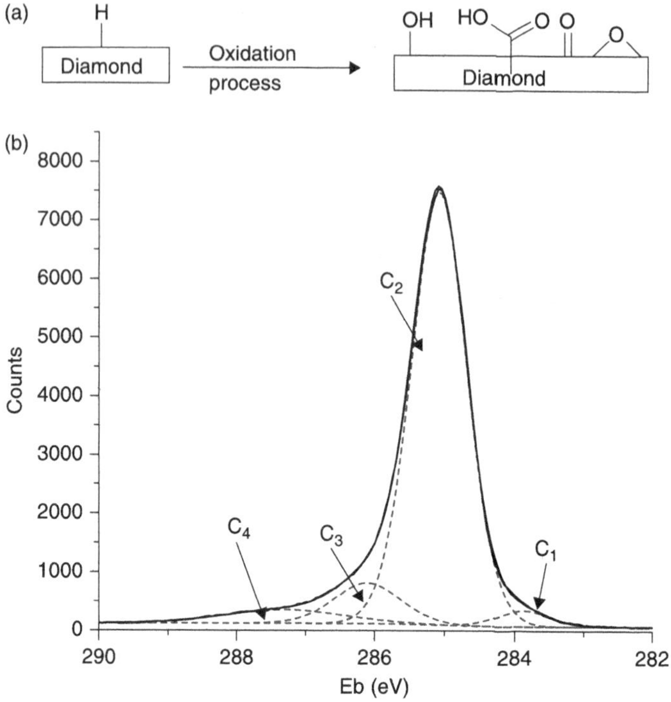

2.6 (a) Different oxygen containing functions after oxidation of hydrogen-terminated polycrystalline diamond. (b) Example of a C1s high resolution XPS spectrum after anodization in H_2SO_4.

The two primary means of organic functionalization of oxygen-terminated diamond surfaces are silanization (Notsu *et al.*, 2001, 2002; Boukherroub *et al.*, 2005; Actis *et al.*, 2006; Kondo *et al.*, 2007a, b) and esterification (Martin *et al.*, 1999; Delabouglise *et al.*, 2003; Bouvier *et al.*, 2005; Szunerits *et al.*, 2007; Das *et al.*, 2009; Wang *et al.*, 2009; Marcon *et al.*, 2010; Szunerits *et al.*, 2010; Wang *et al.*, 2010). Both necessitate the presence of surface hydroxyl groups. Silanization is a versatile approach, in which the OH-terminated surface reacts with methoxy (or ethoxy, chloride) groups of organosilane molecules in the presence of water to form interfacial C-O-Si bonds. The diversity of terminal groups that can be used to form a covalent bond with peptides, proteins, etc. makes this method an attractive means of functionalization. Importantly, the silanization reaction shows essentially no reactivity towards surface carbonyl groups and can thus be considered as an indicator for surface hydroxyl groups (Boukherroub *et al.*, 2005; Wang *et al.*, 2010).

Silanization of photochemically oxidized diamond surface with 3-aminopropyltriethoxysilane (APTES) resulted in the formation of a peptide microarray in a multistep process (Fig. 2.7(a)) (Coffinier *et al.*, 2007b). First, the

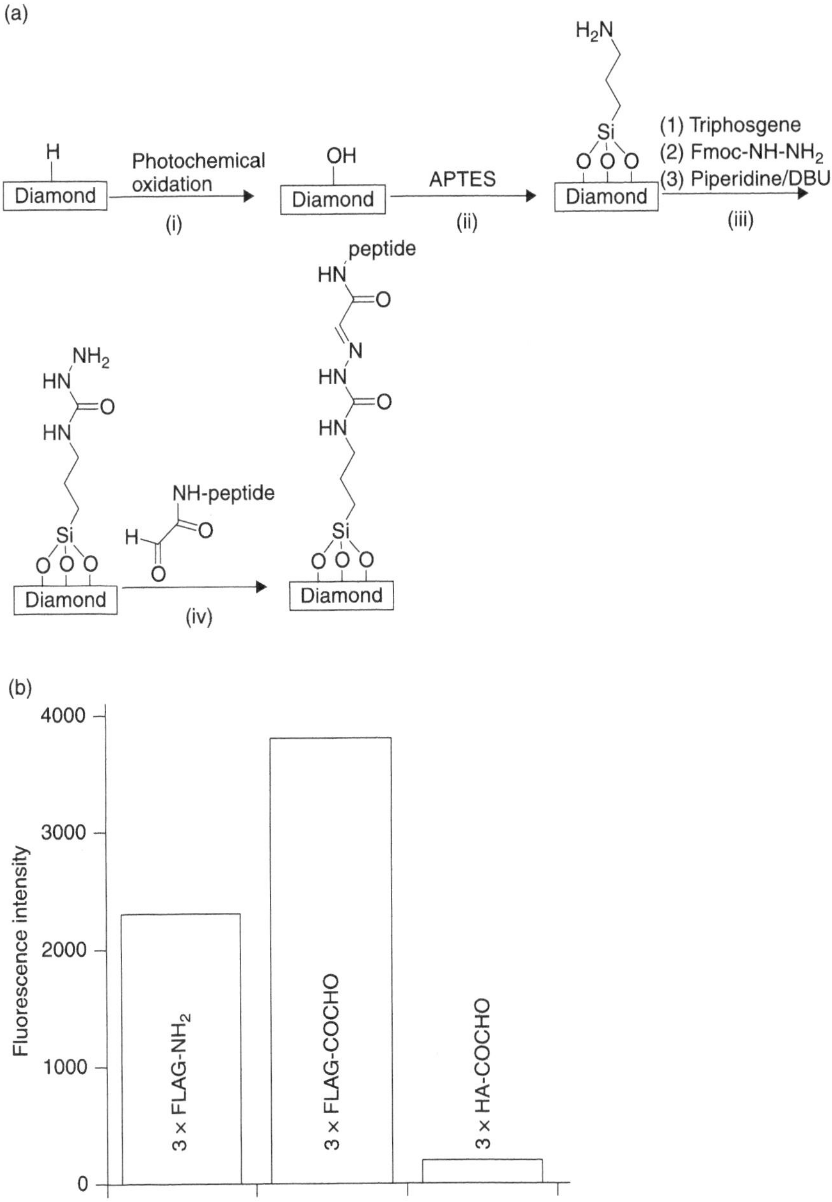

2.7 (a) Schematic illustration of the formation of semicarbazide termination on amine-terminated BDD surfaces and subsequent immobilization of glyoxylyl peptides through semicarbazone ligation. (b) Fluorescence intensity of peptide micro array prepared from semicarbazide-modified diamond surfaces when incubated in the presence of antibody antipeptide FLAG labelled with tetramethylrhodamine (10^{-2} mg/mL). Peptides: 3xFLAG-COCHO, 3xHA-COCHO, 3xFLAG-NH_2.

chemical reaction of the terminal amino groups with triphosgene and Fmoc-protected hydrazine, followed by a deprotection step led to the formation of a semicarbazide termination. The ability of the resulting semicarbazide-terminated diamond surfaces to react chemoselectively with glyoxylyl peptides through the formation of an α-oxo semicarbazone linkage was investigated. Two different glyoxylyl peptides (peptide 1: 3×FLAG-COCHO and peptide 2: 3×HA-COCHO) and a peptide amide (peptide 3: 3×FLAG-NH_2) were printed in a microarray format using a spotting approach. The fluorescence intensities obtained after incubation in the presence of antibody antipeptide FLAG labelled with tetramethylrhodamine are displayed in Fig. 2.7(b). The fluorescence observed from glyoxylyl peptide 1 is more important than that with peptide amide 3 being consistent with specific covalent ligation of peptide 1 with the semicarbazide surface and the non-covalent interaction of peptide 3. Furthermore, the control glyoxylyl peptide 2 (without a FLAG fragment) gives very low fluorescence signal after incubation in the presence of antibody antipeptide FLAG labelled with tetramethylrhodamine. The ratio of fluorescence intensity between peptides 1 and 3 is 2.

The other common route to graft molecules to oxidized diamond surfaces is esterification, in which COOH containing molecules react with surface hydroxyl groups. Like silanization, esterification reactions are often the first step in a cascade of surface functionalization steps. The ester-type linkage is commonly stable in the pH range of 3–10. The linkage is labile in highly acidic and basic media due to protonation and hydrolysis of the ester linkage. Biomolecular interactions are principally performed at pH 6–9, where the ester linkage is chemically stable. For example, 4-benzoylbenzoic acid, activated using N,N-dicyclohexylcarbodiimide (DCC), was linked to photochemically oxidized polycrystalline diamond (Szunerits *et al.*, 2007; Marcon *et al.*, 2010) (Fig. 2.8(a)). The surface-linked benzophenone, a photoreactive probe, can be activated at wavelengths that cause little damage to biomolecules (λ>340 nm) (Dorman and Prestwich, 1994). Upon irradiation, a benzophenone diradicaloid is formed and interacts with weak C-H bonds through H-abstraction. Finally, radical recombination leads to the formation of covalent bonding with molecules such as oligonucleotides, proteins and peptides, having sterically accessible C-H bonds (Fig. 2.8(a)). The fluorescence image of photoimmobilized streptavidin patterns on polyethylene glycol-modified diamond, after reaction with biotin-conjugated quantum dots is shown in Fig. 2.8(b). The strong fluorescence signal indicates that the photochemical linking does not alter the streptavidin molecules, being still capable to interact strongly with biotin.

In the search for new strategies to derivatize diamond surfaces and based on the successful demonstration of 'click' chemistry to covalently attach acetylene-bearing molecules to azide-terminated interfaces (Collman *et al.*, 2004, 2006; Devaraj *et al.*, 2005), 'click' based approaches have been developed to functionalize diamond surfaces (Das *et al.*, 2009; Wang *et al.*, 2009; Ruther, Rigsby *et al.*, 2011)

(a)

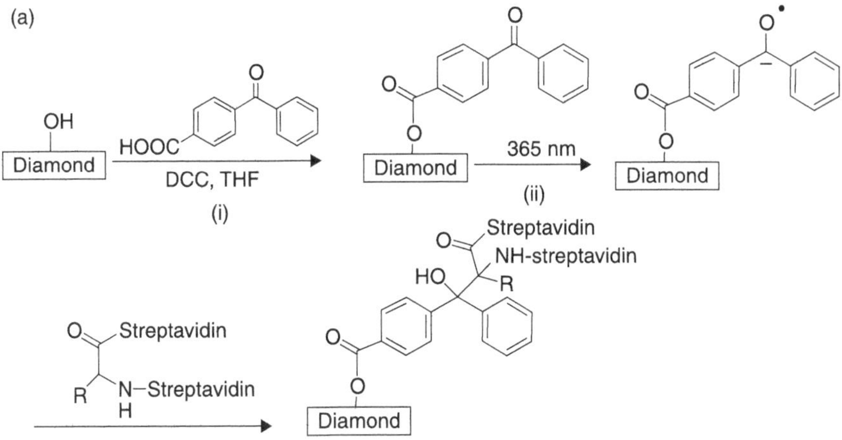

(b)

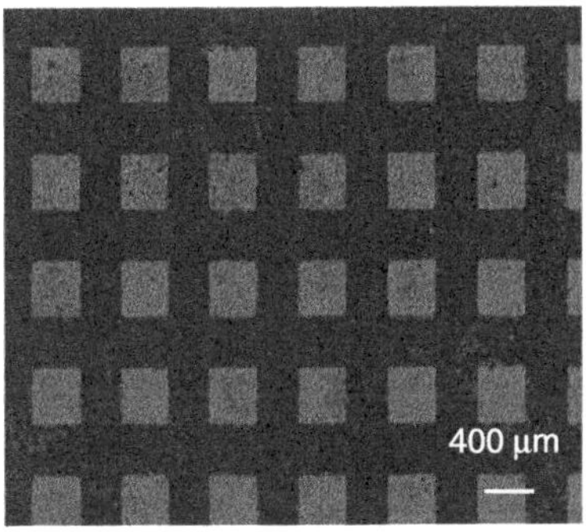

2.8 (a) (i) Schematic illustration of the functionalization of diamond with benzophenone in an esterification reaction (ii) followed by the photoactivation of the benzophenone unit (iii) and H-abstraction reaction to covalently link streptavidin. (b) Fluorescence images after photoimmobilization of streptavidin and revelation with biotin-conjugated Qdots 605; parameters for photochemical linking: $t=30\,min$, $\lambda=365\,nm$, and $P=5\,mWcm^{-2}$.

(Fig. 2.9). The underlying cycloaddition reaction fulfils many of the crucial requirements for mild surface immobilization, including excellent coupling yields, versatility, regioselectivity, excellent functional group tolerance, and stability of the catalytic process in different solvents and pH. Whereas Ruther *et al.* (Ruther, Rigsby *et al.* 2011) attached 1-undecene-1-ol to H-terminated diamond in a photochemical grafting step and converted the alcohol to the azide by first mesylation with mesylchloride followed by treatment with sodium azide, our group used as a first step an esterification reaction of the surface hydroxyl groups of

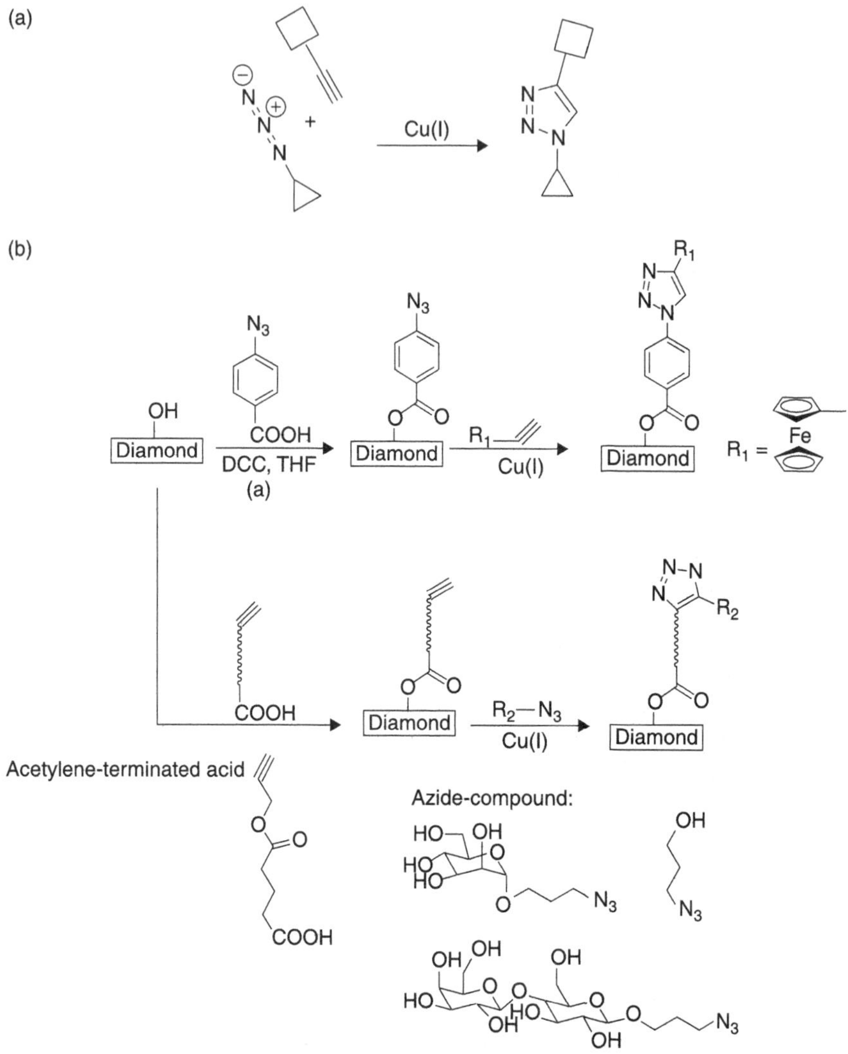

2.9 (a) Schematic illustration of the Huisgen 1,3 dipolar cycloaddition. (b) 'Click' reactions on diamond surfaces.

photochemically oxidized diamond with 4-aziodbenzoic acid, 5-oxo-5-(prop-2-ynyloxy)pentanoic acid or 4-pentynoic acid (Das, Wang *et al.*, 2009; Wang, Das *et al.*, 2009; Ruther *et al.*, 2011). On the one hand, the introduction of an azide (-N_3) group onto the diamond surface allowed covalent linking of alkynyl-modified molecules such as vinylferrocene (Das *et al.*, 2009). On the other hand, functionalization of the diamond surface with a terminal alkynyl function enabled the linkage of azido-terminated glycans (mannose, lactose) via the copper(I) catalyzed triazole formation through the classic Huisgen 1,3-dipolar cycloaddition between azides and alkynes, (Huisgen, 1984; Kim and Laibinis, 1999; Rostovtsev *et al.*, 2002; Szunerits *et al.*, 2010). In addition, the interest in the 'click' chemistry approach for the development of glycan interfaces is the possibility to vary the density of the surface immobilized carbohydrate by clicking the azido-derivatized carbohydrate analogue in the presence of a diluting agent such as azidopropanol. Mixed monolayers (Szunerits *et al.*, 2010) can be formed in an easy and well-controlled fashion, as in the case of thiolated mixed monolayers on gold.

The use of the Cu(I) catalyst in the 'click' chemistry can be avoided by performing thiol-ene or thiol-yne based 'click' reactions (Caipa Campos *et al.*, 2010; Hoyle *et al.*, 2010; Lowe *et al.*, 2010) (Fig. 2.10). Although the 'click' chemistry characteristics such as high yields, regiospecificity, mild reaction conditions and tolerance to a variety of functional groups are preserved, the versatility of the reaction is enhanced by the fact that it does not require any

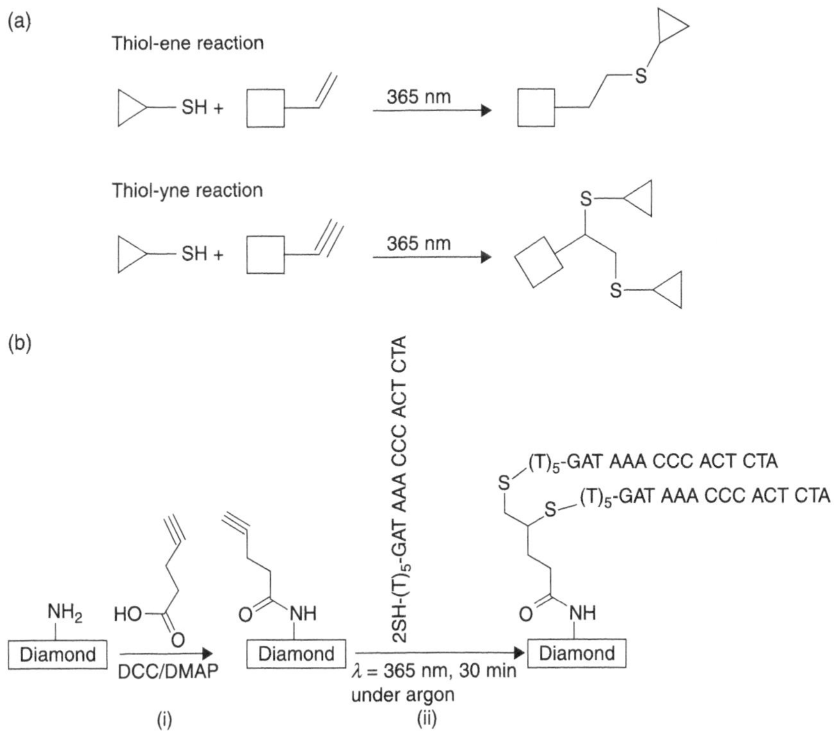

2.10 (a) Reaction mechanism of photoaddition of thiols to alkenes and alkynes. (b) Thiol-yne reaction on diamond: (i) aminolysis of aminated-diamond with 4-pentynoic acid in the presence of N,N'-dicyclohexylcarbodiimide (DCC) and 4-(dimethylamino)-pyridine (DMAP), (ii) thiol-yne coupling of thiolated oligonucleotide molecules.

catalyst as it is initiated thermally or photochemically (Jonkheijm *et al.*, 2008; Bertin and Schlaad, 2009; Caipa Campos *et al.*, 2010; Lin *et al.*, 2010; Weinrich *et al.*, 2010). Similar to alkenes, alkynes can be used for the radical addition of thiols with the main difference being that alkynes can react with two thiol molecules to form a double addition product (Hensarling *et al.*, 2009). Although less investigated than the thiol-ene reaction, thiol-yne chemistry has been employed for the preparation of bifunctional surfaces. This reaction was recently developed on diamond interfaces to immobilize thiolated single-stranded oligonucleotides (Meziane *et al.*, 2012).

2.6 Conclusion and future trends

Over the years, a variety of different surface functionalization schemes have been demonstrated and studied on different diamond interfaces. Versatile strategies such as 'click' chemistry approaches have been revealed to be interesting alternatives for the functionalization of diamond interfaces in an easy, reproducible and mild manner. The knowledge gained on diamond interfaces can be easily transposed to any other type of diamond-based materials. Diamond-based nanomaterials such as nanowires (Yang *et al.*, 2008a,b, 2009; Szunerits *et al.*, 2010), nanoparticles (Barras *et al.*, 2010) or resonate microcantilevers (Bongrain *et al.*, 2011) have shown to be of particular interest. Diamond nanowires are of importance for electrochemical-based sensors and electrolysis, as well as supports for catalysts (Luo *et al.*, 2009; Wei *et al.*, 2009; Yang *et al.*, 2009; Szunerits *et al.*, 2010), due to the relatively large surface area compared to flat diamond. Diamond nanowire electrodes can be currently considered as competitive alternatives to carbon nanotubes (Sun *et al.*, 2005) as they possess all the advantages of diamond together with that of a nanomaterial. Diamond nanowires are mostly formed by oxygen plasma etching of diamond films with and without the use of hard masks (Bai *et al.*, 2000; Yang *et al.*, 2008a,b; Luo *et al.*, 2009; Nebel *et al.*, 2009; Coffinier *et al.*, 2010; Szunerits *et al.*, 2010; Terashima *et al.*, 2011). Reported surface functionalization schemes of such wires are currently limited to electrochemical grafting of diazonium salts (Yang *et al.*, 2009) and silanization reactions (Coffinier *et al.*, 2010). The enhanced electrical field at the very end of the diamond tips resulted in a preferential modification of the tip. This gave rise to optimized hybridization kinetics of DNA, high sensitivity with a detection limit of 2 pM for complementary DNA as well as single-base mismatch discrimination (Yang *et al.*, 2009). We reported that silanization with octadecyltrichlorosilane (OTS) or *1H,1H,2H,2H*-perfluorodecyltrichlorosilane (PFTS) leads to the formation of superhydrophobic diamond surfaces (Coffinier *et al.*, 2010). Under optimized conditions, such surfaces showed water contact angles as high as 160° and quasi null hysteresis. Furthermore, the diamond nanowire interface chemically modified with PFTS displayed oleophobic properties with a contact angle of 94° for hexadecane.

The interest in the use of diamond nanoparticles (NDs) has emerged as these particles are considered particularly well suited for biological applications that require optical transparency, chemical inertness, hardness and high specific area (Kruger, 2006). Surface functionalization is applied to customize the particles for different applications, such as increased solubility in biological media, bioconjugation to antibodies or receptors for drug delivery and diagnostics (Barnard, 2009; Kruger, 2011). As the surface chemistry of NDs is more complex than that of diamond, direct surface functionalization often leads to inhomogeneous and uncontrolled surface chemistry. Intense research efforts have been dedicated to the surface homogenization of the particles and Fento-based reactions to form large numbers of hydroxyl groups on NDs have proven to be of interest (Markovic *et al.*, 1994; Martin *et al.*, 2010; Girard *et al.*, 2011). The attractive features of 'click' chemistry have also been applied to the surface modification of NDs diamond and this opens up an easy way to be used as a general platform for the preparation of functional NDs for various applications (Barras *et al.*, 2010; Meinhardt *et al.*, 2011). Recently, the direct functionalization of hydroxyl-terminated ND with dopamine derivatives has been reported (Barras *et al.*, 2011) taking advantage of the versatility of the catechol anchor and the ease of synthesis of dopamine derivatives bearing functional groups.

2.7 References

Actis P, Manesse M, Nunes-Kirchner C, *et al.* (2006), 'Localized electropolymerization on oxidized boron doped diamond electrodes modified with pyrrolyl units.' *Phys. Chem. Chem. Phys*, 8, 4924–4931.

Ando T, Nishitani-Gamo M, Rawles RE, *et al.* (1996), 'Chemical modification of diamond surfaces using a chlorinated surface as an intermediate state.' *Diamond and Relat. Mater.*, 5, 1136–1142.

Ando T, Yamamoto K, Ishii N, *et al.* (1993), 'Vapour-phase Oxidation of Diamond Surfaces in O_2 studied by Diffuse Reflectance Fourier-transform Infrared and Temperature-programmed Desorption Spectroscopy.' *J. Chem. Soc. Faraday Trans.*, 89, 3635–3640.

Andrieux CP and Pinson J (2003), 'The standard redox potential of the phenyl radical/anion couple.' *J. Am. Chem. Soc*, 125, 14801.

Bai ES, Baik YJ and Jeon DJ (2000), 'Aligned diamond nanowhiskers.' *J. Mater. Res.*, 15, 923.

Barjon J, Habka J, Chevallier J, *et al.* (2011), 'Hydrogen-induced passivation of boron acceptors in monocrystalline and polycrystalline diamond.' *Phys. Chem. Chem. Phys*, 13, 11511.

Barnard AS (2009), 'Diamond standard in diagnostics: nanodiamond biolabels make their mark.' *Analyst*, 134, 1751.

Barras A, Lyskawa J, Szunerits S, *et al.* (2011), 'Direct Functionalization of Nanodiamond Particles using Dopamine Derivatives.' *Langmuir*, 27, 12451.

Barras A, Szunerits S, Marcon L, *et al.* (2010), 'Functionalization of Diamond Nanoparticles using "Click" Chemistry.' *Langmuir*, 26, 13168.

Bertin A and Schlaad H (2009), 'H. Mild and versatile (bio-)functionalization of glass surfaces via thiol-ene photochemistry.' *Chem. Mater.*, 21, 5698.

Bongrain A, Agnes C, Rousseau L, *et al.* (2011), 'High Sensitivity of Diamond Resonant Microcantilvers for Direct Detection in Liquids as probed by Molecular Electrostatic Surface Interactions.' *Langmuir*, 27, 12226.

Boukherroub R, Wallart X, Szunerits S, *et al.* (2005), 'Photochemical oxidation of hydrogenated boron-doped diamond surfaces.' *Electrochem. Commun.*, 7, 937–940.

Bouvier P, Delabouglise D, Denoyell A, *et al.* (2005), 'Photosensitization of boron-doped diamond by surface grafting of pyrene groups.' *Electrochem. Solid-State Lett.*, 8, E57.

Caipa Campos MA, Paulusse JMJ and Zuilhof H (2010), 'Functional monolayers on oxide-free silicon surfaces via thiol –ene click chemistry.' *Chem. Commun.*, 46, 5512.

Chong KF, Loh KP, Vedula SRK, *et al.* (2007), 'Characterization of cell adhesion properties of photochemically functionalized diamond surfaces.' *Langmuir*, 23, 5615.

Coffinier Y, Galopin E, Szunerits S and Boukherroub R (2010), 'Preparation of superhydrophobic and oleophobic diamond nanograss array.' *J. Mater. Chem.*, 20, 10671–10675.

Coffinier Y, Szunerits S, Jama C, *et al.* (2007a), 'Peptide immobilization on amine-terminated boron doped diamond surfaces' *Langmuir*, 23, 4494–4497.

Coffinier Y, Szunerits S, Marcus B, *et al.* (2007b), 'Covalent linking of peptides onto oxygen-terminated boron-doped diamond surfaces.' *Diamond Relat. Mater.*, 16, 892–896.

Colavita PE, Sun B, Tse KY, *et al.* (2006), 'Electrical bias dependent photochemical functionalization of diamond surfaces.' *J. Phys. Chem. B*, 110, 16535.

Collman JP, Devaraj NK and Chidsey CED (2004), ' "Clicking" functionality onto electrode surfaces.' *Langmuir* 20, 1051–1053.

Collman JP, Devaraj NK, Eberspacher TPA and Chidsey CED (2006), 'Mixed Azide-Terminated Monolayers: A Platform for Modifying Electrode Surfaces.' *Langmuir*, 22, 2457.

Das MR, Wang M, Szunerits S, *et al.* (2009), 'Clicking ferrocene groups to boron-doped diamond electrodes.' *Chem. Commun.*, 2753.

Delabouglise D, Marcus B, Mermoux M, *et al.* (2003), 'Biotin grafting on boron doped diamond.' *Chem. Commun.*, 2698–2699.

Devaraj NK, Miller GP, Ebina W, *et al.* (2005), 'Chemoselective Coupling of Oligonucleotides to Self Assembled Monolayers.' *J. Am. Chem. Soc.*, 127, 8600 – 8601.

Dorman G and Prestwich GD (1994), 'Benzophenone Photophores in Biochemistry.' *Biochem.*, 33, 5661.

Fortin E, Chane-Tune J, Mailley P, *et al.* (2004), 'Nucleosides and ODN electrochemical detection onto boron doped diamond electrodes.' *Bioelectrochemistry*, 63, 303–306.

Ghodbane S, Haensel T, Coffinier Y, *et al.* (2010), 'HREELS investigation of the surface of nanocrystalline diamond films oxidized by different processes.' *Langmuir*, 26, 18798–18805.

Girard HA, Petit T, Perruchas S, *et al.* (2011), 'Surface properties of hydrogenated nanodiamonds: a chemical investigation.' *Phys. Chem. Chem. Phys.*, 13, 11517.

Goeting CH, Marken F, Gutiérrez-Sosa A and Compton RC (2000), 'Electrochemically induced surface modification of boron-doped diamond electrodes.' *Diam. Relat. Mater.*, 9, 390–396.

Goodwin DG (1993), 'Scaling laws for diamond chemical-vapor deposition. I. Diamond surface chemistry.' *J. App. Phys.*, 74, 6888.

Hamers RJ, Butler JE, Lasseter T, *et al.* (2005), 'Molecular and biomolecular monolayers on diamond as an interface to biology.' *Diamond Relat. Mater.*, 14, 661–668.

Hartl A, Schmich E, Garrido JA, *et al.* (2004), 'Protein-modified nanocrystalline diamond thin films for biosensor applications.' *Nature Mat.*, 3, 736.
Hensarling RM, Doughty VA; Chan JW and Patton DL (2009), ' "Clicking" polymer brushes with thiol-yne chemistry: indoors and out.' *J. Am. Chem. Soc*, 131, 14673.
Hoeb M, Auernhammer M, Schoell SJ, *et al.* (2010), 'Thermally Induced Alkylation of Diamond.' *Langmuir*, 26, 18862.
Hoyle CE, Lowe AB and Bowman CN (2010), 'Thiol-click chemistry: a multifaceted toolbox for small molecule and polymer synthesis.' *Chem. Soc. Rev.*, 39, 1355.
Huisgen R (1984) *1,3-Dipolar Cycloaddition Chemistry*. New York, Wiley.
Jian W, Firestone MA, Auciello O and Carlisle JA (2004), *Langmuir*, 20, 11450.
John P, Polwart N, Troupe CE and Wilson JIB (2003), 'The Oxidation of Diamond: The geometry and Stretching Frequency of carbonyl on the (111) surface.' *J. Am. Chem. Soc.*, 125, 6600.
Jonkheijm P, Weinrich D, Kohn M, *et al.* (2008), 'Photochemical surface patterning by the thiol-ene reaction.' *Angew. Chem. Int. Ed.*, 47, 4421.
Kanazawa H, Song K-S, Sakai T, *et al.* (2003), 'Effect of iodide ions on the hydrogen-terminated and partially oxygen-terminated diamond surface.' *Diamond Relat. Mater.*, 12, 618–622.
Kim NY and Laibinis PE (1999), 'Improved polypyrrole/silicon junctions by surfacial modification of hydrogen-terminated silicon using organolithium reagents.' *J. Am. Chem. Soc.*, 121, 7162.
Klausner F, Ghodbane S, Boukherroub R, *et al.* (2009), 'Comparison of Different Oxidation Techniques on Single-Crystal and Nanocrystalline Diamond Surfaces.' *Diam. and Relat. Mat.*, 19, 474.
Knickerbocker T, Strother T, Schwartz MP, *et al.* (2003), 'DNA Modified Diamond Surface.' *Langmuir*, 19, 1938–1942.
Kondo T, Aoshima S, Honda K, *et al.* (2007a), 'Fabrication of Covalent SAM/Au Nanoparticle/Boron-Doped Diamond Configurations with a Sequential Self-Assembly Method.' *J. Phys. Chem. C*, 111, 12650.
Kondo T, Honda K, Tryk DA and Fujishima A (2007b), 'Plasma etching treatment for surface modification of boron-doped diamond electrodes.' *J. Electrochem. Soc.*, 152, E18.
Kondo T, Hoshi H, Honda K, *et al.* (2008), 'Photochemical Modification of a Boron-doped Diamond Electrode Surface with Vinylferrocene.' *J. Phys. Chem. C*, 112, 11887.
Kruger A (2011), 'Beyond the shine: recent progress in applications of nanodiamond.' *J. Mater. Chem.*, 21, 12571–12578.
Kruger A (2006), 'Hard and soft: biofunctionalized diamond.' *Angew. Chem. Int. Ed.*, 45, 6426.
Kuga S, Yang J-H, Takahashi H, *et al.* (2008), 'Detection of Mismatched DNA on Partically Negatively Charged Diamond Surfaces by Optical and Potentiometric Methods.' *J. Am. Chem. Soc*, 130, 13251.
Kuo T-C, McCreery RL and Swain GM (1999), 'Electrochemical Modification of boron doped chemical vapor deposited surfaces with covalent bonded monolayers.' *Electrochem. Solid State Lett.*, 2, 288–290.
Lin P-C, Weinrich D and Waldmann H (2010), 'Protein Biochips: Oriented Surface Immobilization of Proteins.' *Macromol. Chem. Phys.*, 211, 136.
Lowe AB, Hoyle CE and Bowman CN (2010), 'Thiol-yne click chemistry: A powerful and versatile methodology for materials synthesis.' *J. Mater. Chem.*, 20, 4745.
Lu MC, Knickerbocker T, Cai W, *et al.* (2004), 'Invasive cleavage reactions on DNA-modified diamond surfaces.' *Biopolymers*, 73, 606.

Lud SQ, Steenackers M, Jordan R, *et al.* (2006), 'Chemical Grafting of Biphenyl Self-Assembled Monolayers on Ultrananocrystalline Diamond.' *J. Am. Chem. Soc.*, 128, 16884.

Luo D, Wu L and Zhi J (2009), 'Fabrication of Boron-doped Diamond Nanorod Forest Electrodes and their application in nonenzymatic amperometric glucose biosensing.' *ACS Nano*, 3, 2121.

Luong JHT, Male KB and Glennon JD (2009), 'Boron-doped diamond electrode: synthesis, characterization, functionalization and analytical applications.' *Analyst*, 134, 1965.

Marcon L, Wang M, Coffinier Y, *et al.* (2010), 'Photochemical Immobilization of proteins and peptides on benzophenone-terminated boron-doped diamond surfaces.' *Langmuir* 26, 1075.

Markovic NM, Adzic RR, Cahan BD and Yeager EB (1994), 'Structural effects in electrocatalysis: oxygen reduction on platinum low index single-crystal surfaces in perchloric acid solutions.' *J. Electroanal. Chem.*, 377, 249.

Martin HB, Argoitia A, Angus JC and Landau U (1999), 'Voltammetry Studies of Single-Crystal and Polycrystalline Diamond Electrodes.' *J. Electrochem. Soc.*, 146, 2959–2964.

Martin R, Alvaro M, Herance JR and Garcia H (2010), 'Fenton-Treated Functionalized Diamond Nanoparticles as Gene Delivery System' *ACSNano*, 4, 65.

Meinhardt T, Lang D, Dill H and Krueger A (2011), 'Pushing the Functionality of Diamond Nanoparticles to New Horizons: Orthogonally Functionalized nanodiamond using click chemistry.' *Adv. Funct. Mater.*, 21, 494.

Meziane D, Kromka A, Boukherroub R and Szunerits S (2012) 'Thiol-yne reaction on boron doped diamond electrodes.' *Anal. Chem.*, 84, 194–200.

Míguez H, Meseguer F, López C, *et al.* (2000), 'Germanium FCC Structure from a Colloidal Crystal Template.' *Langmuir*, 16, 4405.

Miller JB and Brown DW (1995), 'Properties of photochemically modified diamond films.' *Diam. Relat. Mater.*, 4, 435–440.

Miller JB and Brown DW (1996), 'Photochemical Modification of Diamond Surfaces.' *Langmuir*, 12, 5809–5817.

Nakamura T, Suzuki M, Ishihara M, *et al.* (2004), 'Photochemical Modification of diamond films: introduction of perfluorooctyl functional groups on their surface.' *Langmuir*, 20, 5846–5849.

Nebel CE, Nesladek M and Koizumi S (2008), *Physics and Applications of CVD Diamond.* Weinheim, Wiley-VCH.

Nebel CE and Ristein J (2003), *Thin Film Diamond: Semiconductors and Semimetals.* Amsterdam, The Netherlands, Elsevier.

Nebel CE, Shin D, Takeuchi D, *et al.* (2006), 'Alkene/diamond liquid/solid interface characterization using internal photoemission spectroscopy.' *Langmuir*, 22, 5645.

Nebel CE, Yang N, Uetsuka H, *et al.* (2009), 'Diamond nano-wires, a new approach towards next generation electrochemical gene sensor platforms.' *Diamond Relat. Mater.*, 18, 910.

Nichols BM, Butler JE, Russell JN and Hamers RJ (2005), 'Photochemical functionalization of hydrogen-terminated diamond surfaces: A structural and mechanistic study.' *J. Phys. Chem. B.*, 109, 20938.

Nichols BM, Metz KM, Tse K-Y, *et al.* (2006), 'Electrical bias dependent photochemical functionalization of diamond surfaces.' *J. Phys. Chem. B*, 110, 16535.

Notsu H, Fukazawa T, Tatsuma T, *et al.* (2001), 'Hydroxyl Groups on boron-doped diamond electrodes and their modification with a silan coupling agent.' *Electrochem. Solid-State Lett.*, 4, H1–H3.

Notsu H, Tatsuma T and Fujishima A (2002), 'Tyrosinase-modified boron-doped diamond electrodes for the determination of phenol derivatives.' *J. Electroanal. Chem*, 523, 86.

Notsu H, Yagi I, Tatsuma T, *et al.* (1999), 'Surface Carbonyl Groups on Oxidized Diamond Electrodes.' *Electrochem. Solid-State Lett.*, 2, 522.

Notsu H, Yagi I, Tatsuma T, *et al.* (2000), 'Surface carbonyl groups on oxidised diamond electrodes.' *J. Electroanal. Chem.*, 492, 31–37.

Ohta R, Saito N, Inoue Y, *et al.* (2004), 'Organosilan self assembled monolayer linked to the diamond surface.' *J. Vac. Sci. Technol. A*, 22, 2005–2009.

Pehrsson PE and Mercer TW (2000), 'Oxidation of the hydrogenated diamond (100) surface.' *Surf. Sci.*, 460, 49–66.

Pinson J and Podvorica F (2005), 'Attachment of organic layers to conductive or semiconductive surfaces by reduction of diazonium salts.' *Chem. Soc. Rev.*, 34, 429.

Popa E, Notsu H, Miwa T, *et al.* (1999), 'Selective electrochemical detection of dopamine in the presence of ascorbic acid at anodized diamond thin film electrodes.' *Electrochem. Solid State Lett.*, 2, 49–51.

Rezek B, Shin D and Nebel CE (2007), 'Properties of hybridized DNA arrays on single-crystalline undoped and boron-doped (100) diamonds studied by atomic force microscopy in electrolytes.' *Langmuir*, 23, 7626.

Riedel M, Ristein J and Ley L (2004), 'The impact of ozone on the surface conductivity of single crystal diamond.' *Diam. Relat. Mater.*, 13, 746–750.

Rostovtsev VV, Green LG, Fokin VV and Sharpless KB (2002), 'A Stepwise Huisgen cycloaddition process: copper (I) catalysed regioselective "Ligation" of azide and terminal alkyne.' *Angew. Chem. Int. Ed.*, 41, 2596.

Ruther RE, Rigsby ML, Gerken JB, *et al.* (2011), 'Highly Stable Redox-Active Molecular Layers by Covalent Grafting to Conducting Diamond.' *J. Am. Chem. Soc*, 133, 5692.

Sarapuu A, Helstein K, Schiffrin DJ and Tammeveski K (2005), 'Kinetics of oxygen reduction on quinone modified HOPG and BDD electrodes in alkaline solutions.' *Electrochem. Sol.-State Lett.*, 8, E30.

Shin D, Rezek B, Tokuda N, *et al.* (2006a), 'Photo- and electrochemical bonding of DNA to single crystalline CVD diamond.' *Phys. Stat. Sol (a)*, 13, 3245.

Shin D, Tokuda N, Rezek B and Nebel CE (2006b), 'Periodically arranged benzene-linker molecules on boron-doped single-crystalline diamond films for DNA sensing.' *Electrochem. Commun.*, 8, 844.

Shul G, Actis P, Marcus B, *et al.* (2007), 'Solvent-free chemical functionalization of hydrogen-terminated boron-doped diamond electrodes with diazonium salts in ionic liquids.' *Diam. Relat. Mater.*, 17, 1394.

Strother T, Knickerbocker T, Russell JN, *et al.* (2002), 'Photochemical Functionalisation of Diamond Films.' *Langmuir*, 18, 968–971.

Sun B, Baker SE, Butler JE, *et al.* (2007), 'Covalent molecular functionalization of diamond thin-film transistors.' *Diam. Relat. Mater.*, 16, 1608.

Sun LT, Gong JL, Zhu ZY, *et al.* (2005), 'Synthesis and characterization of diamond nanowires from carbon nanotubes.' *Diam. Relat. Mater.*, 14, 749.

Szunerits S, Coffinier Y, Galopin E, *et al.* (2010), 'Preparation of boron-doped diamond nanowires and their application for sensitive electrochemical detection of tryptophan.' *Electrochem. Commun.*, 12, 438–441.

Szunerits S, Jama C, Coffinier Y, *et al.* (2006), 'Direct amination of hydrogenated-terminated boron doped diamond surfaces.' *Electrochem. Commun*, 8, 1185–1190.

Szunerits S, Manesse M, Denault G, *et al.* (2007), 'Investigation of the influence of the surface termination of boron-doped diamond electrodes on the oxygen reduction in basic medium.' *Electrochem. Solid State Lett.*, 10, G43–G46.

Szunerits S, Niedziółka-Jönsson J, Boukherroub R, *et al.* (2010), 'Label-Free Detection of Lectins on Carbohydrate-Modified Boron-Doped Diamond Surfaces.' *Anal. Chem.*, 82, 8203–8210.

Szunerits S, Shirahata N, Actis P, *et al.* (2007), 'Photografting and patterning of oligonucleotides on benzophenone-modified boron-doped diamond.' *Chem. Commun.*, 2793.

Takahashi K, Tanga M, Takai O and Okamura H (2003), 'DNA preservation using diamond chips.' *Diamond and Rel. Mat.*, 12, 572–576.

Terashima C, Arihara K, Okazaki S, *et al.* (2011), 'Fabrication of Vertically aligned diamond wiskers from highly boron doped diamond by oxygen plasma etching.' *ACS App. Mater. Interfaces*, 3, 177.

Tse K-Y, Nichols BM, Yang W, *et al.* (2005), 'Electrical properties of diamond surfaces functionalized with m molecular monolayers' *J. Phys Chem. B*, 109, 8523.

Uetsuka H, Shin D, Tokuda N, *et al.* (2007), 'Electrochemical grafting of boron-doped single crystalline CVD diamond.' *Langmuir*, 23, 3466.

Wang J and Carlisle JA (2006), 'Covalent immobilization of glucose oxidase on conducting ultrananocrystalline diamond thin films.' *Diam. Rel. Mater.*, 15, 279–284.

Wang J, Firestone MA, Auciello O and Carlisle JA (2004), 'Surface Functionalisation of Ultrananocrystalline diamond films by electrochemical reduction of aryldiazonium salts.' *Langmuir*, 20, 11450–11456.

Wang M, Das MR, Li M, *et al.* (2009), ' "Clicking" thiophene on diamond interfaces. Preparation of a conducting polythiophene/diamond hybrid material.' *J. Phys. Chem. C.*, 113, 17082.

Wang M, Simon N, Charrier G, *et al.* (2010), 'Distinction between surface hydroxyl and ether groups on boron-doped diamond electrodes using a chemical approach.' *Electrochem. Commun.*, 12, 351.

Wang M, Simon N, Decorse-Pascanut C, *et al.* (2009), 'Comparison of the chemical composition of boron-doped diamond surfaces upon different oxidation processes.' *Electrochimica Acta*, 54 5818–5824.

Wang Q, Kromka A, Houdkova J, *et al.* (2012), 'Nanomolar Hydrogen Peroxide Detection Using Horseradish Peroxidase Covalently linked to Undoped Nanocrystalline Diamond Surfaces' *Langmuir*, in press.

Wang X, Colavita PE, Metz KM, *et al.* (2007), 'Direct photopatterning and SEM Imaging of molecular monolayers on diamond surfaces: Mechanistic insights into UV-Initiated molecular grafting.' *Langmuir*, 23, 11623.

Wei M, Terashima C, Lv M, *et al.* (2009), 'Boron-doped diamond nanograss array for electrochemical sensors.' *Chem. Commun.*, 3624.

Weinrich D, Lin PC, Jonkheijm P, *et al.* (2010), 'Oriented Immobilization of Farnesylated Proteins by the Thiol-Ene Reaction.' *Angew. Chem. Int. Ed.*, 49, 1252.

Yagi I, Notsu H, Kondo T, *et al.* (1999), 'Electrochemical selectivity for redox systems at oxygen-terminated diamond electrode.' *J. Electroanal. Chem*, 473, 173.

Yan J-H, Song K-S, Zhang G-J, *et al.* (2006), *Langmuir*, 22, 11245.

Yang N, Uetsuka H and Nebel CE (2009), 'Biofunctionalization of Vertically Aligned Diamond Nanowires.' *Adv. Funct. Mater.*, 19, 887.

Yang N, Uetsuka H, Osawa E and Nebel CE (2008), 'Vertically aligned diamond nanowires for DNA sensing.' *Angew. Chem. Int. Ed.*, 47, 5183.
Yang N, Uetsuka H, Osawa E and Nebel CE (2008), 'Vertically aligned nanowires from boron-doped diamond.' *Nano. Lett.*, 8, 3572.
Yang N, Uetsuka H, Watanabe H, *et al.* (2007), 'Photochemical Amine Layer Formation on H-Terminated Single-Crystalline CVD Diamond.' *Chem. Mater.*, 19, 2852.
Yang W, Auciello O, Butler JE, *et al.* (2002), 'DNA-modified nanocrystalline diamond thin-films as stable, biologically active substrates.' *Nature Mat.*, 253–257.
Yang W, Baker SE, Butler JE, *et al.* (2005), 'Electrically addressable biomolecular functionalisation of conductive nanocrystalline diamond films.' *Chem. Mater.*, 17, 938–940.
Zhang G-J, Song K-S, Nakamura Y, *et al.* (2006), 'DNA Micropatterning on Polycrystalline Diamond via One-Step Direct Amination.' *Langmuir* 22, 3728–3734.
Zhong Y-L, Chong KF, May PW, *et al.* (2007), 'Optimizing biosensing properties on undecylenic Acid-functionalized diamond.' *Langmuir*, 23, 5824.
Zhong YL, Loh KP, Midya A and Chen Z-K (2008a), 'Suzuki Coupling of Aryl Organics on Diamond.' *Chem. Mater.*, 20, 3137.
Zhong YL, Midya A, Ng Z, *et al.* (2008b), 'Diamond-Based Molecular Platform for Photoelectrochemistry.' *J. Am. Chem. Soc*, 130, 17218.
Zhong YL, Ng W, Yang J-X and Loh KP (2009), 'Electrostatically self-assembled polyoxometalates on molecular-dye functionalized diamond.' *J. Am. Chem. Soc*, 131, 18293.
Zhou YL and Zhi JF (2006), 'Development of an amperometric biosensor based on covalent immobilization of tyrosinase on a boron-doped diamond electrode.' *Electrochem. Commun.*, 8, 1811.
Zhuang H, Srikanth VVSS, Jiang X, *et al.* (2010), 'Elucidation of Different Steps involved in allylamine functionalization of the diamond surface and its polymerization by time-of-flight secondary ion mass spectrometry.' *Chem. Mater.*, 22, 4414.

3

Biotribology and biological behaviour of nanocrystalline diamond (NCD) coatings for medical applications

M. AMARAL, University of Aveiro, Portugal

DOI: 10.1533/9780857093516.1.48

Abstract: This chapter discusses the application of nanocrystalline diamond (NCD) films as protective coatings for joint replacement. The chapter includes an overview of chemical vapour deposition (CVD) diamond and discusses the influence of hot-filament chemical vapour deposition (HFCVD) parameters on the deposition of NCD on silicon nitride (Si_3N_4) ceramics. The chapter then presents biotribological studies and *in vitro* cell cultures of the deposited NCD coatings.

Key words: nanocrystalline diamond (NCD), coatings, joint replacement, biotribology, biocompatibility.

3.1 Introduction to nanocrystalline diamond (NCD)

Diamond has attracted much interest over the years, partly because of its excellent mechanical, physical and chemical properties, allowing an endless number of possible applications. However, full use of diamond as an engineered material is only possible if the diamond exists in a suitable form with no resource limitations. In the second half of the 1950s, WG Eversole (1962) proposed the chemical vapour deposition (CVD) technique. This method received a great deal of attention because it allowed new applications of diamond, which previously had been either too expensive to implement or too difficult to make. The CVD process makes diamond available in thin sheets or coatings that can cover large areas in a variety of unique shapes. The process is based on decomposition of a reactant gaseous atmosphere near a hot substrate, which in the case of CVD of diamond always includes a carbon source, and typically a hydrogen source (Lee *et al.*, 1999, Spitsyn *et al.*, 2000). The chemical reactions that mediate decomposition of the reactant gas can be activated by different sources: electrical, thermal and chemical (Spitsyn *et al.*, 2000). In the present chapter we focus on thermally activated CVD, known as hot-filament chemical vapour deposition (HFCVD).

3.1.1 Hot-filament chemical vapour deposition (HFCVD)

The HFCVD process was first proposed by Matsumoto and co-workers in 1982 (Matsumoto *et al.*, 1982). A tungsten (W) filament is heated to a temperature above 2000°C and the molecular hydrogen (H_2) that passes through the filament is dissociated into atomic hydrogen (H). The production of H simultaneously with hydrocarbon pyrolysis leads to diamond deposition, while formation of graphite is suppressed. The HFCVD technique is very popular as it allows coating of complex shapes and internal surfaces, with a low operating cost (Lee *et al.*, 1999).

3.1.2 Varieties of chemical vapour deposition (CVD) diamond

Diamond growth by CVD typically starts with nucleation on nanocrystalline seeds. During growth, diamond crystallites can remain in the nano-size regime or increase to micron-size. As a result, diamond films can be deposited with different grain sizes and are usually called microcrystalline (MCD) for sizes between 1 and 10 μm, or nanocrystalline (NCD) if the crystallites are between 10 and 100 nm and do not increase with the film thickness (Gruen, 1999, Krauss *et al.*, 2001, Tjong and Chen, 2004). Furthermore, a new term, 'ultrananocrystalline diamond' (UNCD), has been introduced to distinguish diamond films with grain sizes below 10 nm (usually between 2 and 5 nm) (Gruen, 1999). These films differ from NCD, not only because of smaller grain size, but also because they have little or no graphitic impurities at the grain boundaries (May and Mankelevich, 2006, Williams *et al.*, 2006). In the present work, our focus will be on NCD films.

3.1.3 Nanocrystalline diamond

In the last decade, publications with NCD as the main topic have seen a tremendous boom, exceeding 200 publications in 2008 and 2009 (Williams, 2011). Two main reasons support the ever-increasing study of NCD. Firstly, NCD overcomes one of the great problems of standard CVD polycrystalline diamond (MCD), the surface roughness. Whereas the faceted morphology of MCD prevents some applications in tribology, optics and biomedicine, where smooth surfaces are a requirement, with NCD all these applications are viable without the need for time-consuming and costly post-polishing operations. Secondly, NCD retains many of the fundamental properties of diamond, like mechanical hardness, chemical inertness and biological compatibility (Gruen, 1999, Tjong and Chen, 2004, Kulisch and Popov, 2006), and presents unique features when compared to conventional MCD films, such as higher toughness, wide band gap and higher electron emission efficiency (Jiang *et al.*, 2000, Sharda *et al.*, 2001, Hong *et al.*, 2002, Griffin and Ray, 2006). These properties open the door for new application areas like biomedicine, advanced optics and electronics.

The use of NCD as a wear-resistant and biocompatible coating for orthopaedic prostheses is now discussed.

3.2 NCD-coated silicon nitride ceramics as new materials for joint replacement

Every year almost two million people worldwide, suffering from arthritic diseases or trauma due to accidents, are subjected to hip and knee joint replacements, improving their quality of life considerably. Recent efforts have been made to identify new materials that can assist with reducing wear of the implants and avoiding adverse biological reactions with the surrounding tissues. Coating the implants with NCD is one possibility.

3.2.1 Inspiration

Total hip replacement is one of the most challenging types of human implants from the point of view of materials science (Tiainen, 2001). Selection of materials for an artificial hip joint is not always straightforward and mechanical properties (strength, elasticity, toughness and ductility), tribological features (low friction and low wear), biocompatibility and corrosion resistance are just some aspects that must be considered (Santavirta *et al.*, 2003, Borruto *et al.*, 2005). The commercial options for the hip prosthesis usually include metallic alloys (stainless steel, CoCr or some Ti-based alloys) or ceramics (Al_2O_3 or ZrO_2) for the femoral head component and ultra-high molecular weight polyethylene (UHMWPE), alumina (Al_2O_3), zirconia (ZrO_2), or CoCr alloys for the acetabular cup. These prostheses last 10–15 years and then must be replaced, with the patient having to undergo a revision surgery with a much lower success rate than the first surgery. As life expectancy increases, the development of long-lasting prostheses is mandatory.

It is known that one of the main causes of failure of hip prostheses is related to production of wear debris particles (Tiainen, 2001, Borruto *et al.*, 2005, Liang *et al.*, 2004, Katti, 2004, Jin *et al.*, 2006), which enhance the wear rate through a three-body wear mechanism when deposited between the two bearing surfaces. These residues are responsible for severe inflammatory responses, leading to osteolysis and aseptic loosening of the implant (Liang *et al.*, 2004, Katti, 2004, Jin *et al.*, 2006).

The search for new materials that could potentially improve the wear resistance and minimize generation of harmful debris, thereby increasing the prosthesis lifetime, has been an objective over recent years. Coating the implants with protective functional films could provide a way of reducing wear and avoiding adverse biological reactions with the surrounding tissues. NCD coatings have the required properties to perform this function. Their super hardness combined with the low surface roughness of this film ensures low wear rates, while the innocuous nature of any wear debris prevents inflammatory responses.

However, we go further and, besides suggesting NCD as a coating for artificial joints, we also propose a structural material for the prostheses. Silicon nitride

(Si_3N_4) is a high-tech ceramic material with excellent mechanical properties, namely high hardness and high fracture toughness, which fulfil the requirements for being a bulk material for joint prostheses. Some reports attest the biocompatibility of this ceramic, which is a prerequisite for use in the human body. Human osteoblastic cells proliferated on polished surfaces of Si_3N_4 (Kue *et al.*, 1999) and porous intramedullary Si_3N_4 rods implanted in rabbit femurs supported bone ingrowth (Howlett *et al.*, 1989). Furthermore, Si_3N_4-bioglass composites proved to have an inductive effect on the proliferation of MG63 osteoblast-like cells and were able to allow complete expression of the osteoblastic phenotype (Amaral *et al.*, 2002).

Si_3N_4 is also one of the most suitable substrates for diamond deposition, ensuring excellent film adhesion, a crucial requirement for biomedical applications. Adhesion is sometimes difficult to obtain, because during the CVD cooling step a large amount of thermal stress can be induced, which can cause the delamination of the coating. However, this stress can be reduced with the use of substrates with thermal expansion coefficients close to that of diamond. Si_3N_4 is one of those substrates owing to the similarity of the thermal expansion coefficients of both materials: $0.8\times10^{-6}\,K^{-1} < \alpha > 4.5\times10^{-6}\,K^{-1}$ for $20 < T > 800°C$, diamond (Ralchenko *et al.*, 1995); $2.9\times10^{-6}\,K^{-1} < \alpha > 3.6\times10^{-6}\,K^{-1}$ for $20 < T > 1500°C$, Si_3N_4 (Ziegler *et al.*, 1997).

Si_3N_4 ceramics coated with CVD diamond are frequently used as cutting tools. The diamond films are very useful at protecting the Si_3N_4 tools from the failure mechanism associated with oxidation and fracture by crack propagation.

3.3 Growth and characterization of NCD films deposited on Si_3N_4 substrates

The key for NCD growth is to increase the secondary nucleation rate of diamond while disabling the growth of crystallites to sizes reaching the micrometre scale. This may be accomplished by the use of carbon-rich C_xH_y/H_2 mixtures, the partial or complete replacement of hydrogen (H_2) by argon (Ar), helium (He), nelium (Ne) or nitrogen (N_2), and the use of low pressures or low temperatures (Li *et al.*, 2000, Yang *et al.*, 2001, Zhang *et al.*, 2001, Haubner and Lux, 2002, Rabeau *et al.*, 2004). Nevertheless, because of insufficient atomic H to etch the non-diamond carbon forms, care must be taken because graphitic material appears promptly at high C/H ratios (Connell *et al.*, 1995, Smith *et al.*, 2001, Zhang *et al.*, 2001, Haubner and Lux, 2002).

3.3.1 Study of HFCVD parameters

Amaral *et al.* (2004, 2006) discussed the influence of NCD growth parameters on Si_3N_4 substrates using the HFCVD technique, with Ar-CH_4-H_2 gas mixtures.

Parameters such as gas composition (Ar/H_2 and CH_4/H_2 ratios), total gas pressure (P), total mass flow (F) and substrate (T_s) and filament temperatures (T_f), were studied to assess their effect on NCD growth kinetics as well as on film quality and morphology (Amaral *et al.*, 2004, 2006).

Scanning electron microscopy (SEM), μ-Raman spectroscopy (Ar^+ 514.5 nm line), atomic force microscopy (AFM), transmission electron microscopy (TEM) and low incident beam angle diffraction (LIBAD) were used to characterize the NCD films. The LIBAD measurements allowed calculation of the diamond crystallite size, being made for the 2θ range = 41–47°, to identify the most intense diamond peak corresponding to the (111) plane.

Different NCD coatings were grown by adjusting the CH_4/H_2 and Ar/H_2 ratios, keeping constant the remaining parameters: P=50 mbar, F=50 mL·min^{-1}, T_s=650°C, T_f=2200°C (Amaral *et al.*, 2006). The optimal NCD films, concerning the combination of crystallite size (15 nm), growth rate (0.7 μm·h^{-1}) and film quality (less graphitic material) were obtained for Ar/H_2=0.1 and CH_4/H_2=0.04. Smaller diamond crystallite sizes, of about 8 nm, were achieved for the largest amount of Ar tested (55 vol.%), corresponding to an Ar/H_2 ratio of 1.25. This reduced grain size results from the dilution of the diamond growth species, methyl radical (CH_3) and atomic hydrogen (H), with the increment of Ar concentration, increasing diamond re-nucleation instead of crystallite growth (Zhang *et al.*, 2001). Although the grain size is very small, this type of NCD film grows very slowly, 0.1 μm·h^{-1}. Therefore, longer deposition times are required to grow an effective protective coating for biomedical applications, particularly joint prostheses, of 10–20 μm thick. Deposition conditions were sought for a practicable growth rate and a balance between grain size, film quality and surface roughness (Amaral *et al.*, 2006). Continuous NCD coatings with a remarkable growth rate of 1.6 μm·h^{-1} and 28 nm of crystallite size, were obtained using the following parameters: Ar/H_2=0.1, CH_4/H_2=0.04, P=50 mbar, F=50 mL·min^{-1}, T_s=750°C, T_f=2300°C (Amaral *et al.*, 2006). The increase in the growth rate is mainly due to increasing T_f from 2200°C to 2300°C; however, it is achieved at the expense of a larger crystallite size (15 nm and 28 nm at 2200°C and 2300°C, respectively), which is probably linked to an increase in atomic H concentration (Connell *et al.*, 1995).

In Fig. 3.1(a) a representative cross-section SEM image is shown of the NCD film obtained under the above referred conditions. An equivalent, but highly magnified, observation in bright-field TEM is given in Fig. 3.1(b), showing the interface coating/substrate. A dark-field image of the NCD film, Fig. 3.1(c), provides direct evidence of the nanometric diamond grain size. The correspondent electron diffraction pattern corroborates the crystallinity of the coating (inset of Fig. 3.1(c)). The SEM top view micrograph, Fig. 3.1(d), shows the typical morphology of the film of NCD, which is composed by tiny agglomerates of diamond nanocrystals.

AFM scans of 100×100 μm^2 size performed in tapping mode assessed the surface topography and determined a root-mean-square (RMS) surface roughness value of 41 nm (Fig. 3.2(a)). A representative μ-Raman spectrum is given in Fig. 3.2(b).

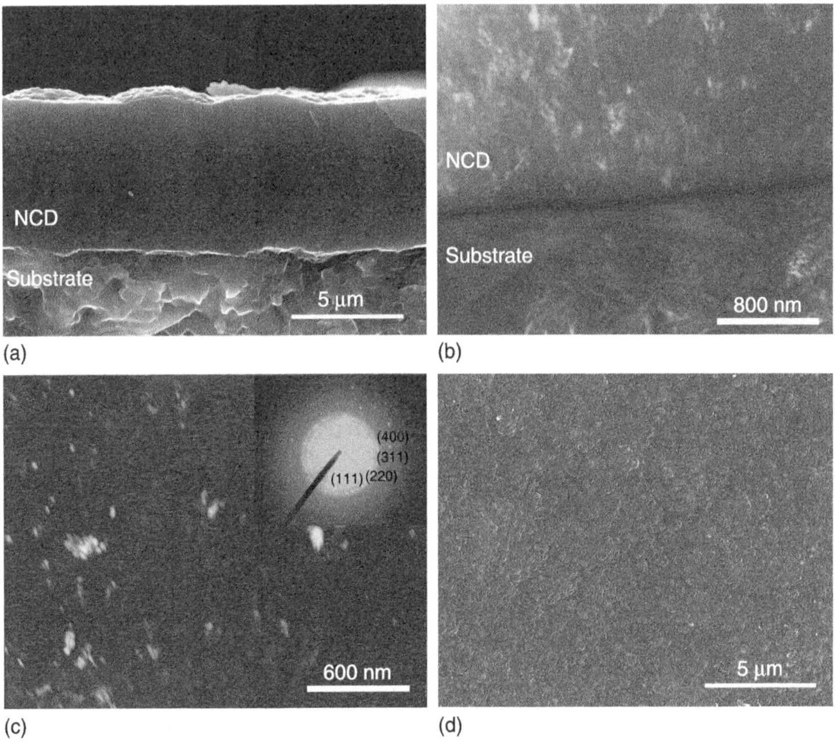

3.1 (a) SEM and (b) TEM cross-sectional views of the substrate/NCD interface, (c) dark-field TEM micrograph and electron diffraction patterns (inset) of the NCD film and (d) SEM plan view of NCD film (Amaral *et al.*, 2006).

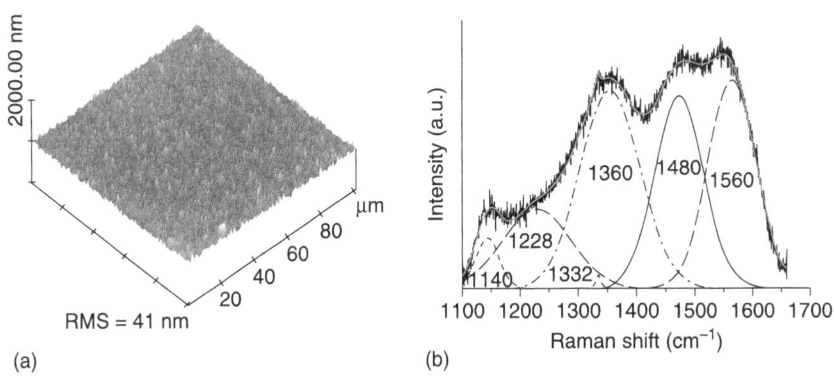

3.2 (a) AFM image and (b) μm-Raman spectrum (514.5 nm) of the as-grown NCD films.

The 1140 cm^{-1} and 1480 cm^{-1} shoulders, usually attributed to trans-polyacetylene, are indirect proof of the presence of NCD (Ferrari and Robertson, 2001, Pfeiffer *et al.*, 2003). Also, a band is visible at 1228 cm^{-1}, which appears to be conjugated with vibration modes of C-H chains characteristic of nano- and ultrananocrystalline diamond (Fernandes *et al.*, 2007). Furthermore, the 1332 cm^{-1} diamond band is visible, as well as the D (1360 cm^{-1}) and G (1560 cm^{-1}) graphite bands.

Considering the excellent topographic, morphological and quality features of the NCD film described above, further characterization is required to assess its ability to perform as a protective coating on joint prostheses. Biotribological and biological studies are mandatory.

3.4 Biotribology of NCD coatings

Joint replacement is undoubtedly a great challenge concerning all the items that should be considered in the choice of materials for hip prosthesis. The most important requirements are biocompatibility, and suitable mechanical and tribological properties. Therefore, it is of vital significance in the search for new materials to assure that these requirements are satisfied. Several tests need to be made, namely biotribological tests.

3.4.1 Biotribology concept

Biotribology is the science of tribology applied to functioning biological systems, in particular, the synovial joints and their artificial replacements (Hall *et al.*, 2001). Tribology is defined as the science and technology of interacting surfaces in relative motion (Hall *et al.*, 2001, Jin *et al.*, 2006), and comprises three related areas: friction, wear and lubrication.

Understanding the wear mechanism is important in design of appropriate strategies to reduce wear debris and associated problems, like aseptic loosening. A wide range of laboratory equipment, test methods and measuring systems have been developed for study of the wear mechanisms in total hip replacement. For example, screening analysis, where pin-on-disc and pin-on-plate machines are used to assess the wear behaviour of new combinations of materials at an early phase; and joint simulation, using equipment that simulates the functioning of a human joint.

Pin-on-disc machines are widely used in tribology to evaluate the nature of wear and friction of material pairs under well-controlled steady-state conditions of load, sliding speed and environment. Pin-on-plate machines sacrifice the steady sliding speed between specimens, but partially simulate the reciprocating action broadly associated with the hip joint.

Joint simulators reproduce the three-dimensional loading and motion patterns experienced by hip joints and provide a lubricant environment similar to synovial fluid. This kind of equipment allows a comparative performance evaluation of hip joints of different designs and material combinations.

As this chapter was being written, only the results of pin-on-plate tests of NCD coatings were available. The experiments on the hip simulator were being carried out.

3.4.2 Pin-on-plate experiments

Friction and wear coefficient values of NCD-coated Si_3N_4 substrates, under simulated physiological conditions, were assessed using a pin-on-plate test configuration (Amaral *et al.*, 2008a). The tribological experiments described are self-mated as it was considered that the articulating surfaces of the hip prosthesis, acetabular cup and femoral head, could both be coated with NCD films.

Si_3N_4 square plates ($10\times10\times3\,mm^3$) and cylindrical- and flat-ended pins (diameter = 4 mm; thickness = 3 mm) were polished with colloidal silica until a mirror-like surface was obtained. Two sets of samples were used in the tribological tests: one composed only of polished samples (P) and one composed of polished and tetrafluoromethane (CF_4) plasma etched substrates (PE). These two types of surface finishing are supposed to have an effect on the surface roughness, adhesion and even on the growth rate of NCD (Abreu *et al.*, 2006).

NCD films were grown for 22 hours using the optimum conditions described in Section 3.1: Ar/H_2=0.1, CH_4/H_2=0.04, P=50 mbar, F=50 $mL\cdot min^{-1}$, T_s=750°C, T_f=2300°C.

The tribological tests were performed in a reciprocating sliding tribometer (Plint TE67/R), under lubricated conditions at room temperature. The liquids used were: Hank's balanced salt solution (HBSS, Cambrex, Belgium) containing $8g\cdot L^{-1}$ NaCl, $1g\cdot L^{-1}$ glucose, $0.4g\cdot L^{-1}$ KCl, $0.35g\cdot L^{-1}$ $NaHCO_3$, $0.09g\cdot L^{-1}$ $Na_2HPO_4\cdot 7H_2O$ and $0.06\,g\cdot L^{-1}$ KH_2PO_4 as the main components; and fetal bovine serum (FBS, Cambrex, Belgium) diluted to 50% to contain $18.5\,mg\cdot mL^{-1}$ of protein, which is the concentration present in the synovial fluid, plus 0.2 wt% of a biocide (NaN_3, Merck, Germany).

A constant stroke of 6 mm and frequency of 1 Hz were imposed to give a sliding velocity that lies in the range typically found for a working hip joint (Dumbleton, 1981, Widmer *et al.*, 2001). The tests lasted for 500 000 cycles, giving a total sliding distance in the order of 6 km, under 45 N of normal load, with the friction coefficient being continuously recorded. The use of flat-ended pins on the tribotests lowers the nominal contact stresses to approximately 3.5 MPa, a value compatible with *in vivo* hip and knee joint stress conditions (Dumbleton, 1981). However, due to difficulties in warranting a perfect parallelism between the pin and flat specimens, a full contact could not be achieved and thus only a portion of the flat pin area truly contacted the plate. By measuring this area after testing, the real contact stresses were calculated, yielding values of about 25 MPa. This value corresponds to the upper limit measured in hip and knee joints when testing different loading axes (Szivek *et al.*, 1996).

As-deposited and worn surfaces were studied using SEM and AFM, in order to characterize the microstructure and the wear process and to assess topographical features and wear volume, respectively. Wear rates were calculated using the AFM bearing function for volume loss quantification, the procedure for which is described elsewhere (Amaral *et al.*, 2007).

In Fig. 3.3, SEM micrographs show the microstructure of as-deposited NCD films on polished (P) (Fig. 3.3(a)), and on etched (PE) ceramics (Fig. 3.3(b)). The P samples exhibit lower surface roughness (RMS=70–130 nm) than the PE samples (RMS=200–400 nm), which is confirmed by AFM analysis (Fig. 3.3(c) and (d)). The insets of Fig. 3.3(a) and (b) also reveal differences in the growth rate of NCD, due only to distinct substrate surface finishing, as the deposition conditions are the same. For P samples the measured growth rate is about 0.6 $\mu m \cdot h^{-1}$, whereas it is nearly double (~1 $\mu m \cdot h^{-1}$) for PE plates and pins. The fracture surface of both NCD films (inset Fig. 3.3(a) and (b)), reveal also that P samples have a smaller crystallite size.

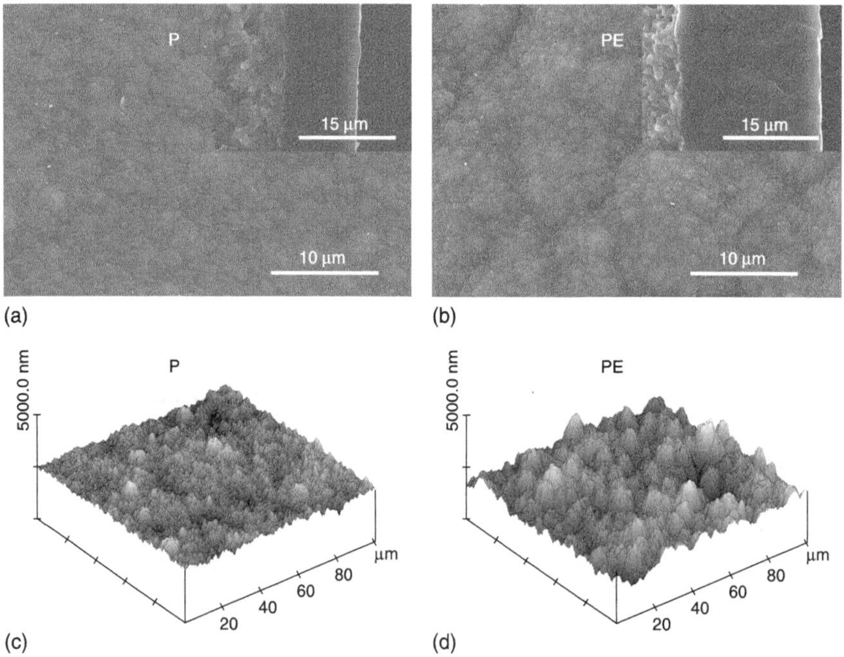

3.3 SEM micrographs of NCD-coated samples with inset micrographs of fracture cross-section showing the thickness of the NCD films for (a) P samples and (b) PE samples. AFM micrographs evidencing the surface roughness differences between P (c) and PE (d) NCD-coated substrates (Amaral *et al.*, 2008a).

The NCD films deposited on PE samples present higher initial friction peaks than the ones deposited on P substrates (Fig. 3.4). This corresponds to the truncation of surface asperities in the first moments of sliding, which are rougher in the case of PE, as seen by AFM (Fig. 3.3(c) and (d)). During the running-in stage, there are little differences between the coefficient of friction of the NCD-coated PE and P samples, when tested under the same physiological fluid, as illustrated by the graphs in Fig. 3.4. However, for P samples, after testing with both liquids, HBSS and FBS, cracks perpendicular and parallel to the sliding direction are detected by SEM (Fig. 3.5). This fracture of the NCD film was not perceptible in the friction coefficient evolution as no abrupt change was observed during the pin-on-flat tests (Fig. 3.4). The fracture of the films at nominal loads as low as 25 MPa is due to low adhesion that induces interfacial failure and finally breakage. One way of increasing adhesion is to chemically attack the Si_3N_4 grains by radiofrequency-induced CF_4 plasma. This increases the surface roughness at the micrometre level, enabling mechanical interlocking between coating and

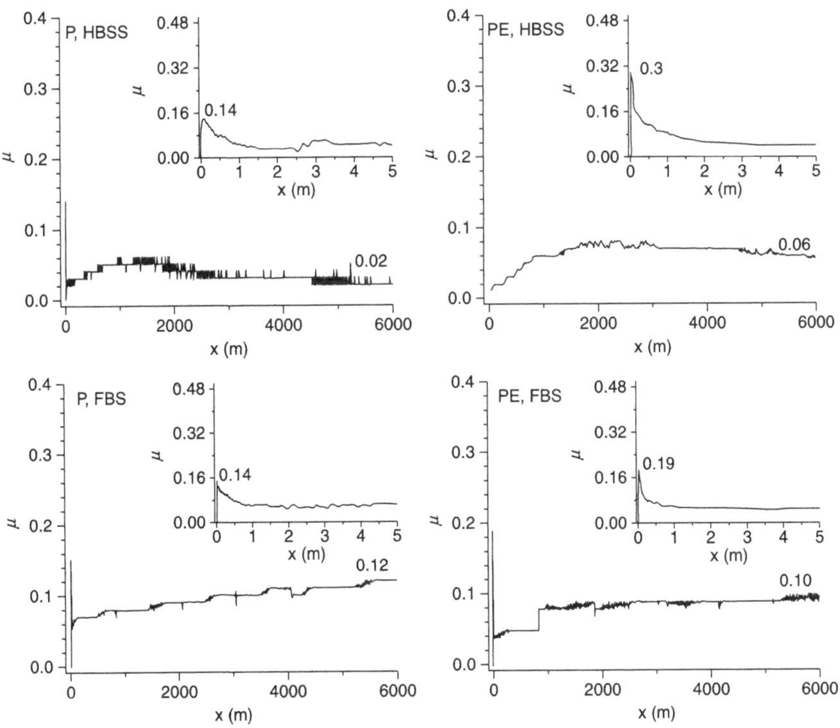

3.4 Evolution of the friction coefficient of NCD self-mated contacts tested under HBSS and under FBS. Inset charts evidence the effect of increased surface roughness of PE samples relative to P samples (Amaral *et al.*, 2008a).

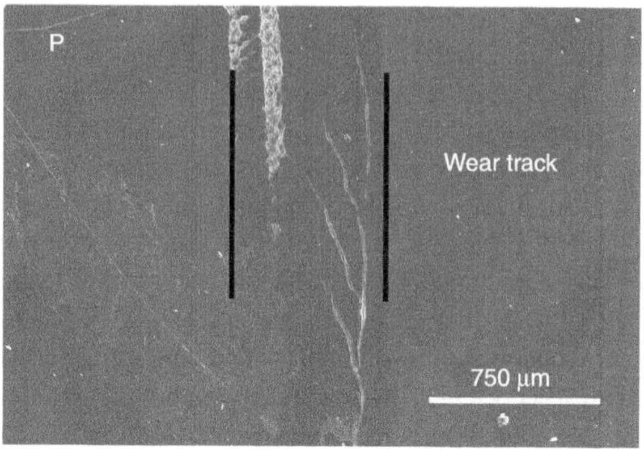

3.5 SEM micrograph of the wear track showing the cracks of the film deposited on P samples (Amaral *et al.*, 2008a).

substrate. The adhesion improvement allowed the tribological tests, using the PE samples, to run the entire 500 000 cycles without evidence of fracture, as was later confirmed by SEM and AFM analysis. Similar NCD coatings on optimized substrates could withstand up to 3.5 GPa of nominal load in dry sliding self-mated experiments using a ball-on-flat geometry (Abreu *et al.*, 2006).

It was verified that for both sets of samples (P and PE) the steady-state friction value is always larger when the tribological tests are carried out with the FBS liquid (Fig. 3.4). This effect is thought to be due to protein attachment (Scholes *et al.*, 2000, Gispert *et al.*, 2006). In order to clarify this point, a scanning electron microscope operating at 1 mbar total pressure, was used to observe one pair pin/plate tribologically tested with FBS. This technique allows microstructural and chemical characterization without the need for an electrically conductive coating that would latter mask the AFM data, where a well-cleaned surface is needed in order to assess the wear volume loss. The SEM micrographs shown in Fig. 3.6, illustrate the morphology of a NCD-coated PE sample after tribological testing with FBS. Figure 3.6(a) and (b) allows comparison of the as-tested and cleaned surfaces of the worn tracks of the NCD plates. An extensive film covering the wear zone (a), contrasts with the clean surface in (b) where only the flat plateaus of the NCD clusters and unfilled valleys are observed. The inset of (a) shows in detail the deformed layer of material that covers the NCD surface. In Fig. 3.6(c), a higher magnification of those deposits is depicted and the corresponding EDS analysis is shown in Fig. 3.6(d), evidencing the presence of carbon (C), nitrogen (N), oxygen (O), and sodium (Na) as major components. The C is mostly from the NCD film, whereas N and O are possibly from the amino acids that constitute the protein structure. Sources of Na are the biocide (0.2 wt% NaN_3) but, most likely, the aqueous saline solution that constitutes the serum base. Therefore, there is direct evidence of serum material attachment, proteins and salts, on the NCD

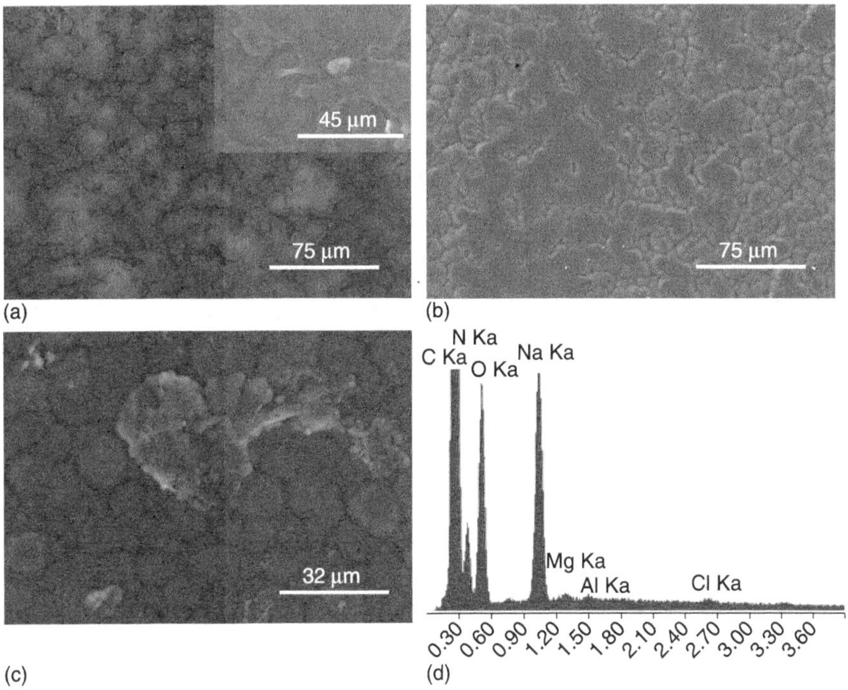

3.6 SEM micrographs of NCD-coated PE substrates after tribological testing under FBS showing the presence of a surface smeared film (a and c) rich in N, 0 and Na as detected by EDS (d) and after cleaning in acetone and ethanol (b) (Amaral *et al.*, 2008a).

surface that can explain the higher coefficient of friction verified with the use of FBS fluid. This trend has been already observed with other material combinations, namely alumina-on-alumina and alumina-on-UHMWPE (Scholes *et al.*, 2000, Hall *et al.*, 2001, Gispert *et al.*, 2006). The reasons for this increase are not fully understood because for metal-on-metal bearings, the friction coefficient is smaller when using protein-containing fluids than when using protein-free fluids. Some explanations are based on wetting differences, as proteins tend to adsorb more strongly on hydrophobic surfaces producing more stable adsorbed layers (Gispert *et al.*, 2006). Alumina is less hydrophobic than metals and thus proteins are less stable and may contribute to the increase of friction. Another possible explanation is that adsorbed proteins act to increase the surface roughness of the originally smooth ceramic surface, leading to a predominantly mixed lubrication regime and therefore to an increase of the friction coefficient (Scholes *et al.*, 2000).

The tribological tests of NCD-coated P and PE samples assessed values of 0.02 and 0.06, respectively, for the long-term friction coefficient under HBSS lubrication and 0.12 and 0.10 when using FBS as can be seen in Fig. 3.4. These values are slightly higher than values found for bearings for artificial hip joints in the presence of bovine serum, namely ceramic-on-ceramic and ceramic-on-metal (0.002–0.07), but are considerably lower than the values for metal-on-metal combinations (0.22–0.27) (Jin *et al.*, 2006). The main reason for the observed differences between the present NCD/NCD tribosystem and those involving ceramics lies in the high starting surface roughness values when compared to 5–10 nm for the ceramics (Jin *et al.*, 2006). However, as already explained, a compromise between surface roughness and adhesion had to be found for NCD coatings. In the case of the metallic bearing surfaces, the relatively high friction coefficients are related to corrosion induced surface modification.

It is worth mentioning that for a given couple, low friction does not imply low wear and vice versa (Hall *et al.*, 2001). For example, NCD-coated PE substrates undergo higher friction in FBS but lower wear when compared to HBSS lubrication (Fig. 3.7). A different behaviour is seen for NCD-coated P samples where higher friction corresponds with higher wear for FBS. The only significant differences between the two diamond films are the thickness and the roughness, so it is believed that smooth surfaces are more exposed to protein attachment effects than rough surfaces. In fact, the latter have more pronounced peaks and valleys, and proteins can remain partly below the surface where wear is taking place.

The bar graphs in Fig. 3.7 also show that NCD-coated PE samples present higher wear coefficients than NCD-coated P substrates, because of their rougher surface. For both samples, the wear of the plates is always higher than the wear of pins as a result of a fatigue effect. The wear coefficients measured for NCD-on-NCD bearings are in the order of ~10^{-9}–10^{-8} mm^3·N^{-1}m^{-1} (ultra-mild wear regime), values that are equal to or better than the wear factors assessed in similar

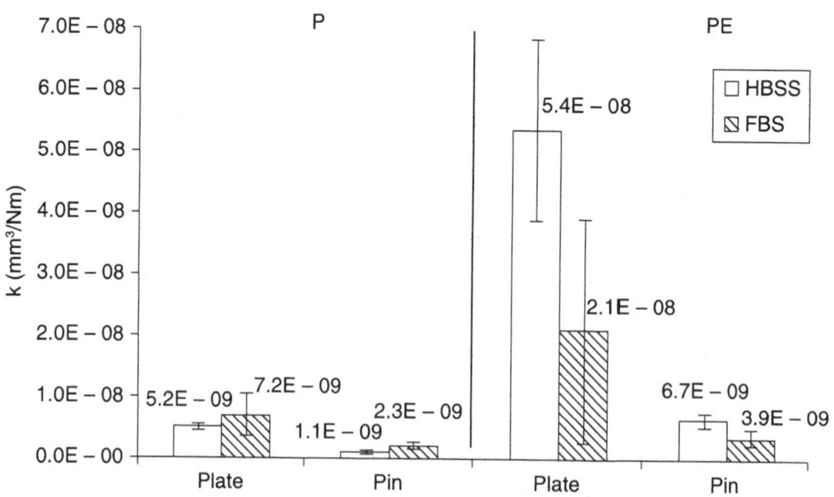

3.7 Wear coefficients of the self-mated NCD-coated P and PE substrates tested under HBSS and FBS fluids (Amaral *et al.*, 2008a).

test conditions for metal-on-metal (~10^{-7} $mm^3 \cdot N^{-1}m^{-1}$), UHMWPE-on-metal (~10^{-7} $mm^3 \cdot N^{-1}m^{-1}$) and ceramic-on-ceramic (~10^{-8} $mm^3 \cdot N^{-1}m^{-1}$) contacts (Jin *et al.*, 2006).

These results foresee the reduction of the amount of wear debris and the increase of the prosthesis lifetime, if NCD-coated Si_3N_4 ceramics are used as materials for joint replacement. However, the type of surface finishing of the ceramic substrates is crucial to determine the adhesion and the wear coefficient of NCD coatings. The tests reported in the present work contribute only to a screening analysis, and further tests conducted in hip joint simulators are needed to confirm the applicability of NCD as a new coating for biotribological applications.

3.5 Biological behaviour of NCD-coated Si_3N_4 ceramics

Research into novel materials for orthopaedic implants had been focused on the incorporation of a certain degree of nanostructured surface features that mimic the nanometric structures and molecules found in bones. In particular, these appear to reduce the chances of rejection of the hip or knee prosthesis (Shane *et al.*, 2002, 2003). Most of the studies reported that nanophase topography fosters cell adhesion on polymers, ceramics and metals, and suggested a positive effect on osteoblasts metabolic activities (Webster *et al.*, 1999, Price *et al.*, 2003, Palin *et al.*, 2005, Perla and Webster, 2005). NCD films are able to mimic the bone surface roughness and are also capable of controlling the biological response with precision. NCD can be used as a template for the immobilization of active molecules for biological or biosensoric applications (Yang and Hamers, 2004, Siew *et al.*, 2005, Wenmackers *et al.*, 2005, Retama *et al.*, 2006, Kulisch *et al.*, 2007, Popov *et al.*, 2007). One example is functionalization of NCD with bone morphogenetic protein-2 (BMP-2), creating a biomimetic coating that results in improved osseointegration, which is a powerful strategy in tissue engineering and in the context of bone tissue regeneration (Steinmuller-Nethl *et al.*, 2006). The NCD surface can also be modified with the linking of an antibody, human immunoglobulin G (IgG), which provides biomolecular recognition capability, turning out a biologically sensitive field-effect transistor (Bio-Fet) (Yang and Hamers, 2004).

Despite all the referenced reports of NCD bioproperties, the biocompatibility of this coating can differ to some extent in surface and bulk properties depending on the deposition method and parameters applied (Kulisch *et al.*, 2007). Besides, biocompatibility refers to the ability of a material to execute a specific application with an appropriate host response (Williams, 2003). Therefore, the biocompatibility must be assessed for each type of NCD and respective application, considering adequate *in vitro* and *in vivo* biological systems to evaluate specific cell and tissue responses.

Amaral *et al.* (2008b, 2009) reported *in vitro* cytotoxicity and biocompatibility studies of NCD films grown on Si_3N_4 substrates, considering their future application as a coating for joint and dental implants. In the present chapter only the assays related to biocompatibility assessment for the first application (articular prostheses) are presented. In the first step of this study, NCD coatings were exposed to MG63 osteoblast-like cells for screening toxicity (Amaral *et al.*, 2008b). Then, in a later phase, the NCD films were seeded with human bone marrow cells to assess the effects of the material in cell growth and expression of the osteoblastic phenotype, that is the formation of a mineralized extracellular matrix (Amaral *et al.*, 2008b).

3.5.1 Screening of acute toxicity by *in vitro* cell cultures

MG63 cells were cultured in α-Minimal Essential Medium (supplemented with foetal bovine serum, ascorbic acid, gentamicin and fungizone), at 37°C in a humidified atmosphere of 5% CO_2 in air, for 7 days in control conditions (absence of materials, standard plastic culture plates) and on the surface of the sterilized NCD-coated samples. The medium was changed every 2–3 days. Control cultures and seeded material samples were evaluated at days 1, 3 and 7 for cell viability/proliferation (MTT assay) and observed by SEM. Further experimental details can be found elsewhere (Amaral *et al.*, 2008b).

The results of the viability/proliferation assay determined by a colorimetric method, the MTT test, are plotted in Fig. 3.8. MTT (3-[4,5-dimethylthiazol-2-

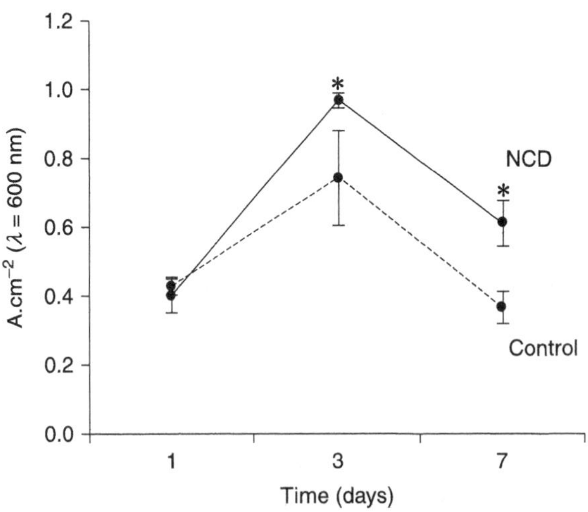

3.8 Cell viability/proliferation of MG63 cells cultured on NCD-coated Si_3N_4 substrates for 7 days, estimated by the MTT assay (* statistically different from the control).

yl]–2,5-diphenyltetrasodium bromide) is metabolized to a purple formazan salt by mitochondrial enzymes in living cells and the absorbance is proportional to the number of viable cells. Compared to control cultures, MTT reduction values for the seeded material samples were similar at day 1 and statistically significantly higher at days 3 and 7.

As can be seen in Fig. 3.9(a), at day 1 of culture the MG63 osteoblast-like cells were already well attached and completely spread, displaying a flat configuration and a typical morphology (central spherical body with the cytoplasm extending away from the central area in all directions and adhering to the material surface). Neighbouring cells have extensive connections with each other through cytoplasmic extensions. After three days of culture, the cells formed multilayers of flattened sheets, covering the material surface completely. No deleterious or cytotoxic responses were observed for the entire time of culture. Control cultures showed a similar behaviour on SEM.

From these cytotoxicity results (Fig. 3.8 and 3.9), one can conclude that the NCD surface allows an excellent proliferation of osteoblast-like cells, while keeping a normal cellular morphology.

3.5.2 Osteoblastic biocompatibility of NCD coating

The clinical success of a bone tissue implant relies on its osseointegration reflected by a proper bone metabolism at the bone/implant interface. This represents a dynamic process involving the migration of osteoprogenitor cells from the adjacent bone marrow and the subsequent adhesion to the material surface, and their proliferation and differentiation with the production of a mineralized matrix around the implant material.

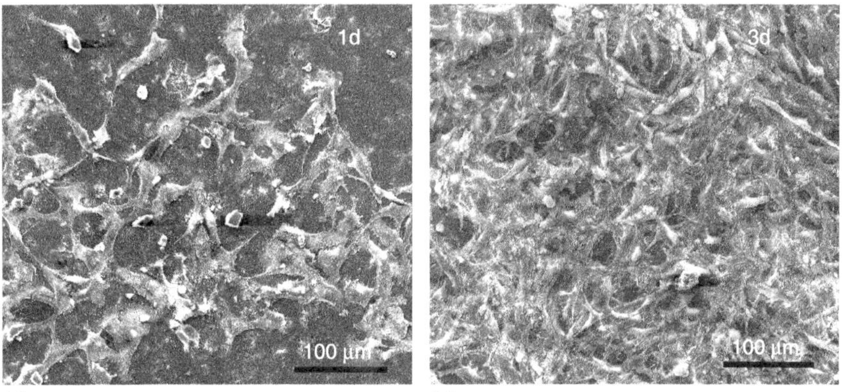

3.9 SEM photographs of MG63 cells cultured on NCD-coated Si_3N_4 substrates for days 1 (a) and 3 (b) (Amaral *et al.*, 2008b).

Human bone marrow (HBM), obtained from orthopaedic surgery procedures after patient informed consent, was cultured in the same experimental conditions as those used in the culture of MG63 cells. Control and seeded material samples were cultured for 21 days in the experimental conditions described elsewhere (Amaral *et al.*, 2008b) and characterized at days 3, 7, 14 and 21 for cell viability/proliferation (MTT assay), total protein content, alkaline phosphatase (ALP) activity, and observation by SEM to evaluate cell morphology and matrix mineralization (Amaral *et al.*, 2008b). The results are presented in Fig. 3.10–3.12.

HBM cells grown in control conditions proliferated during the first two weeks presenting a high cell growth rate during the first week, as evident in the MTT assay (Fig. 3.10(a)). Seeded NCD coating showed a similar pattern, but MTT values were significantly higher at days 7, 14, and 21. Similar results were assessed by the total protein content measurements (Fig. 3.10(b)), which are also an indicator of cell proliferation. HBM cells increased the production of ALP during the first two weeks, attaining the maximum level by day 14, and decreasing later (Fig. 3.10(c)). ALP is a membrane-linked polypeptide, synthesized by the osteoblasts, that is thought to promote crystal formation in matrix vesicles by removing nucleation inhibitors, mediating the calcification process (Sikavitsas *et al.*, 2001). ALP activity, normalized as a function of the protein content, was higher on the cultures grown on NCD surface, which may suggest that NCD is able to stimulate osteoblast metabolic differentiated activities.

SEM (Fig. 3.11 and 3.12) observations of seeded NCD samples confirmed the favourable profile of the NCD coating suggested by the biochemical assays. After 7–14 days (Fig. 3.11(a) and (b)), cells were well spread presenting a homogenous distribution on the NCD surface and, by day 21, mineralized globular structures were observed interspersed within the cell layer (Fig. 3.11(c)). At low magnification (Fig. 3.12(a)), an elevated number of those mineralized deposits were present. Mineralized structures were intimately associated with the fibrillar matrix (Fig. 3.12(b)), and the X-ray spectrum from EDS analysis (labelled with an asterisk in Fig. 3.12(b)) proves the inorganic nature of these structures by showing strong Ca and P peaks. This sequence of events was similar to that occurring on standard polystyrene culture plates (Fig. 3.11(d)–3.11(f)). Quantitative assessment of the relative abundance of mineral structures on the cell layer was not evaluated, but SEM qualitative analysis strongly suggested that mineral deposition density was higher on the NCD coating. This might be related to the presence of increased cell number on the coating (as suggested by the MTT assay), presenting an identical activity regarding matrix mineralization. Also, induction of this phenotype feature by the NCD coating might be hypothesized, taking into account the increased ALP activity measured on the coating. However, the results of this study do not provide information regarding the subjacent mechanism.

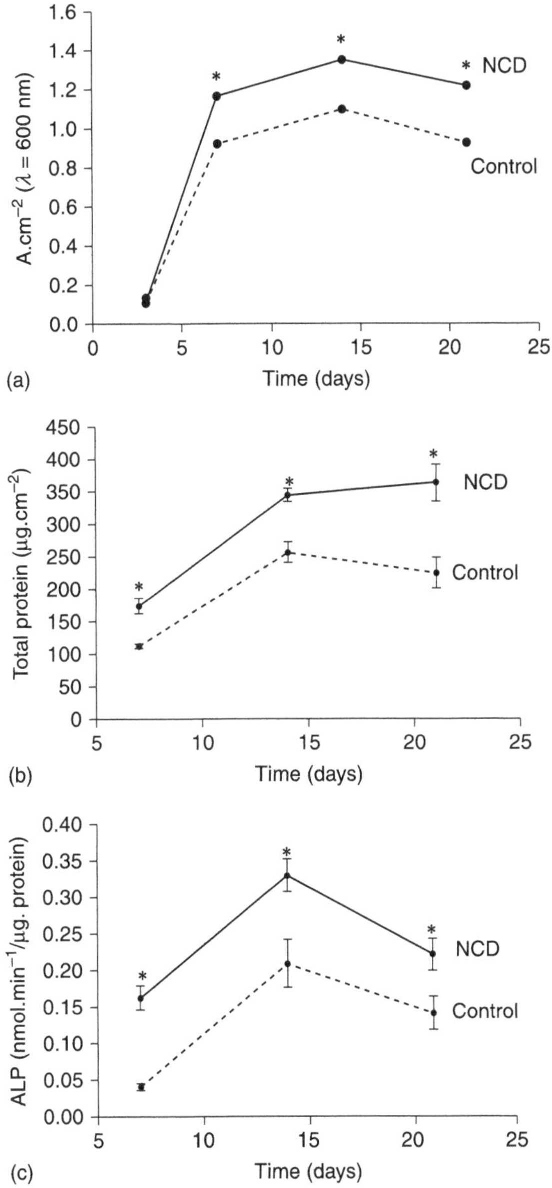

3.10 Cell viability/proliferation (a), total protein content (b), and ALP activity (c) of human bone marrow osteoblast cells grown on NCD-coated Si_3N_4 for 21 days. *Statistically different from control.

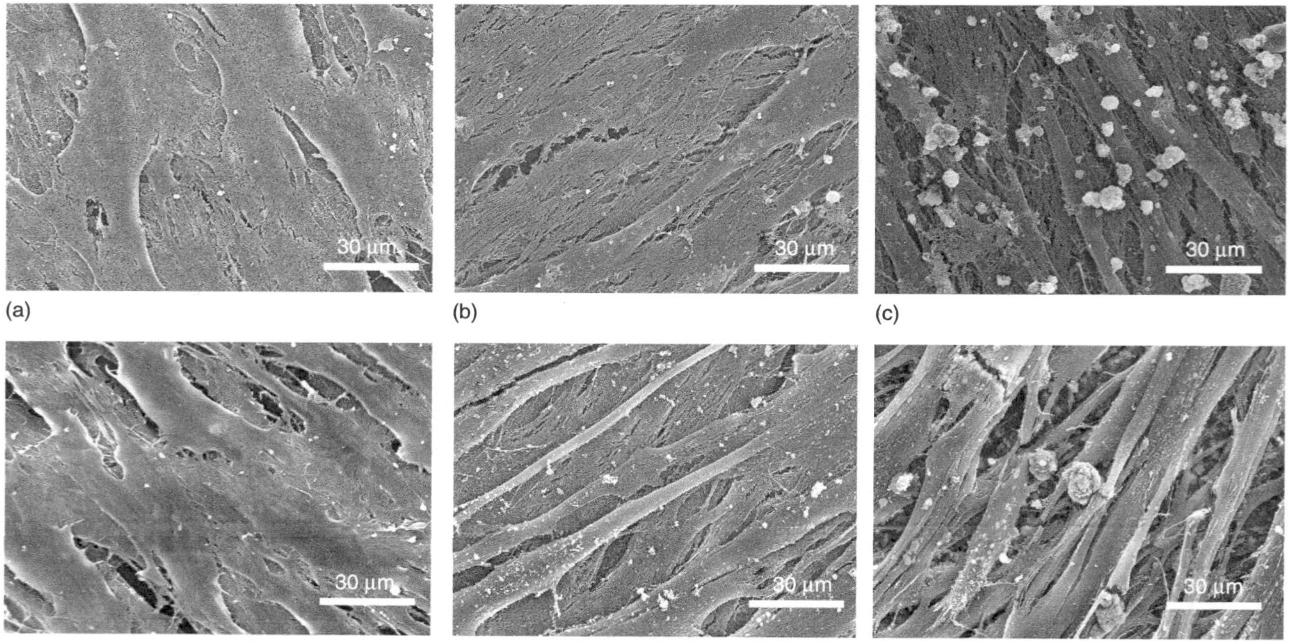

(a) (b) (c) (d) (e) (f)

3.11 SEM photographs of the time-course behaviour of human bone marrow osteoblast cell cultures grown over NCD-coated Si_3N_4 substrates at days 7 (a), 14 (b) and 21 (c). For comparison, the cell behaviour observed on standard polystyrene culture plates is also shown (SEM): (d), (e) and (f), respectively, for 7, 14 and 21 days.

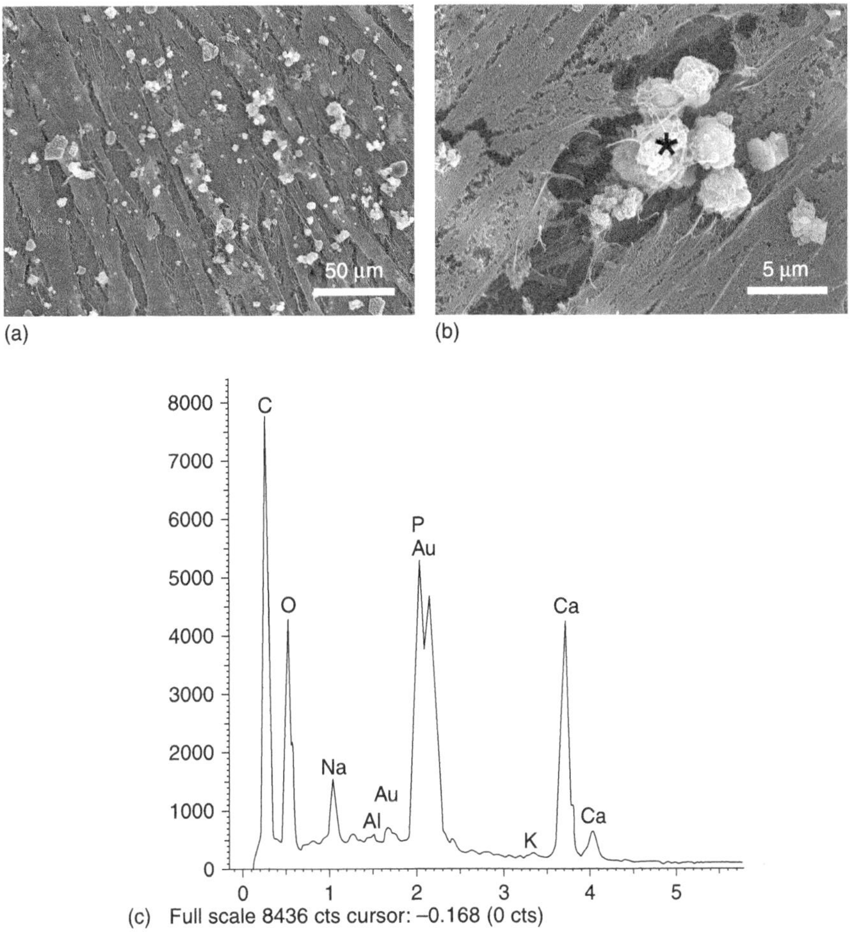

3.12 Matrix mineralization by human bone marrow osteoblast cell cultures grown over the NCD films at day 21. SEM: low magnification (a), detail of the mineralized structures (b), and EDS spectrum of the mineralized deposits (c).

In vitro study strongly suggests that the prepared NCD coating presented improved features for osteoblast proliferation and function. *In vivo* experiments in animals, including histological studies and push-out strength measurements, are now imperative for a complete characterization of NCD as a biomaterial.

3.6 References

Abreu CS, Amaral M, Oliveira FJ, *et al.* (2006), 'Enhanced performance of HFCVD nanocrystalline diamond self-mated tribosystems by plasma pretreatments on silicon nitride substrates', *Diam. Relat. Mater.*, 15, 2024–2028.

Amaral M, Costa MA, Lopes MA, *et al.* (2002), 'Si_3N_4-bioglass composites stimulate the proliferation of MG63 osteoblast-like cells and support the osteogenic differentiation of human bone marrow cells', *Biomaterials*, 23, 4897–4906.

Amaral M, Oliveira FJ, Fernandes AJS, *et al.* (2004), 'Hot-filament chemical vapour deposition of nanodiamond on silicon nitride substrates', *Diam. Relat. Mater.*, 13, 643–647.

Amaral M, Fernandes AJS, Vila M, *et al.* (2006), 'Growth rate improvements in the hot-filament CVD deposition of nanocrystalline diamond', *Diam. Relat. Mater.*, 15, 1822–1827.

Amaral M, Abreu CS, Oliveira FJ, *et al.* (2007), 'Biotribological performance of NCD coated Si_3N_4 – bioglass composites', *Diam. Relat. Mater.*, 16, 790–795.

Amaral M, Abreu CS, Oliveira FJ, *et al.* (2008a), 'Tribological characterization of NCD in physiological fluids', *Diam. Relat. Mater.*, 17, 848–852.

Amaral M, Gomes PS, Lopes MA, *et al.* (2008b), 'Nanocrystalline diamond: in vitro biocompatibility assessment by MG63 and human bone marrow cells cultures', *J. of Biomedical Mater. Res.*, 87A, 91–99.

Amaral M, Gomes PS, Lopes MA, *et al.* (2009), 'Cytotoxicity evaluation of nanocrystalline diamond (NCD) coatings by fibroblast cell cultures', *Acta Biomaterialia*, 5, 755–763.

Borruto A, Marrelli L and Palma F (2005), 'The difference of material wettability as critical factor in the choice of a tribological prosthetic coupling without debris release', *Tribology Letters*, 20, 1–10.

Connell LL, Fleming JW, Chu H-N, *et al.* (1995), 'Spatially resolved atomic hydrogen concentrations and molecular hydrogen temperature profiles in the chemical vapour deposition of diamond', *J. Appl. Phys.*, 78, 3622–3634.

Dumbleton JH (1981), 'Tribology of natural and artificial joints', Tribology Series – 3, Amsterdam, Elsevier.

Eversole WG (1962) *Synthesis of diamond.* U.S. Patent 3030188 1962-April-17.

Fernandes AJS, Neto MA, Almeida FA, *et al.* (2007), 'Nano- and micro-crystalline diamond growth by MPCVD in extremely poor hydrogen uniform plasmas', *Diam. Relat. Mater.*, 16, 757–761.

Ferrari AC and Robertson J (2001), 'Origin of the 1150 cm^{-1} Raman mode in nanocrystalline diamond', *Phys. Rev. B*, 63, 121405-1–121405-4.

Gispert MP, Serro AP, Colaço R and Saramago B (2006), 'Friction and wear mechanisms in hip prosthesis: Comparison of joint materials behaviour in several lubricants', *Wear*, 260, 149–158.

Griffin J and Ray PC (2006), 'Role of inert gas in the low-temperature nano-diamond chemical vapour deposition process', *Nanotechnology*, 17, 1225–1229.

Gruen DM (1999), 'Nanocrystalline diamond films', *Annu. Rev. Mater. Sci.*, 29, 211–259.

Hall RM, Bankes MJK and Blunn G (2001), 'Biotribology for joint replacement', *Current Orthopaedics*, 15, 281–290.

Haubner R and Lux B (2002), 'Deposition of ballas diamond and nano-crystalline diamond', *Internat. J. of Refract. Metals & Hard Mater.*, 20, 93–100.

Hong SP, Yohikawa H, Wazumi K and Koga Y (2002), 'Synthesis and tribological characteristics of nanocrystalline diamond film using CH_4/H_2 microwave plasmas', *Diam. Relat. Mater.*, 11, 877–881.

Howlett C, McCartney E and Ching W (1989), 'The effects of silicon nitride ceramic on rabbit skeletal cells and tissues', *Clin. Orthop.*, 244, 296–301.

Jiang N, Kujime S, Ota I, *et al.* (2000), 'Growth and structural analysis of nano-diamond films deposited on Si substrates pretreated by various methods', *J. Cryst. Growth*, 218, 265–271.

Jin ZM, Stone M, Ingham E and Fisher J (2006), 'Biotribology', *Current Orthopaedics*, 20, 32–40.

Katti KS (2004), 'Biomaterials in total joint replacement', *Colloids and Surfaces B: Biointerfaces*, 39, 133–142.

Kue R, Sahrabi A, Nagle D, *et al.* (1999), 'Enhanced proliferation and osteocalcin production by human osteoblast-like cells on silicon nitride ceramic discs', *Biomaterials*, 20, 1195–1201.

Kulisch W and Popov C (2006), 'On the growth mechanisms of nanocrystalline diamond films', *Phys. Stat. Sol. (a)*, 203, 203–219.

Kulisch W, Popov C, Bliznakov S, *et al.* (2007), 'Surface and bioproperties of nanocrystalline diamond/amorphous carbon nanocomposite films', *Thin Solid Films*, 515, 8407–8411.

Krauss AR, Auciello O, Gruen DM, *et al.* (2001), 'Ultrananocrystalline diamond thin films for MEMS and moving mechanical assembly devices', *Diam. Rel. Mater.*, 10, 1952–1961.

Lee Tong S, Lin Z and Jiang X (1999), 'CVD diamond films: nucleation and growth', *Mater. Sci. and Eng. R: Reports*, 25, 123–154.

Li T, Yu GY, Wee TS, *et al.* (2000), 'Compositional mapping of the argon–methane–hydrogen system for polycrystalline to nanocrystalline diamond film growth in a hot-filament chemical vapor deposition system', *Appl. Phys. Lett.*, 77, 2692–2694.

Liang H, Shi B, Fairchild A and Cale T (2004), 'Applications of plasma coatings in artificial joints: an overview', *Vacuum*, 73, 317–326.

May PW and Mankelevich YA (2006), 'Experiment and modeling of the deposition of ultrananocrystalline diamond films using hot filament chemical vapor deposition and $Ar/CH_4/H_2$ gas mixtures: A generalized mechanism for ultrananocrystalline diamond growth', *J. Appl. Phys.*, 100, 024301-1–024301-9.

Matsumoto S, Sato Y, Tsutsimi M and Setaka N (1982), 'Growth of diamond particles from methane-hydrogen gas', *J. Mat. Sci.*, 17, 3106–3112.

Palin E, Liu H and Webster TJ (2005), 'Increased osteoblast adhesion on polymer casts of nanostructured ceramics', *Nanotechnology*, 16, 1828–1836.

Perla V and Webster TJ (2005), 'Better osteoblast adhesion on nanoparticulate selenium – A promising orthopedic implant material', *J. Biomed. Mater. Res.*, 75A, 356–364.

Pfeiffer R, Kuzmany H, Knoll P, *et al.* (2003), 'Evidence for trans-polyacetylene in nano-crystalline diamond films', *Diam. Relat. Mater.*, 12, 268–271.

Popov C, Kulisch W, Reithmaier JP, *et al.* (2007), 'Bioproperties of nanocrystalline diamond/amorphous carbon composite films', *Diam. Relat. Mater.*, 16, 735–739.

Price RL, Haberstroh KM and Webster TJ (2003), 'Enhanced functions of osteoblasts of nanostructure surfaces of carbon and alumina', *Med. Biol. Eng. Comput.*, 41, 372–375.

Rabeau JR, John P, Wilson JIB and Fan Y (2004), 'The role of C_2 in nanocrystalline diamond growth', *J. Appl. Phys.*, 96, 6724–6732.

Ralchenko VG, Smolin AA, Pereverzev VG, *et al.* (1995), 'Diamond deposition on steel with CVD tungsten intermediate layer', *Diam. Relat. Mater.*, 4, 754–758.

Retama JR, Hernando J, Lopez-Ruiz B, *et al.* (2006), 'Synthetic nanocrystalline diamond as a third-generation biosensor support', *Langmuir*, 22, 5837–5842.

Santavirta S, Böhler M, Harris WH, *et al.* (2003), 'Alternative materials to improve total hip replacement tribology', *Acta Orthop. Scand.*, 74, 380–388.

Scholes SC, Unsworth A, Hall RM and Scott R (2000), 'The effects of material combination and lubricant on the friction of total hip prostheses', *Wear*, 241, 209–213.

Shane AC, Marc DF, Yogesh KV, *et al.* (2002), 'Nanostructured Ceramics for Biomedical Implants', *J. of Nanoscience and Nanotechnology*, 2, 293–312.

Shane AC, Monique C, Yogesh KV, *et al.* (2003), 'Surface crystalline phases and nanoindentation hardness of explanted zirconia femoral heads', *J. Mater. Sci.: Mater. in Medicine*, 14, 863–867.

Sharda T, Rahaman MM, Nukaya Y, *et al.* (2001), 'Structural and optical properties of diamond and nano-diamond films grown by microwave plasma chemical vapor deposition', *Diam. Relat. Mater.*, 10, 561–567.

Siew PS, Loh KP, Poh WC and Zhang H (2005), 'Biosensing properties of nanocrystalline diamond film grown on polycrystalline diamond electrodes', *Diam. Relat. Mater.*, 14, 426–431.

Sikavitsas VI, Temenoff JS and Mikos AG (2001), 'Biomaterials and bone mechanotransduction' *Biomaterials*, 22, 2581–2593.

Smith JA, Cameron E, Ashfold MNR, *et al.* (2001), 'On the mechanism of CH_3 radical formation in hot filament activated CH_4/H_2 and C_2H_2/H_2 gas mixtures', *Diam. Relat. Mater.*, 10, 358–363.

Spitsyn BV, Bouilov LL and Alexenko AE (2000), 'Origin, State of the Art and Some Prospects of the Diamond CVD', *Braz. J. Phys.*, 30, 471–481.

Steinmuller-Nethl D, Kloss FR, Haq MNU, *et al.* (2006), 'Strong binding of bioactive BMP-2 to nanocrystalline diamond by physisorption', *Biomaterials*, 27, 4547–4556.

Szivek JA, Anderson PL and Benjamin JB (1996), 'Average and peak contact stress distribution evaluation of total knee arthroplasties', *J. Arthropl.*, 11, 952–963.

Tiainen V (2001), 'Amorphous carbon as a bio-mechanical coating – mechanical properties and biological applications', *Diamond Relat. Mater.*, 10, 153–160.

Tjong SC and Chen H (2004), 'Nanocrystalline materials and coatings', *Mater. Sci. Eng. R*, 45, 1–88.

Webster TJ, Siegel RW and Bizios R (1999), 'Osteoblast adhesion on nanophase ceramics', *Biomaterials*, 20, 1221–1227.

Wenmackers S, Christiaens P, Daenen M, *et al.* (2005), 'DNA attachment to nanocrystalline diamond films', *Phys. Status Solidi A – Appl. Mater. Sci.*, 202, 2212–2216.

Widmer MR, Heuberger M, Vörös J, and Spencer ND (2001), 'Influence of polymer surface chemistry on frictional properties under protein-lubrication conditions: implications for hip-implant design', *Tribology Lett.*, 10, 111–116.

Williams D (2003), 'Revisiting the definition of biocompatibility', *Medical Device Technology*, 14, 10–13.

Williams OA, Daenen M, D'Haen J, *et al.* (2006), 'Comparison of the growth and properties of ultrananocrystalline diamond and nanocrystalline diamond', *Diam. Relat. Mater.*, 15, 654–658.

Williams OA (2011), 'Nanocrystalline diamond', *Diam. Relat. Mater.*, 20, 621–640.

Yang TS, Lai JY, Cheng CL and Wong MS (2001), 'Growth of faceted, ballas-like and nanocrystalline diamond films deposited in $CH_4/H_2/Ar$ MPCVD', *Diam. Relat. Mater.*, 10, 2161–2166.

Yang W and Hamers RJ (2004), 'Fabrication and characterization of a biologically sensitive field-effect transistor using a nanocrystalline diamond thin film', *Appl. Phys. Lett.*, 85, 3626–3628.

Zhang YF, Zhang F, Gao QJ, *et al.* (2001), 'The roles of argon addition in the hot filament chemical vapor deposition system', *Diam. Relat. Mater.*, 10, 1523–1527.

Ziegler G, Heinrich J and Wötting G (1987), 'Relationships between processing, microstructure and properties of dense and reaction-bonded silicon nitride', *J. Mater. Sci.*, 22, 3041–3086.

4

Blood compatibility of diamond-like carbon (DLC) coatings

M. FEDEL, University of Trento, Italy

DOI: 10.1533/9780857093516.1.71

Abstract: Diamond-like carbon (DLC) films offer numerous functional characteristics that make them particularly attractive as potential wear resistant coatings for biomedical applications. This chapter first discusses the blood compatibility of various forms of plain and doped DLCs, and evaluates possible correlations with film structure and surface properties. The chapter then considers the application of DLC coatings to different typologies of implants and medical devices, with special regard to cardiovascular prostheses.

Key words: diamond-like carbon, coatings, blood compatibility, cardiovascular applications.

4.1 Introduction

Carbon is a highly versatile element. Various allotropes originate from the multiple possible hybridization states of its orbitals, including graphite, diamond and fullerene, and each of these materials offers different properties dependent on its particular structure.

Development of a special class of carbon-based materials called diamond-like carbon (DLC) began during the 1970s and has rapidly gained the interest of the scientific community due to the outstanding qualities and performance exhibited.

The term DLC is used to define a large family of amorphous carbon-based materials containing both sp^3 and sp^2 carbon bonds in variable amounts, and potentially including hydrogen or other alloying elements, such as nitrogen, fluorine, silicon or phosphorous. DLC forms isotropic disordered thin films, which exhibit some extreme properties similar to those of diamond, including hardness, elastic modulus and chemical inertness (Robertson, 2002).

Different deposition techniques have been proposed that give origin to a large selection of amorphous carbons with varying sp^3 and hydrogen content. The fraction of sp^3 bonds and the hydrogen content significantly contribute to determining the structure and, consequently, the final properties of DLC films.

DLC coatings are characterized by a high level of hardness, low friction coefficient, high resistance to corrosion and smooth surface finishing. These properties make them attractive as potential wear resistant coatings for several interesting applications, including optical, mechanical, microelectronic and biomedical applications. Another big advantage of DLC coatings is that they can be produced at low deposition temperatures on various substrates and can therefore be used in coating heat-sensitive materials such as polymers.

Since its discovery, DLC has been the object of intensive research studies, leading to greater knowledge of its properties and facilitating the development of different deposition techniques that can be used to tailor its characteristics.

DLC was first produced in 1953 by Schmellenmeier using C_2H_2 gas in glow-discharge plasma (Donnet and Erdemir, 2008). This was followed in the early 1970s by Aisenberg and Chabot, who used an ion beam deposition system to produce amorphous carbon films with remarkable mechanical properties (Aisenberg and Chabot, 1971; Donnet and Erdemir, 2008). However, it was not until the early 1990s that interest in DLCs really began to increase. Their properties and processing techniques started to be studied and improved, and a variety of possible applications began to be identified (Boehm *et al.*, 2011; Donnet and Erdemir, 2008).

Due to their unique properties, DLC coatings have been used for various industrial applications, including optics and microelectronics, manufacturing and transportation, and have been employed in the production of items ranging from razor blades and eyeglasses to magnetic storage media, fuel injectors and critical engine components (Table 4.1).

Alongside their other key characteristics, DLCs demonstrate superior bio- and blood-compatibility properties, and are therefore being used as coatings for a wide range of biomedical implants, devices and tools (Roy and Lee, 2007; Lackner and Waldhauser, 2010; Donnet and Erdemir, 2008; Dearnaley and Arps, 2005;

Table 4.1 Applications of diamond-like carbon coatings

Biomedical	Other
Hip, knee and shoulder joints	Magnetic recording systems
Coronary stents and guidewires	Optical storage devices
Vascular prostheses	Sliding/friction parts
Heart valves, blood pumps for ventricular assistance and artificial hearts	Engine components (e.g. cylinders and pistons, fuel injectors, etc.)
Sutures	Drill bits
Catheters	Precision gauges
Breast implants	Razor blades
Orthodontic archwires	Antireflective and wear protective coating for infrared optics and windows
Cochlear implants	Microelectronics
Surgical instruments (e.g. laparoscopic instruments and needles for corneal surgery)	Thin film cathodes for field emission displays
Orthopaedic screws	

Arps and Dearnaley, 2004). The deposition of a thin DLC layer on the surface of medical device components can considerably increase their biocompatibility, improving materials interaction with the biological environment. Their use decreases, for example, the probability of thrombus formation in the case of blood environment, and stimulates cell adhesion and proliferation.

Moreover, a hard and wear resistant coating like DLC can act as a protective barrier contributing to a reduction in corrosion, formation of wear debris and release of toxic elements (e.g. Ni, Co, Cr, Al and V), thus preventing possible allergic, inflammatory or carcinogenic reactions.

The first tentative application of DLC coatings to blood-contacting devices originated from the knowledge of the excellent blood compatibility properties demonstrated by pyrolytic carbon, which can in some ways be considered the antenate of DLC. Pyrolytic carbon, a turbostratic form of isotropic carbon, is currently used for mechanical heart valves and other implantable prosthetic devices due to its blood compatibility, first largely investigated by Bokros, Gott *et al.* in the 1970s.

Bio- and blood-compatibility of various forms of DLC have been investigated by *in vitro* and *in vivo* analysis, and the influence of deposition parameters on the properties of the coatings has been studied. In particular, several studies have demonstrated that DLC coatings can improve the thromboresistance of cardiovascular implants by reducing platelet adhesion and activation (Fedel *et al.*, 2009; Jones *et al.*, 2000), whereas hydrogenated DLC films showed a tendency to prolong clotting time and suppress the platelet and complement convertase activation (Nurdin *et al.*, 2003). Moreover, DLC do not seem to induce haemolytic effects in whole blood (Jones *et al.*, 1999), nor provoke macrophage activation or inflammatory signals from monocytic cells (Linder *et al.*, 2002).

Tentative descriptions of DLC blood compatibility as a function of material properties (for example sp^3/sp^2 fraction, wettability and surface energy) have been formulated with some contrasting results.

At present, DLC coatings are applied to devices for total joint replacement, orthopaedic screws, dental prostheses and surgical needles for corneal surgery, as well as to medical and surgical instrumentation. Application in the field of cardiovascular devices is of particular interest, and DLC coatings have been employed for vascular prostheses, heart valves, rotary pumps for ventricular assistance, dialysis membranes, stents and guidewires (Table 4.1).

In the following paragraphs DLC structure, properties and production technologies are examined, and the great influence that these features can have on the biological response of materials considered. Extensive analysis of the scientific literature related to the response of DLCs to the biological environment follows, discussing in detail DLC blood compatibility properties and considering both *in vitro* and *in vivo* performance. The influence of doping elements on the properties and haemocompatibility of DLC is explored, and current applications of DLCs as coatings for implants and medical devices are described.

4.2 Diamond-like carbon (DLC) structure, properties and applications

The term 'diamond-like carbon' commonly describes a family of metastable amorphous carbon films obtained via different deposition processes and characterized by a variable but significant fraction of sp^3 type C-C bonds along with an absence of long-range order in a dense amorphous structure (Robertson, 2002).

To clarify the terminology used for different forms of amorphous carbons as a function of their content of sp^2 and sp^3 bonding and of their hydrogenation degree, we can refer to the ternary phase diagram reported in Fig. 4.1. The type, structure and final properties of the amorphous carbon film depend on both the deposition method and the hydrogen content. We can, therefore, have amorphous carbon (a-C), hydrogenated amorphous carbon (a-C:H), tetrahedral amorphous carbon (ta-C) or hydrogenated tetrahedral amorphous carbon (ta-C:H), depending on the fraction of sp^3 bonding and on the presence of H in the carbon film. Hydrogen free ta-C has a C-C sp^3 content higher than 60–80%, whereas ta-C:H features a hydrogen content of around 25–30 at.% with a very high percentage of sp^3 bonding (up to 70% or higher if deposited at high ion energies) (Chhowalla *et al.*, 1997). Hydrogenated and non-hydrogenated a-C films have a lower sp^3 content with respect to tetrahedral amorphous carbons, and a variable amount of H ranging from less than 1% for a-C up to 50 at.% for a-C:H (Robertson, 2002; Grill, 1999; Lifshitz, 1999; Dongping and Baoxiang, 2006; Casiraghi *et al.*, 2007).

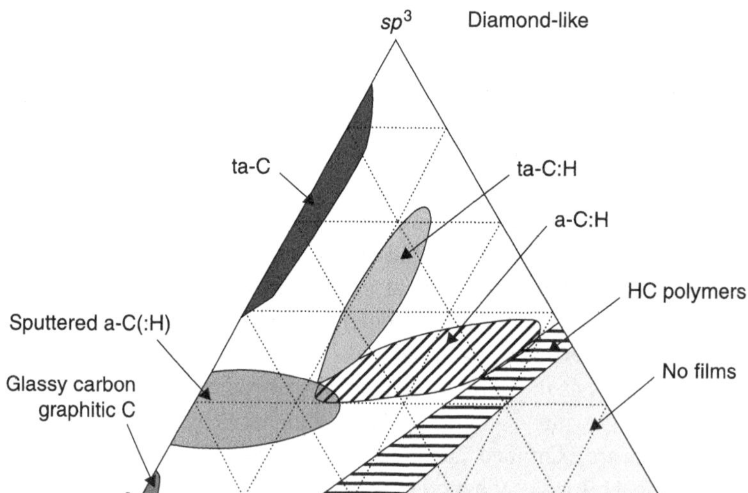

4.1 Amorphous carbon regions in a ternary phase diagram of bonding in carbon-hydrogen alloys. Reprinted from *Materials Science and Engineering: R: Reports*, 37(4–6), Robertson J, 'Diamond-like amorphous carbon', pages 129–281. Copyright (2002), used with permission from Elsevier.

The use of the term 'diamond-like' is justified by the high presence of tetrahedral sp^3-hybridized carbon atoms. This high presence contributes to several interesting properties of the film similar to the properties of diamond, including high hardness and elastic modulus, excellent wear resistance and chemical inertness. As shown in Table 4.2, DLC films offer a range of very attractive characteristics, including exceptional mechanical, tribological, chemical, electronic, optical and biological properties, making them suitable candidates for several applications. In Table 4.3 the main structural and mechanical properties of different types of DLCs are presented and compared to the properties of diamond and graphite, as well as to pyrolytic carbon.

Mechanical properties and density of DLC depend mainly on the presence of C-C sp^3 bonds. In general, DLC films are characterized by high hardness and high

Table 4.2 Main properties of DLC films

High density
High hardness and elastic modulus
Smoothness
Low friction coefficient and high wear resistance
Chemical inertness and corrosion resistance
Optical transparency (mainly infrared)
Good thermal conductivity
Wide band gap semiconductor
Low dielectric constant
Possible deposition at low temperature
Biocompatibility and blood compatibility

Table 4.3 Structural and mechanical properties of different diamond-like carbon (DLC) films compared to crystalline carbon allotropes (diamond and graphite), and to pyrolytic carbon

	sp^3 content	H content	Density (g cm^{-3})	Young's modulus	Hardness
Diamond	100%	0%	3.52	1000–1200 GPa	100 GPa
ta-C	>80%	0%	3.1–3.5	800 GPa	80 GPa
ta-C:H	70%	30%	2.4	n.a.	50 GPa
a-C:H soft	60%	40–50%	1.2–1.6	n.a.	<10 GPa
a-C:H hard	40%	30–40%	1.6–2.2	n.a.	10–20 GPa
Graphite	0%	0%	2.3	686 GPa (//a) low (⊥a)	–
Pyrolytic carbon	–	–	1.5–2.1	28 GPa	>230 (DPH 500 g)

Source: Data obtained from Grill, 1999; Koidl *et al.*, 1990; Lifshitz, 1999; More *et al.*, 2004.

elastic modulus. Typical hardness values of a-C:H films are in the range of 10–30 GPa (Grill, 1999) and can increase up to 40–80 GPa in the case of hydrogen-free ta-C. As expected, increasing hardness and elastic modulus correlate with an increasing sp^3 percentage and a decreasing hydrogen content. Furthermore, the properties of DLC films can be varied over a wide range by changing the deposition conditions. Mechanical characteristics, in particular, depend on the substrate temperature and usually improve with increasing ion energy per condensing carbon atom.

Thanks to their special properties, DLCs have manifold applications in different areas, including, the automotive and transportation industry, optics and electronics fields. They are often used for data storage (hard discs and heads, tape-recording heads and guides, for example), or as wear protective coatings on components requiring superior mechanical and tribological qualities, as in the case of engines or sliding parts.

Moreover, due to the combination of their physico-chemical and mechanical properties with specific bio- and blood-compatibility properties, DLCs present a valuable success in the biomedical field, and particular importance can be attributed to the properties of DLC films that can be exploited for the improvement of medical implants and devices. Hardness and wear resistance are particular requirements for several implant components, for example orthopaedic joints, mechanical heart valves and other devices which are subjected to fatigue and repetitive cyclical stresses. The presence of a biocompatible carbon-based coating on the surface of a metallic component (Co-Cr alloys, Ti-6Al-4V, NiTi, etc.) can protect the organism from contact with toxic or potentially allergenic, inflammatory or carcinogenic elements. It can also help prevent the release of metal ions and the detachment from polymeric (e.g. HDPE) or metallic components of dangerous debris with the potential to cause an adverse response of the host organism through foreign body reaction.

Chemical inertness and corrosion resistance are also especially important characteristics. The human body presents a range of very aggressive, hostile environments, and body fluids could easily trigger corrosion, etching or oxidation phenomena. DLC films therefore represent ideal coatings for metallic or polymeric bulk materials for the avoidance of corrosion, degradation or oxidation phenomena on the surface of devices inserted in the human body.

Besides a great number of advantageous properties, DLC films feature a small number of critical characteristics. In particular, they are subject to high internal compressive stresses, mainly resulting from the quenching of the impinging species during film growth (Donnet and Erdemir, 2008). This reduces their adhesion to the substrate and prevents the growth of thick coatings, limiting film thickness to less than 1 μm (Grill, 1999).

DLCs have been reported to adhere well on substrates containing carbide-forming elements (for example silicon or titanium), but often intermediate layers need to be deposited on different substrates to improve the deposition and adhesion of DLC films (Donnet and Erdemir, 2008). Critical adhesion and delamination properties represent one of the main limitations related to DLC films and to their industrial applications, especially for biomedical applications.

4.3 Deposition techniques for DLC films

Diamond-like carbon coatings can be deposited using a number of different techniques. These techniques can generally be divided in two categories: chemical vapour deposition (CVD) and physical vapour deposition (PVD).

In general, a carbonaceous precursor and an energy source are required. The carbon source may be an ionized carbon-containing gas or a solid carbon target that can be activated by, for example, thermal evaporation, ion sputtering or laser ablation. Most of the processes upon which DLC deposition is based are physical in nature, as the sp^3 bonds are produced by the impact of carbon (or hydrocarbon) ions on the growing film. The physical processes that have been proposed to deposit DLC thin films include direct ion beam (IB) and ion beam assisted deposition (IBAD), filtered cathodic vacuum arc (FCVA), DC and RF sputtering, pulsed laser deposition (PLD), and plasma immersion ion implantation (PIII). Other techniques involving chemical processes include plasma enhanced chemical vapour deposition (PECVD) and electron cyclotron resonance plasma chemical vapour deposition (ECR-CVD).

The first DLC films produced by Aisenberg and Chabot were obtained by direct IB deposition. In this method, the target surface is bombarded under vacuum conditions by energetic carbon ions, produced by plasma activation from a graphite cathode or from a hydrocarbon gas such as methane. Mass selected ion beam (MSIB) represents a more controllable deposition technique, which allows the flux ratio of ions to be increased to neutral species, and permits the fine adjustment of DLC properties, despite holding a low deposition rate. In this case, carbon ions C^+ are produced with a very sharp ion energy distribution (1–10 eV), accelerated to a high voltage (20–30 kV) and passed through a magnetic filter, which removes from the beam neutral unionized particles and/or contaminants. The ion beam, which diverges due to Coulomb repulsion, is then focused and decelerated by an electrostatic lens so that it impacts the substrate surface with a controlled energy, typically in the range from 5 eV to 20 keV (Lifshitz, 1999; Robertson, 2002).

Cathodic arc deposition involves generation of an electric discharge between a graphite cathode and an anode. This produces highly energetic plasma, with very high carbon fluxes and high deposition rates. As the plasma can contain, besides carbon ions, neutral carbon and particulate, these films may present a variable amount of graphitic bonding. In FCVA, a toroidal magnetic filter is used, helping to remove micro- and macro-particles and thereby increasing the purity of cathodic arc deposited DLC films. The films obtained by FCVA deposition, which can be virtually hydrogen-free, offer particularly beneficial properties, including high smoothness and hardness (Arps and Dearnaley, 2004). Cathodic arc and FCVA are frequently used on an industrial scale. The advantages of these systems include high deposition rates and the potential use as coating for insulating materials, thanks to the neutral nature of the plasma.

In pulsed laser ablation, an excimer laser (ArF) is used to vaporize carbon species from a carbon target using very short, intense laser pulses. Depending on the source (e.g. graphite or polycarbonate), ta-C or a-C:H can be produced (Robertson, 2002; Arps and Dearnaley, 2004).

Sputtering is a very typical method used for the production of DLC films and, as a very versatile and controllable process, is frequently exploited at the industrial level. Non-hydrogenated DLC films are produced by DC or RF sputtering of pure graphite targets using an Ar plasma. In magnetron sputtering, magnets are placed behind the target and used to increase the ionization degree of the plasma, thus increasing the deposition rate of DLC film on the substrate by PVD. In some cases, dual ion beam sputtering (also called IBAD) is used to produce relatively pure DLC films. This involves the simultaneous use of two ion guns: one Ar gun is used to sputter carbon from a graphite target, and a second gun is used to bombard the substrate, encouraging sp^3 bond formation in the growing film.

In PIII, the substrate is immersed in plasma and periodic high-voltage pulses are applied to form an electric sheath between the substrate and the plasma. Carbon ions from the plasma are thus accelerated to the substrate by the expanding sheath's electric field (Anders, 2000). PIII deposited carbon films typically present high hardness and low friction coefficients, occasionally with high compressive stress values (Arps and Dearnaley, 2004).

A different method frequently used for the laboratory production of DLC films is PECVD. Based on a CVD process, PECVD involves the decomposition of a selected precursor (such as methane, ethane, ethylene, acetylene, etc.) at high temperature and low pressure to maximize the ion radical fraction. In PECVD the energy for the chemical reaction is supplied by plasma, generally created by RF frequency or DC discharge between two electrodes in a chamber filled with the reacting gases. Several process parameters can be varied, including composition, pressure and flow rate of the source gas, or frequency and intensity of the RF power source. These modifications can influence such film characteristics as adhesion, hydrogen content, density and mechanical properties. By using PECVD, hydrogenated DLC films can be obtained, as the presence of hydrogen (10–50%) is required to passivate the dangling bonds in the amorphous structures (Grill, 1999). Doped films can also be produced using opportune gas mixtures. PECVD is particularly interesting as it allows the deposition of thin films at a much lower temperature than that commonly used in conventional CVD reactors. With this technique, good film adhesion and high growth rates can be achieved.

As reported, a number of different methods have been proposed to fabricate DLC coatings, and the composition (sp^3-to-sp^2 fraction and H content), microstructure and related properties can vary significantly depending on the technique, deposition parameters, substrate temperature and carbon precursor used (Cho *et al.*, 1992).

Recent advances in DLC film deposition and characterization facilitate the production of materials with controlled properties, tailored to suit specific requirements. In some cases, further film modifications (gas plasma treatments or laser irradiation, for example) can be introduced following deposition, in order to improve some characteristics of the coating and obtain the desired performance for specific applications.

4.4 DLC blood compatibility

Implants, prostheses and some medical devices are engineered to enter the human body and work in particular physiological environments, dependent on the specific function they are required to fulfil. In the case of cardiovascular implants, in particular, the specific biological environment is represented by the complex blood system. When a biomaterial is placed in contact with blood, it is recognized as a foreign element by the host, and key reactions such as thrombosis, inflammation and fibrosis can take place (Gorbet and Sefton, 2004). Thrombosis is the major and most frequent complication related to devices for cardiovascular applications. This can take place when blood contacts a foreign surface, triggering platelet adhesion and activation of the coagulation cascade through the intrinsic pathway.

Protein adsorption assumes a particularly critical role in blood compatibility, as it is the first event that rapidly occurs on all surfaces exposed to blood, and is finally responsible for the haemocompatibility of a material. Within seconds of contact between the material and the blood, the surface is covered by a layer of proteins whose composition, relative concentration and conformation guide the subsequent host response, therefore playing a key role in determining the fate of the material. Blood plasma contains various molecular species and hundreds of proteins in a wide range of molecular weights, charges, structures, and concentrations. About a dozen proteins, 'the big twelve,' are considered to dominate plasma protein adsorption. These include albumin (HSA), immunoglobulins (IgG, IgA, IgM), C3 complement component, fibrinogen (Fng), haptoglobin, α1-antitrypsin and α2-macroglobulin, as well as low and high density lipoproteins (Andrade and Hlady, 1987). In particular albumin, fibrinogen and, to a lesser extent, fibronectin, assume a prominent role in leading blood–material interactions.

A series of biological reactions, such as platelet adhesion/activation, triggering of coagulation and complement systems, and activation of leucocytes, are strongly dependent on protein adsorption. Thus the adsorption of contact phase proteins, for example, may be responsible for the activation of the intrinsic coagulation system (Gorbet and Sefton, 2004), whereas platelet adhesion is likely to take place thanks to the role of adsorbed adhesive plasma proteins, including fibrinogen, von Willebrand factor, fibronectin and vitronectin.

Due to the complexity of the blood system and of possible blood–material interaction mechanisms, various aspects have to be considered for a complete assessment of DLC haemocompatibility, including protein adsorption, platelet adhesion/activation, triggering of coagulation and complement systems, activation of leucocytes and haemolysis. As such, several studies have been presented in the literature analyzing diverse aspects of the blood compatibility of different types of DLC coatings.

In our previous work, we studied the properties of commercially available DLC films deposited at low temperature by PVD on different substrata, including a Co-Cr alloy used for heart valve components and silicon chips (Fedel *et al.*, 2009; Fedel *et al.*, 2010). DLC films were compared to uncoated substrata and to pyrolytic carbon, an isotropic carbon coating used for biomedical applications (More *et al.*, 2004). Protein adsorption kinetics and binding strength, as well as platelet adhesion/activation on the sample surfaces were analyzed *in vitro*.

As a general rule, the results showed that the protein mainly adsorbed on the carbon-coated surfaces was albumin, whereas the control materials presented more rich and complex protein adsorption profiles. DLC surfaces revealed a weak and reversible interaction with a small amount of mid- and high-MW plasma proteins, whereas a preferential and tenacious albumin adsorption was enhanced.

The fibrinogen-to-albumin adsorption ratio was studied as a measure of the blood compatibility of a material, as surface competition between these two plasma proteins can contribute to defining the thrombogenic/non-thrombogenic behaviour of artificial blood-contacting materials (Cui and Li, 2000). Human serum albumin (HSA, 66 kDa) and fibrinogen (Fng, 340 kDa) are two of the most abundant plasma proteins, and present opposite haemocompatibility potential, as Fng is a pro-adhesive protein (Grunkemeier *et al.*, 2000; Wu *et al.*, 2005) which stimulates platelet activation, whereas HSA seems to inhibit the initial blood platelet adhesion (Young *et al.*, 1982).

A low fibrinogen-to-albumin ratio was observed for DLC deposited on Co-Cr alloy and silicon at all the residence intervals tested, in particular at high incubation times (Fig. 4.2). This was a result of lower Fng adsorption for these samples in relation to control materials.

Platelet activation on the sample surfaces has been assessed by analyzing the morphology of adherent platelets, as the activation process is characterized by platelet change from the typical resting discoid shape to varying degrees of spreading (Goodman *et al.*, 1996).

According to our findings, all of the carbon-coated materials presented a significantly lower level of platelet adhesion and activation after 15 and 25 minute incubation periods with platelet-poor plasma and a lower propensity to form

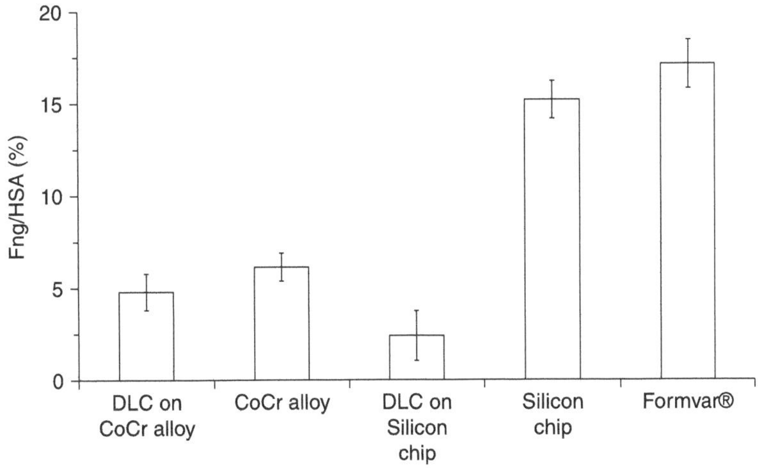

4.2 Protein adsorption on DLC-coated and uncoated samples and on Formvar positive control. Fibrinogen-to-albumin surface adsorption ratio after 25 minutes incubation with platelet-poor plasma (Fedel *et al.*, 2009).

three-dimensional (3-D) platelet aggregates in comparison to the respective non-coated substrata and control materials (Fig. 4.3). A specific relationship was found between the degree of platelet activation and the amount of Fng-to-HSA adsorbed on the tested surfaces. Minimum platelet spreading was evident on the surfaces presenting lower Fng-to-HSA adsorption ratios from plasma, whereas the highest degree of platelet spreading was reported in the case of higher Fng/HSA adsorption (Fedel *et al.*, 2009).

According to our work, DLC blood compatibility seems to be related to surface chemical heterogeneity more than to the absolute hydrophilicity/hydrophobicity degree of materials. Blood compatibility may be guided by a favourable disposition of the acid/base and dispersive sites on the amorphous carbon film surface (Fedel *et al.*, 2009). Moreover, the smooth topography of DLC films may contribute to inhibit the adsorption and retention of mid- and high-MW proteins (Fedel *et al.*, 2010).

Our studies support the hypothesis that rapid and tenacious binding of albumin globular molecules to carbon-based materials through 'domain-match' mechanisms contributes to passivation of the surfaces. The tightly bound albumin layer prevents the adsorption of Fng and higher MW proteins on DLC surfaces, thus rendering the coating more thromboresistant and less adhesive and activating for platelets.

In agreement with our studies, various authors reported a typical propensity of DLC films produced by several different deposition technologies to limit platelet adhesion and activation. DLC films have been compared to numerous materials,

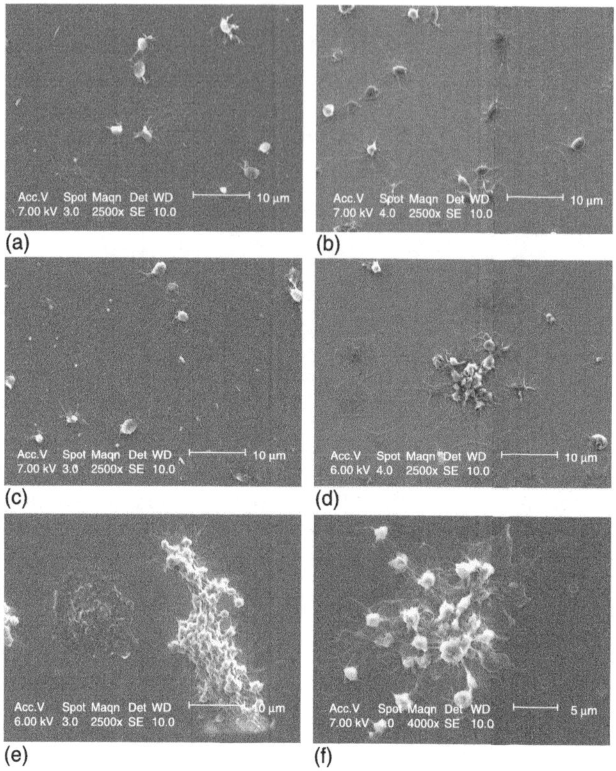

4.3 Platelet adhesion and spreading on DLC-coated (a, c) and uncoated substrata after 25 minutes incubation with platelet-rich plasma. DLC on CoCr alloy (a), uncoated CoCr alloy (b), DLC on silicon chip (c), silicon chip (d), Formvar® positive control (e, f). Adapted from Fedel *et al.* (2009).

including polymers, metals, oxides and thin layers, demonstrating, in most cases, superior properties in terms of thromboresistance (Nurdin *et al.*, 2003; Alanazi *et al.*, 2000; Jones *et al.*, 2000; Dion *et al.*, 1993; Cui and Li, 2000; Sui *et al.*, 2006) (Table 4.4).

Alanazi *et al.* evaluated the blood compatibility of DLC deposited on polycarbonate in comparison with polycarbonate substrata (PC), PC coated with heparin (Heparin-PC) and 2-hydroxyethylmethacrylathe/styrene (HEMA/St), with a different level of platelet adhesion observed on the various materials (HEMA/St < DLC < Heparin-PC < PC) (Alanazi *et al.*, 2000).

A quantitative study using I-125 labelled platelets under dynamic conditions reported a considerably reduced platelet adhesion on PECVD-deposited DLC coatings with respect to titanium samples (Krishnan *et al.*, 2002), and showed the dependence of platelet adhesion on the shear rate exerted by blood fluids on the

Table 4.4 Blood compatibility of DLC films discussed for different deposition techniques and physico-chemical characteristics and compared to different control materials

Material	Deposition technique	Main characteristics	Control materials	Blood compatibility with respect to control materials	References
a-C:H	PECVD	Smooth coating Water contact angle 56° ca	Ti TiN TiC	Good haemocompatibility Higher HSA/Fng ratio Low platelet spreading	Jones *et al.*, 1999 Jones *et al.*, 2000
DLC	IBAD?		CN PMMA	Higher HSA/Fng ratio Lower platelet adhesion	Cui *et al.*, 2000
a-C:H	Magnetron sputtering	Smooth surface Intermediate hydrophobicity	SiC MS PDMS LDPE PMMA SiR	Delay of clotting time Inhibition of platelet adhesion, activation and aggregation Absence of activated complement factor adsorption	Nurdin *et al.*, 2003
a-C:H @ different deposition conditions	PIII-D + annealing		SS LTIC	Platelet adhesion and activation on a-C:H is affected by annealing Platelets are strongly activated by – C:H deposited at high bias, and the situation worsens after annealing	Yang *et al.*, 2004
a-C a-C:H ta-C @ different deposition conditions	RF magnetron sputtering FCVA			Haemocompatibility improves with sp^3 content on sputtered a-C films a-C:H films exhibit better haemocompatibility than a-C Platelets activate and aggregate on biased a-C:H films Higher HSA/Fng ratio and round platelets on floating a-C:H films	Logothetidis *et al.*, 2007

(*Continued*)

Table 4.4 Continued

Material	Deposition technique	Main characteristics	Control materials	Blood compatibility with respect to control materials	References
a-C:H @ different deposition conditions	RF magnetron sputtering	Film density increases by the increase of sp^3 and decreases by the incorporation of hydrogen		a-C:H films grown with floating substrates and with 10 at.% H_2 showed the highest HSA/Fng ratio Rougher protein layers are formed on films deposited under floating conditions	Lousinian *et al.*, 2007
a-C:H(CH_4) a-C:H(C_2H_2) ta-C	PECVD FCVA	sp^3 fraction: a-C:H(CH_4) < a-C:H(C_2H_2)<ta-C H content: ta-C< a-C:H(C_2H_2)<a-C:H(CH_4) Surface energy:a-C:H(CH_4)< a-C:H(C_2H_2)<ta-C Surface roughness: a-C:H(CH_4)< a-C:H(C_2H_2)<ta-C	Si Thermanox	DLC suppressed macrophage attachment Macrophage viability: Thermanox <a-C:H(CH_4)< a-C:H(C_2H_2)<ta-C<Si HSA/Fng ratio: a-C:H(CH_4)< a-C:H(C_2H_2)<ta-C The higher the H content, the lower the HSA/Fng adsorption ratio	Ma *et al.*, 2007
Carbofilm™ on different substrata	PVD	Low surface roughness Moderate hydrophilicity High hysteresis between advancing and receding contact angle	Stellite Si PET Formvar ®	Tenacious HSA binding Low Fng/HSA adsorption Low platelet adhesion and activation	Fedel *et al.*, 2009
DLC	PVD	Equilibrium contact angle: DLC ≤ PyC < F < S	PyC Formvar ®	Rapid and tight binding of HSA globular molecules passivate DLC surfaces, inducing low platelet adhesion and activation	Fedel *et al.*, 2010

Note: FCVA: filtered cathodic vacuum arc; IBAD: ion beam assisted deposition; PIII-D: plasma immersion ion implantation and deposition; PVD: physical vapour deposition; PECVD: plasma enhanced chemical vapour deposition; CN: carbon nitride; HEMA/St: 2-hydroxyethylmethacrylathe/styrene; Heparin-PC: polycarbonate coated with heparin; LDPE: low density polyethylene; LTIC: low temperature isotropic carbon; MS: medical steel; PDMS: polydimethylsiloxane; PET: polyethylene terephthalate; PMMA: polymethyl methacrylate; PyC: pyrolytic carbon; Si: silicon; SiC: silicon carbide; SiR: silicone rubber; SS: stainless steel; Ti: titanium; TiC: titanium carbide; TiN: titanium nitride; Fng: fibrinogen; HSA: human serum albumin.

material surface. In many cases, a low degree of platelet adhesion or activation was related to a high albumin-to-fibrinogen adsorption ratio on DLC films in comparison to different materials commonly used for biomedical applications, such as medical grade silicone elastomer (Dion *et al.*, 1993), carbon nitride (CN) or poly(methyl methacrylate) (PMMA) (Cui and Li, 2000).

Jones *et al.* (2000) analyzed the HSA/Fng ratio as a possible marker of haemocompatibility, and reported a favourable blood compatibility of DLC coatings with respect to Ti substrate, TiN and TiC layers. Although the authors could not find a direct correlation between material surface energy and protein adsorption, they suggested that the high HSA/Fng ratio on DLC coatings contributed to reduce platelet activation and spreading, even in cases where platelet attachment was not reduced.

In a previous work, Jones *et al.* reported the absence of a DLC-induced haemolytic effect when compared to a medical-grade polystyrene control, and related the lower platelet degree of spreading to the hydrophobic nature of DLC surfaces (Jones *et al.*, 1999). The hydrophobic character of DLC coatings, as well as low surface energy and low surface roughness, were formerly defined by McLaughlin *et al.* as possible causes of DLC haemocompatibility (McLaughlin *et al.*, 1996).

In a comprehensive work, Nurdin *et al.* (2003) evaluated the haemocompatibility of DLC and SiC films deposited by the PECVD technique through the analysis of coagulation, platelets and complement activation. The authors demonstrated that clotting was delayed on DLC surfaces, and complement convertases adsorbed on DLC surfaces were inactive as a result. Moreover, DLC-coated materials presented strongly reduced platelet adhesion and activation, while generally showing good *in vitro* blood compatibility when compared to other materials like PMMA, LDPE, PDMS and medical steel. According to Nurdin and co-authors, the chemically inert nature and smoothness of the DLC coating appears to control protein adsorption and blood compatibility (Nurdin *et al.*, 2003).

Haemolysis has also been tested as one of the factors concurring to DLC blood compatibility. A lower tendency to induce haemolysis was found in the case of DLC films with respect to LTI-carbon (Yu *et al.*, 2000). This result, combined with low platelet density on ta-C films produced by FCVA deposition, was ascribed to material work function (Yu *et al.*, 2000).

It is reasonable to think that deposition techniques and parameters used for DLC film preparation can influence the surface physico-chemical properties, and, consequently, the biological response of the coatings belonging to the large DLC family. Among various parameters, sp^3 and sp^2 bonding fractions and hydrogen content may be important factors influencing the biological response of DLC films. Various authors have tried to investigate the dependence of blood compatibility on the intrinsic properties of DLC films, providing a set of variable results. In particular, the dependence of HSA/Fng protein adsorption and of platelet adhesion/activation on DLC structural and compositional properties has been studied. However, a univocal response has not been determined.

Better blood compatibility of a-C:H and ta-C films deposited by PIII (Chen *et al.*, 2002; Cheng and Zheng, 2006) or by PECVD (Huang *et al.*, 2004) has been reported at minimum I_D/I_G ratio in the Raman spectra, that is to say for films with lower sp^3 content (Leng *et al.*, 2003). Some authors have shown the opposite behaviour, claiming higher haemocompatibility for DLC films with higher sp^3/sp^2, as in the case of DLC deposited on NiTi alloys by PIII (Sui *et al.*, 2006) or in the case of magnetron sputtered DLC films (Logothetidis *et al.*, 2005). Lousinian *et al.* (Lousinian *et al.*, 2008) described a lower possibility of thrombus formation for a-C:H films with 40–45% sp^3 content, whereas, according to Vinnichenko *et al.*, sp^3 content does not correlate to the amount of adsorbed albumin, but more likely to surface wetting properties (Vinnichenko *et al.*, 2004).

According to Logothetidis *et al.*, the higher HSA/Fng ratio was related to higher hydrogen content in the amorphous carbon film, as well as to positive bias of the substrate (Logothetidis *et al.*, 2005), resulting in better haemocompatibility for films with a higher polymeric component. The same authors, in a more recent work, performed a careful characterization and comparison of carbon based thin films (Logothetidis, 2007). a-C and a-C:H films were deposited by RF magnetron sputtering at room temperature, varying the substrate bias, whereas ta-C films were produced by FCVA deposition. In this study, the authors analyzed the dependence of deposition conditions and H content on the blood compatibility of DLC films, concluding that the haemocompatibility increased with sp^3 content on magnetron sputtered a-C films, even if a-C:H exhibited better haemocompatibility properties. On the whole, biased a-C:H films induced small values of HSA/Fng ratio as well as platelet spreading and aggregation. In contrast, a-C:H films grown under floating conditions presented round resting platelets and a higher albumin-to-fibrinogen ratio, demonstrating an overall higher blood compatibility.

Other DLC surface characteristics have been analyzed, such as wettability, surface energy, roughness and bias, in order to evaluate possible effects on blood compatibility. Hasebe studied the effects of surface roughness on platelets, demonstrating that platelet surface coverage on DLC and F-DLC was not affected by coating roughness at the nanoscale (Hasebe *et al.*, 2007). Deposition conditions have also been analyzed, generally showing that platelet activation increases with high bias and annealing temperature (Yang *et al.*, 2004; Karagkiozaki *et al.*, 2008).

Last but not least, the structure and composition of DLC coatings also appear to influence the inflammatory response. In fact, *in vitro* studies showed a different response to the attachment and viability of macrophages depending on film sp^3 fraction and hydrogen content. In general, DLC coatings showed the ability to suppress the inflammatory response, generating lower monocyte/macrophage attachment in relation to uncoated Si surfaces (Ma *et al.*, 2007), as well as presenting reduced hydrogen peroxide production compared to stainless steel, thermanox and polyurethane-coated stainless steel (Ball *et al.*, 2004). Ma *et al.* tested different types of DLC films. Besides having a low HSA/Fng ratio, a-C:H with the highest H content, lower sp^3 fraction, lowest surface roughness and surface energy revealed a lower propensity towards macrophage adhesion and viability (Ma *et al.*, 2007).

In general, some dominant trends guiding DLC haemocompatibility have been identified. But the description of material blood compatibility is highly complex as many factors concur to determine the behaviour of a material. Moreover, the various interlinked aspects related to blood compatibility, including platelet activation, protein adsorption and coagulation and leucocyte activation, have to be considered.

As a general rule, good blood compatibility properties can be claimed for DLC films. However, specific materials must be tested on a case-by-case basis, as deposition techniques and parameters used, as well as source material and possible surface treatments, could significantly affect the final haemocompatibility of the films.

4.5 Modified DLC films

Since the early 1990s, DLC coatings have become increasingly attractive to both industry and the scientific community. In the meantime, novel types of DLC films have been formulated in an attempt to improve the properties of these promising materials and to widen their fields of application, tailoring DLCs to produce specific responses and to meet specific requirements.

Recently, several new carbon-based films have been synthesized and tested, including hydrogenated or non-hydrogenated forms of DLC films doped with nitrogen, silicon, phosphorous, fluorine, calcium, boron, as well as metal ions such as tungsten, chromium or titanium. Such modifications have been introduced to modulate the mechanical, tribological, electrical and biological properties of films. As an example, N, Si or metal incorporation has been introduced to reduce the typically high internal compressive stresses of DLCs, whereas F or Si–O have been used to decrease surface energy and friction coefficients. The doped DLC films are deposited by the same techniques as carbon films (see Section 4.3), adding the doping-carrier species to the deposition environment (Grill, 1999). Other types of surface modification, such as gas plasma treatments, infrared or ultraviolet irradiation by nanosecond laser, have also been used to change the surface properties of DLC films (Mochizuki *et al.*, 2011; Grigonis *et al.*, 2011).

Systematic studies have been carried out to characterize the new modified DLC coatings, providing detailed information about their chemistry, mechanical and tribological properties, as well as bio- and blood-compatibility (Table 4.5). The effects of fluorine doping on DLC properties have been investigated, showing reduced film surface energy and Young's modulus, as well as increased flexibility.

Table 4.5 Blood compatibility of modified DLC films discussed for different deposition techniques and physico-chemical characteristics in comparison with DLC and different control materials

Material	Deposition technique	Main properties	Control materials	Blood compatibility with respect to control materials	References
a-C:N	PIII-D	Graphitization induced degradation of the wettability properties	a-C LTIC	The amount of N is critical to the haemocompatibility of the materials The blood compatibility of hydrogen-free a-C films is better than that of LTIC and it can be further improved by the addition of nitrogen	Kwok *et al.*, 2004
F-DLC	RF-PECVD	Contact angle: Si < DLC < F-DLC	DLC Si	Low platelet adhesion and activation: F-DLC < DLC < Si	Saito *et al.*, 2005
Ca-DLC CaP-DLC P-DLC	PIII-D	Contact angle: P-DLC< CaP-DLC<LTIC<Ca-DLC	LTIC	P-DLC and Ca-DLC exhibited lower platelet adhesion and activation P-DLC and Ca-DLC high interfacial energy seems to inhibit albumin adhesion and cause Fng conformational changes	Kwok *et al.*, 2006
F-DLC	RF-PECVD	Contact angle: SUS316L <DLC<F-DLC	DLC SUS316L PC	F-DLC low thrombogenicity *in vitro* Absence of inflammatory response HSA/Fng ratio: PC < DLC < F-DLC Reduction of platelet activation and coagulation biomarkers Greater suppression of platelet adhesion and activation with increasing F doping in the F-DLC films	Hasebe *et al.*, 2006 Hasebe *et al.*, 2007
a-C(Si)	Magnetron sputtering	Si doping decreases the fraction of sp^2 carbon bonds	a-C	The number of adherent platelets diminished with increasing Si concentration	Ong *et al.*, 2007

ta-C:P	FCVA	Contact angle: ta-C:P < ta-C γ_S: ta-C < ta-C:P γ^p_S/γ^d_S: ta-C < ta-C:P	ta-C	Low platelet adhesion and activation Phosphorus incorporation improved the wettability and blood compatibility of ta-C film	Liu *et al.*, 2008
Plasma-treated (CF_4, N_2, O_2) Si-DLC	RF-PECVD	Contact angle: Si-DLC(O_2) < Si ≤ Si-DLC(N_2) < Si-DLC < Si-DLC(CF_4)	Si NiTi	Improved haemocompatibility (protein adsorption, activated partial thromboplastin time, platelet adhesion) of N_2- or O_2-plasma treated surfaces	Roy *et al.*, 2009
F-DLC	RF-PECVD	C-F bonds increased with increasing CF_4/CH_4	DLC PTFE	Adsorbed BSA decreased with increasing CF_4 ratio Fng and γ-globulin adsorption increased with the CF_4 ratio	Ozeki *et al.*, 2010

Note: FCVA: filtered cathodic vacuum arc; PIII-D: plasma immersion ion implantation and deposition; RF-PECVD: radio frequency plasma enhanced chemical vapour deposition; LTIC: low temperature isotropic carbon; NiTi: nickel-titanium; PC: polycarbonate; PTFE: polytetrafluoroethylene; Si: silicon; BSA: bovine serum albumin; Fng: fibrinogen; HSA: human serum albumin.

These characteristics permit significant improvements to the films as candidate coatings for biomedical devices. Saito *et al.* demonstrated improved antithrombogenicity of F-DLC in relation to DLC films showing significantly lower platelet adhesion and activation compared to more hydrophilic silicon substrata (Saito *et al.*, 2005).

Hasebe *et al.* compared the properties of fluorinated and conventional DLC films prepared by RF-CVD. They demonstrated that the more hydrophobic F-DLC surface was less thrombogenic if compared to conventional DLC or stainless steel (SUS316L) (Hasebe *et al.*, 2006a). A higher HSA/Fng adsorption ratio was observed on F-DLC in comparison to DLC and polycarbonate films, while the increase of F doping in the F-DLC films induced greater suppression of platelet adhesion and activation (Hasebe *et al.*, 2007).

In the work of Ozeki *et al.*, F-DLC coatings have been deposited on polytetrafluoroetilene (PTFE) using RF plasma enhanced CVD (Ozeki *et al.*, 2010). In contrast to other authors, Ozeki and colleagues showed that the amount of adsorbed albumin on the F-DLC films decreased with increasing F/C ratio, whereas the amount of adsorbed fibrinogen and γ-globulin increased. From these results the authors hypothesized that the non-doped films had higher antithrombogenicity with respect to the fluorinated carbon coatings.

Phosphorus incorporation was shown to improve the wettability and blood compatibility of tetrahedral amorphous carbon films (Liu *et al.*, 2008). Kwok *et al.* analyzed calcium and phosphorous-doped a-C:H films synthesized by PIII, assessing that both P-DLC and Ca-DLC films presented a smaller number of adhered and unactivated platelets in relation to LTIC, whereas, in contrast, a higher number of platelets was found on DLC doped with a combination of Ca and P (Kwok *et al.*, 2005; Kwok *et al.*, 2006). The same authors demonstrated that the amount of nitrogen is critical for the haemocompatibility of N-DLC films (Kwok *et al.*, 2004). Comparing a-C:N with varying nitrogen content, they showed variable adhesion and activation of platelets, depending on the fraction of sp^2 bonding. Other *in vitro* tests on nitrogen-doped hydrogenated amorphous carbon (a-C:H:N) films fabricated by PIII showed no cytotoxicity on human micro-vascular endothelial cells (HMEC), and better antithrombotic properties with respect to a-C:H films (Yang *et al.*, 2006).

Silicon incorporation in amorphous carbon coatings has been performed by various authors (Okpalugo *et al.*, 2004; Ong *et al.*, 2007; Roy *et al.*, 2009). Okpalugo *et al.* showed that a modification of microstructure, surface energy and electron conduction was induced by Si incorporation in DLC films (Okpalugo *et al.*, 2004). A lower level of platelet aggregation on Si-doped a-C:H synthesized by PE-CVD was revealed when compared to undoped DLC.

A recent study investigated the haemocompatibility of Si-incorporated DLC films, surface-modified by gas plasma treatments (O_2, N_2 and CF_4). The authors demonstrated that plasma treatments mostly affected the polar component of surface energy, and argued that the negatively charged polarity induced on Si-DLC by N_2 and O_2 plasma treatments improved the haemocompatibility of the films, suppressing fibrinogen adsorption and platelet adhesion (Roy *et al.*, 2009). Similarly, the decrease of platelet adhesion with Si concentration onto Si-DLC films was reported as a consequence of decreased sp^2 carbon bonding fraction, and of an increased polar component of the surface energy (Ong *et al.*, 2007).

DLC films treated by different gas plasmas (O_2, Ar, C_2H_2 and NH_3) under either low- or high-vacuum conditions showed excellent compatibility with blood platelets (low adhesion) regardless of the gas plasma used in comparison to polyethylene terephthalate (PET), stainless steel or untreated DLC (Mochizuki *et al.*, 2011). The films treated with ammonia plasma showed better performance with regard to the generation of thrombin-antithrombin complex (TAT) and kallikrein-like plasma activity. Alternatively, the surfaces treated with oxygen plasma presented higher surface concentration of carboxyl groups and activated the coagulation system via the intrinsic pathway.

Besides improved haemocompatibility, some modified DLC films presented promising antifouling properties and showed a significant inhibition of bacterial adhesion, as in the case of Si, N or F-doped DLC coatings (Shao *et al.*, 2010; Zhao *et al.*, 2009; Su *et al.*, 2010).

The work of Choi *et al.* showed that modifications at different levels are introduced by the incorporation of Ag into DLC films, suggesting possible use of Ag-DLCs for biomedical applications to exploit Ag antibacterial properties. The same authors showed changes of microstructure (increase of sp^2 C bonds in the amorphous carbon) and wetting, gradual decrease of surface energy, and an intensification of the HSA/Fng protein adsorption ratio with increasing Ag concentration (from 0.1 to 9.7 at.%) (Choi *et al.*, 2008).

4.6 Biomedical applications of DLC coatings

A high percentage of the implants and medical devices currently used in clinical practice exhibit specific characteristics and advanced qualities. In the development of these highly demanding medical products, scientists and medical engineers must consider numerous parameters that can concur to ensure the success or failure of the device. The use of materials for applications in the human body must, in fact, take into account various aspects, such as the suitability of mechanical, tribological and chemical properties of the materials with respect to their specific application, as well as their biocompatibility (Ruckenstein and Gourisankar, 1986).

In particular, surface properties are very important as biomaterials cross-talk with the surrounding biological environment through their surface. Biomaterials interact with different tissues and organs in the living organism, coming into contact with body fluids containing ions, proteins and other biomolecules, as well as with cells from different tissues. The performance and fate of a medical device are highly dependent on its interaction with the specific biological environment it is intended to work in. Various adverse events can cause the failure of medical implants, including mechanical failure (wear, tear, cracking or fatigue), degradation, corrosion or oxidation. Other possible problems could include thrombosis, infection, formation of a fibrotic capsule, release of debris and sensitization reactions.

Surface modification of biomaterials can appropriately contribute to the limitation of such adverse events and significantly improve the performance and probability of success of numerous implants and medical devices.

Due to their singular properties, DLC coatings are exploited in a wide range of highly demanding biomedical applications (Fig. 4.4), for example where high hardness, low friction, or resistance to wear and corrosion are required. One of the advantages of DLCs is that they can be deposited at low temperature, thus allowing the coating of heat-sensitive and insulating materials. DLCs are applied to metallic (stainless steel, Al, Co-Cr, NiTi or Ti-6Al-4V alloys), polymeric (PET, PTFE, silicone, polyurethanes) or ceramic materials for medical devices. Amorphous carbon films are often used to protect implants against bio-deterioration and corrosion, and to serve as diffusion barriers, significantly decreasing the probability of toxic element release (Ni, Cr, V, Co, for example) or wear particulate into the tissues (Santavirta, 2003). In addition, coatings can reduce the effects of body fluids on implants, protecting them from corrosion and potential structural failure (Sheeja *et al.*, 2001; Tiainen, 2001).

DLC are exploited to coat orthopaedic prostheses for total joint replacement, such as hip (both femoral heads and/or acetabular cups), knee and shoulder, as well as transcutaneous prostheses and orthopaedic screws. Because of their

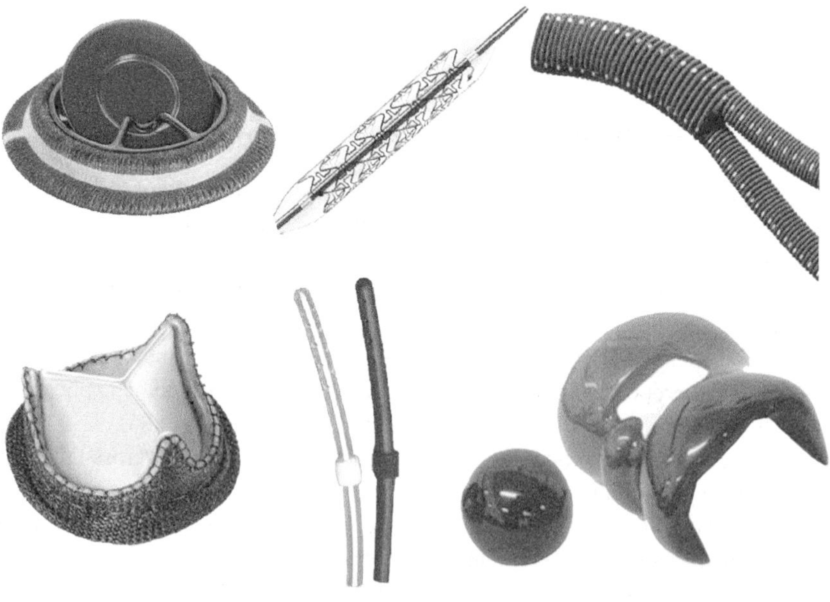

4.4 DLC-coated implants and medical devices.

ultralow roughness and chemical resistance to saliva, carbon coatings are also used for dental prostheses and orthodontic NiTi wires, showing limited Ni ion release and low bacterial biofilm adhesion (Kobayashi *et al.*, 2005).

The deposition of DLC coatings on cutting tools was reported to improve performance and energy efficiency (Zolgharni *et al.*, 2008). DLCs are also used on surgical instruments where, alongside biocompatibility, criteria such as functional performance, sterility and cleanability, structural integrity and fatigue resistance must be satisfied (for example in arthroscopic instrumentation and scissors). They can be employed in devices for urological dialysis, surgical needles for corneal surgery and in coating intraocular lenses. Their excellent smoothness and low friction make DLCs suitable candidates for coating urinary catheters. Moreover, their recognized antiadhesive properties can help decreasing the probability of microbial biofilm adhesion on catheter surfaces.

DLCs are particularly utilized in the case of cardiovascular devices. They have been employed for coating vascular prostheses, vascular stents and guidewires, heart valves, rotary blood pumps for ventricular assistance, artificial hearts and dialysis membranes.

The major requirements for materials used for cardiovascular applications are good surface mechanical properties and blood compatibility. DLCs can assure excellent mechanical and tribological properties, like wear and fatigue resistance (which are fundamental for high-demand implants such as heart valves), or smoothness and stability (required for vascular stents).

The main complication related to the use of cardiovascular devices is thrombosis, a crucial event that can consequently induce thromboembolism in the case of heart valves or occlusion and restenosis at the site of stent implantation. Both thromboembolism and thrombotic occlusion are related to platelet activation and aggregation on contact with the foreign surface of an implant. The use of carbon-based coatings has been adopted to decrease the risk of thrombosis, stenosis and thromboembolism.

Since the 1970s, pyrolytic carbon (PyC) has been used to improve the haemocompatibility of graphite occluders in mechanical heart valves (HV). The subsequent development, in the mid-1980s, of new deposition technologies allowed the coating of many different types of substrates with thin carbon films, overcoming intrinsic PyC manufacturing limits (such as process temperature). Because of their excellent structural characteristics, good biocompatibility and haemocompatibility, these carbon films were suitable for cardiovascular implantable devices. The use of low temperature deposition techniques encouraged the deposition on metallic and polymeric materials, and was then applied to stents (Fig. 4.5) and vascular prostheses, as well as to the polymeric fibres (PTFE, PET) of heart valve sewing rings.

As reported in the previous paragraphs, the blood compatibility of conventional and modified DLC films has been extensively demonstrated by *in vitro* tests. *In vivo* studies on DLC-coated implants are, in contrast, quite scarce. However, the research conducted so far has revealed no adverse reactions to DLC films.

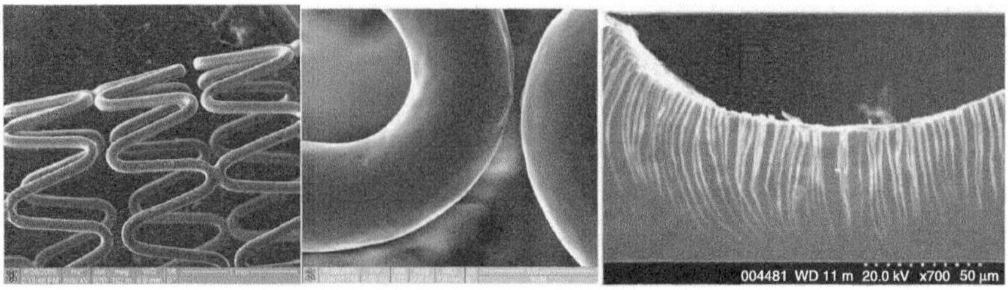

(a) (b) (c)

4.5 (a) DLC-coated stent, (b) smooth integral expanded film, (c) film microcracking. Elaborated from *Diamond and Related Materials*, 17(4c5), McLaughlin J A and Maguire P D, 'Advances on the use of carbon based materials at the biological and surface interface for applications in medical implants', pages 873–877. Copyright (2008), used with permission from Elsevier.

Tran *et al.* showed that DLC coating of mechanical heart valve components may render the surfaces of mechanical HV more thromboresistant in the vascular system, due to various effects, including surface cleaning of organic and inorganic debris, generation of reactive and functional groups, improved adhesion of endothelial cells and albumin, and decreased platelet adhesion (Tran *et al.*, 1999).

Carbofilm™-coated cylinders (Sorin Biomedica Cardio S.p.A.) implanted in the cubital bone of sheep were histologically evaluated at 3 and 12 months. Coated cylinders showed a better biological response (lower osteoclastic erosion and connective-tissue formation) in comparison to uncoated samples (Vallana *et al.*, 1993).

Thrombosis can be triggered by the activation of platelets as a consequence of shear stress, contact with foreign materials or release of metal ions. The effects of metallic stent coating by DLC were investigated by Gutensohn and colleagues (2000). During a thorough *in vitro* study the authors compared ion release and platelet activation on carbon-coated and stainless steel uncoated stents. The results of the study showed that coating intracoronary stents with DLC significantly reduced thrombogenicity. In particular, the release of metal ions (Cr, Ni, Mo and Mn) was significantly higher for stainless steel uncoated stents, and corresponded to a lower level of platelet activation in the case of DLC-coated stents. The authors thus concluded that DLC coatings improve the blood compatibility of vascular stents (Gutensohn *et al.*, 2000).

Analyzing the mechanical stability, corrosion resistance and bioresponse of DLC coatings for stents and guidewires, Maguire and colleagues showed that Si doping and use of an a-Si:H interlayer can help minimize the risk of adhesion failure or film cracking (Maguire *et al.*, 2005) (Fig. 4.6). Moreover, Si doping improved barrier properties (McLaughlin and Maguire, 2008) and reduced platelet adhesion, while increasing the attachment of human microvascular endothelial cells in comparison to undoped a-C.

Korkmaz and colleagues evaluated the consequences of stent carbon coating on inflammatory response, comparing carbon-coated and uncoated MAC stents (AMG®, Raesfeld-Erle, Germany) (Korkmaz *et al.*, 2002). They analyzed the plasma concentration of C-reactive protein (CRP), fibrinogen and several cytokines (TNF, IL-1b, IL-6, IL-8) as well as leukocyte counts. These showed no significant differences when compared to patients treated with carbon-coated or stainless steel uncoated stents. According to this study, coating stainless steel stents with carbon film does not affect the inflammatory response.

The biocompatibility of two diamond-like stent coatings (Dylyn, Bekaert, Belgium) was tested in a porcine coronary stent model, demonstrating that the films contributed to decrease thrombogenicity and neointimal hyperplasia (De Scheerder *et al.*, 2000).

Although the antithrombogenic properties of DLCs seem to be well established, some clinical trials report conflicting results for carbon-coated stent performance with regard to neointimal formation and in-stent restenosis. For example, in a study on 112 patients, Antoniucci *et al.* proved very low 6-month restenosis (11%) and reintervention (10%) rates with a Carbofilm™-coated stent (Sorin Biomedica Cardio, Saluggia, Italy) (Antoniucci *et al.*, 2000). With a randomized trial including 196 patients, Salahas and colleagues provided clinical evidence that DLC-coated

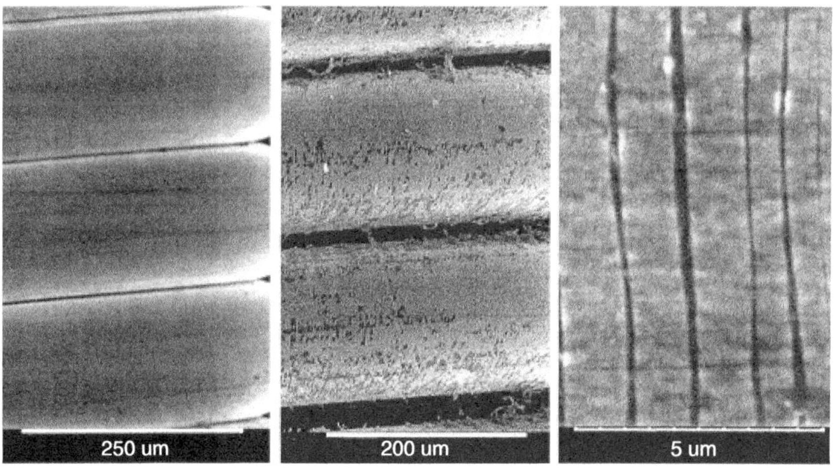

(a) (b) (c)

4.6 (a) Conformal DLC coating with minimal cracking after winding, (b) DLC-coated guidewire showing adhesion and cracking failure after winding, (c) transverse cracking of DLC after winding. Elaborated from *Diamond and Related Materials*, Vol 14, Issue 8, Maguire P D, McLaughlin J A, Okpalugo T I T, Lemoine P, Papakonstantinou P, McAdams E T, Needham M, Ogwu A A, Ball M and Abbas G A, 'Mechanical stability, corrosion performance and bioresponse of amorphous diamond-like carbon for medical stents and guidewires', Pages 1277–1288, Copyright (2005), used with permission from Elsevier.

stent implantation correlated with high success rates, safety and efficacy both in the hospital and six months after the interventional procedure (Salahas *et al.*, 2007). In contrast, other studies showed no significant improvements of DLC-coated versus uncoated stents as regards restenosis rate, major adverse cardiac events (Haase *et al.*, 2003; Airoldi *et al.*, 2004) or angiographic results (Sick *et al.*, 2004).

Thanks to their lubricating properties, DLC films are promising candidates for the coating of intravascular guidewires and catheters (Hasebe, *et al.*, 2006b). Good adherence, good friction coefficient and better haemocompatibility were reported in the case of DLC-coated stainless steel guidewires in relation to other coatings, such as PTFE (McLaughlin *et al.*, 1996). Moreover, it has been reported that DLC and heparin based coatings are the coatings most commonly used for ventricular assistance devices (VAD), owing to their elevated haemocompatibility, durability and technical maturity (Sin *et al.*, 2009).

Since its discovery, researchers have made great efforts to better understand DLC properties, as well as to evaluate and develop possible medical applications. The high number of patents involving DLC coatings is a testament to this intensive research (Table 4.6). At present, DLCs represent an important class of materials

Table 4.6 Some of the patents involving carbon coatings for medical applications

US patent #	Description	Authors	Original assegnee	Issue date
3952334	Biocompatible carbon prosthetic devices	Bokros J.C., Horsley J.B.	General Atomic Company	Apr 27, 1976
4537791	Carbon coating of grafts or catheters	Tarjan P.P.	Cordis Corporation	Aug 27, 1985
5370684	Prosthesis of polymeric material coated with biocompatible carbon	Vallana F. *et al.*	Sorin Biomedica S.p.A.	Dec 6, 1994
5387247	Prosthetic device having a biocompatible carbon film thereon and a method of and apparatus for forming such device	Vallana F., Arru P.	Sorin Biomedica S.p.A.	Feb 7, 1995
5423886	Cyclically deformable haemocompatible and biocompatible devices coated with biocompatible carbonaceous material	Arru P. *et al.*	Sorin Biomedica S.p.A.	Jun 13, 1995
5725573	Medical implants made of metal alloys bearing cohesive diamond like carbon coatings	Dearnaley G., Lankford, J.	Southwest Research Institute	Mar 10, 1998
6761736	Medical article with a diamond-like carbon coated polymer	Woo Y. *et al.*	St. Jude Medical, Inc.	Jul 13, 2004

with exceptionally attractive properties, which are already exploited for numerous biomedical products commercially available on the market, and hold the potential to be used in many more.

4.7 Conclusion and future trends

DLC films exhibit several exceptional characteristics, such as elevated hardness, low friction, high wear resistance and chemical inertness, making them particularly attractive for various high-demand applications in different fields.

Although DLC films have been developed relatively recently, the scientific literature about the blood compatibility of this class of materials is quite extensive. Several studies have investigated the degree of haemocompatibility of DLC films produced by different deposition techniques in different working conditions in relation to their specific structural and surface characteristics. *In vitro* and *in vivo* tests have been used to evaluate the feasibility of employing these materials in the biomedical field, finding in general a good response of DLCs in the blood environment.

Despite belonging to the same family, the large variety of materials and wide range of different properties they display means that it is not possible to generalize in describing the bioresponse of DLCs. Thus, each specific material must be considered and tested individually. Nevertheless, it is well established that, in general, this class of materials presents extraordinary properties with regard to their mechanical, tribological and chemical performances, as well as a superior blood compatibility in comparison to many other materials. For this reason, pure or doped DLC coatings represent ideal materials for coating prostheses components and medical devices in the cardiovascular, orthopaedic, ophthalmic and orthodontic fields.

One of the key issues that may limit the usefulness of DLCs in biomedical applications is the low degree of adhesion of this material to common biomedical alloys. This problem may be overcome in a number of ways, including reducing high internal stress by introducing doping elements in the DLC films.

Research should continue to further optimize DLC films, trying to improve critical aspects like interfacial adhesion, uniformity and integrity of DLC coatings on medical devices, especially in the case of complex geometric substrates.

4.8 References

Airoldi F, Colombo A, Tavano D, *et al.* (2004), 'Comparison of diamond-like carbon-coated stents versus uncoated stainless steel stents in coronary artery disease', *The American Journal of Cardiology*, 93(4), 474–477.

Aisenberg S and Chabot R (1971), 'Ion Beam Deposition of Thin Films of Diamondlike Carbon', *Journal of Applied Physics*, 42(7), 2953–2958.

Alanazi A, Nojiri C, Kido T, *et al.* (2000), 'Engineering analysis of diamond-like carbon coated polymeric materials for biomedical applications', *Artificial Organs*, 24(8), 624–627.

Anders A (2000), *Handbook of plasma immersion ion implantation and deposition* Anders A, New York/Chichester/Weinheim/Brisbane/Singapore/Toronto, John Wiley & Sons.

Andrade J and Hlady V (1987), 'Plasma Protein Adsorption: The Big Twelve', *Annals Of The New York Academy Of Sciences*, 516(1), 158–172.

Antoniucci D, Bartorelli A, Valenti R, *et al.* (2000), 'Clinical and angiographic outcome after coronary arterial stenting with the carbostent', *The American Journal of Cardiology*, 85(7), 821–5.

Arps J H and Dearnaley G (2004), 'Diamond and Diamond-Like Carbons', *Encyclopedia of Biomaterials and Biomedical Engineering*, 446–455.

Ball M, O'Brien A, Dolan F, *et al.* (2004), 'Macrophage responses to vascular stent coatings', *Journal of Biomedical Materials Research Part A*, 70A(3), 380–390.

Boehm R D, Jin C and Narayan R J (2011), 'Carbon and Diamond', in Ducheyne P, Healy K, Hutmacher D, Grainger D and Kirkpatrick C, *Comprehensive biomaterials*, Amsterdam, Oxford, Waltham, Elsevier Ltd., 115–119.

Casiraghi C, Robertson J and Ferrari A C (2007), 'Diamond-like carbon for data and beer storage', *Materials Today*, 10(1–2), 44–53.

Chen J Y, Wang L P, Fu K Y, *et al.* (2002), 'Blood compatibility and sp3/sp2 contents of diamond-like carbon (DLC) synthesized by plasma immersion ion implantation-deposition', *Surface and Coatings Technology*, 156, 289–294.

Cheng Y and Zheng Y F (2006), 'The corrosion behavior and hemocompatibility of TiNi alloys coated with DLC by plasma based ion implantation', *Surface and Coatings Technology*, 200(14–15), 4543–4548.

Chhowalla M, Robertson J, Chen C W, *et al.* (1997), 'Influence of ion energy and substrate temperature on the optical and electronic properties of tetrahedral amorphous carbon (ta-C) films', *Journal of Applied Physics*, 81(1), 139–145.

Cho N H, Veirs D K, Ager J W, *et al.* (1992), 'Effects of substrate temperature on chemical structure of amorphous carbon films', *Journal of Applied Physics*, 71(5), 2243.

Choi H, Dauskardt R, Lee S, *et al.* (2008), 'Characteristic of silver doped DLC films on surface properties and protein adsorption', *Diamond and Related Materials*, 17(3), 252–257.

Cui F and Li D (2000), 'A review of investigations on biocompatibility of diamond-like carbon and carbon nitride films', *Surface and Coatings Technology*, 131(1–3), 481–487.

Dearnaley G and Arps J (2005), 'Biomedical applications of diamond-like carbon (DLC) coatings: A review', *Surface and Coatings Technology*, 200(7), 2518–2524.

Dion I, Roques X, Baquey C, *et al.* (1993), 'Hemocompatibility of diamond-like carbon coating', *Biomedical Materials Engineering*, 3, 51–55.

Dongping L and Baoxiang C (2006), 'Structures of Diamond-Like Carbon Films', *Plasma Science and Technology*, 8(3), 285–291.

Donnet C and Erdemir A (2008), 'Diamond-like Carbon Films: A Historical Overview', in Donnet C and Erdemir A, *Tribology of diamond-like carbon films: fundamentals and applications*, New York, Springer.

Fedel M, Motta A, Maniglio D and Migliaresi C (2010), 'Carbon Coatings for Cardiovascular Applications: Physico-Chemical Properties and Blood Compatibility', *Journal of Biomaterials Applications*, 25, 57–74.

Fedel M, Motta A, Maniglio D and Migliaresi C (2009), 'Surface properties and blood compatibility of commercially available diamond-like carbon coatings for cardiovascular devices', *Journal of Biomedical Materials Research. Part B, Applied Biomaterials*, 90(1), 338–349.

Goodman S L, Tweden K S and Albrecht R M (1996), 'Platelet interaction with pyrolytic carbon heart-valve leaflets', *Journal of Biomedical Materials Research*, 32(2), 249–258.

Gorbet M B and Sefton M V (2004), 'Biomaterial-associated thrombosis: roles of coagulation factors, complement, platelets and leukocytes', *Biomaterials*, 25(26), 5681–703.

Gott V L and Furuse A (1973), 'The current status of in vivo screening of carbon for use in bioengineering', *Medical Instrumentation*, 7, 121–129.

Grigonis A, Marcinauskas L, Vinciunaite V and Raciukaitis G (2011), 'Modification of the amorphous carbon films by the ns-laser irradiation', *Central European Journal of Physics*, 9(5), 1344–1350.

Grill A (1999), 'Diamond-like carbon: state of the art', *Diamond and Related Materials*, 8 (July 1998), 428–434.

Grunkemeier J M, Tsai W B, McFarland C D and Horbett T A (2000), 'The effect of adsorbed fibrinogen, fibronectin, von Willebrand factor and vitronectin on the procoagulant state of adherent platelets', *Biomaterials*, 21(22), 2243–2252.

Gutensohn K, Beythien C, Bau J, *et al.* (2000), 'In vitro analyses of diamond-like carbon coated stents. Reduction of metal ion release, platelet activation, and thrombogenicity', *Thrombosis Research*, 99(6), 577–85.

Haase J, Storger H, Hofmann M, *et al.* (2003), 'Comparison of stainless steel stents coated with turbostratic carbon and uncoated stents for percutaneous coronary interventions', *The Journal of Invasive Cardiology*, 15(10), 562–565.

Hasebe T, Ishimaru T, Kamijo A, *et al.* (2007), 'Effects of surface roughness on anti-thrombogenicity of diamond-like carbon films', *Diamond and Related Materials*, 16(4–7), 1343–1348.

Hasebe T, Matsuoka Y., Kodama H, *et al.* (2006a), 'Lubrication performance of diamond-like carbon and fluorinated diamond-like carbon coatings for intravascular guidewires', *Diamond and Related Materials*, 15(1), 129–132.

Hasebe T, Shimada A, Suzuki Tetsuya, *et al.* (2006b), 'Fluorinated diamond-like carbon as antithrombogenic coating for blood-contacting devices', *Journal of Biomedical Materials Research. Part A*, 76(1), 86–94.

Huang N, Yang P, Leng YX, *et al.* (2004), 'Surface Modification for Controlling the Blood-Materials Interface', *Key Engineering Materials*, 288–289, 295–298.

Jones M I, McColl I R, Grant D M, *et al.* (1999), 'Haemocompatibility of DLC and TiC–TiN interlayers on titanium', *Diamond and Related Materials*, 8(2–5), 457–462.

Jones M I, McColl I R, Grant D M, *et al.* (2000), 'Protein adsorption and platelet attachment and activation, on TiN, TiC, and DLC coatings on titanium for cardiovascular applications', *Journal of Biomedical Materials Research*, 52(2), 413–421.

Karagkiozaki V, Logothetidis S, Laskarakis A, *et al.* (2008), 'AFM study of the thrombogenicity of carbon-based coatings for cardiovascular applications', *Materials Science and Engineering: B*, 152(1–3), 16–21.

Kobayashi S, Ohgoe Y, Ozeki K, *et al.* (2005), 'Diamond-like carbon coatings on orthodontic archwires', *Diamond and Related Materials*, 14(3–7), 1094–1097.

Koidl P, Wild C, Dischler B, *et al.* (1990), 'Plasma deposition, properties and structure of amorphous hydrogenated carbon films', *Materials Science Forum*, 52–53, 41–70.

Korkmaz M E, Tayfun E, Muderrisoglu H, *et al.* (2002), 'Carbon Coating of Stents Has No Effect on Inflammatory Response to Primary Stent Deployment', *Angiology*, 53(5), 563–568.

Krishnan L K, Varghese N, Muraleedharan C V, *et al.* (2002), 'Quantitation of platelet adhesion to Ti and DLC-coated Ti in vitro using (125)I-labeled platelets', *Biomolecular Engineering*, 19(2–6), 251–253.

Kwok S C H, Ha P C T, McKenzie D R, *et al.* (2006), 'Biocompatibility of calcium and phosphorus doped diamond-like carbon thin films synthesized by plasma immersion ion implantation and deposition', *Diamond and Related Materials*, 15(4–8), 893–897.

Kwok S C H, Yang P, Wang J, *et al.* (2004), 'Hemocompatibility of nitrogen-doped, hydrogen-free diamond-like carbon prepared by nitrogen plasma immersion ion implantation-deposition', *Journal of Biomedical Materials Research. Part A*, 70(1), 107–114.

Kwok S, Wang J and Chu P (2005), 'Surface energy, wettability, and blood compatibility phosphorus doped diamond-like carbon films', *Diamond and Related Materials*, 14(1), 78–85.

Lackner J M and Waldhauser W (2010), 'Diamond and Diamond-like Carbon Coated Surfaces as Biomaterials', *BHM*, 155(11), 528–533.

Leng YX, Chen JY, Yang P, *et al.* (2003), 'Mechanical properties and platelet adhesion behavior of diamond-like carbon films synthesized by pulsed vacuum arc plasma deposition', *Surface Science*, 531(2), 177–184.

Lifshitz Y (1999), 'Diamond-like carbon – present status', *Diamond and Related Materials*, 8, 1659–1676.

Linder S, Pinkowski W and Aepfelbacher M (2002), 'Adhesion, cytoskeletal architecture and activation status of primary human macrophages on a diamond-like carbon coated surface', *Biomaterials*, 23(3), 767–773.

Liu Aiping, Zhu J, Liu M, *et al.* (2008), 'Platelet adhesion on phosphorus-incorporated tetrahedral amorphous carbon films', *Applied Surface Science*, 255(2), 279–281.

Logothetidis S (2007), 'Haemocompatibility of carbon based thin films', *Diamond and Related Materials*, 16(10), 1847–1857.

Logothetidis S, Gioti M, Lousinian S and Fotiadou S (2005), 'Haemocompatibility studies on carbon-based thin films by ellipsometry', *Thin Solid Films*, 482(1–2), 126–132.

Lousinian S, Kalfagiannis N and Logothetidis S (2008), 'Albumin and fibrinogen adsorption on boron nitride and carbon-based thin films', *Materials Science and Engineering: B*, 152(1–3), 12–15.

Ma W J, Ruys A J, Mason R S, *et al.* (2007), 'DLC coatings: effects of physical and chemical properties on biological response', *Biomaterials*, 28(9), 1620–1628.

Maguire P D, McLaughlin J A, Okpalugo T I T, *et al.* (2005), 'Mechanical stability, corrosion performance and bioresponse of amorphous diamond-like carbon for medical stents and guidewires', *Diamond and Related Materials*, 14(8), 1277–1288.

McLaughlin JA, Meenan B, Maguire P and Jamieson N (1996), 'Properties of diamond like carbon thin film coatings on stainless steel medical guidewires', *Diamond and Related Materials*, 5, 486–491.

McLaughlin JA and Maguire PD (2008), 'Advances on the use of carbon based materials at the biological and surface interface for applications in medical implants', *Diamond and Related Materials*, 17(4–5), 873–877.

Mochizuki A, Ogawa T, Okamoto K, *et al.* (2011), 'Blood compatibility of gas plasma-treated diamond-like carbon surface—Effect of physicochemical properties of DLC surface on blood compatibility', *Materials Science and Engineering: C*, 31(3), 567–573.

More R B, Sines G, Ma L and Bokros J C (2004), 'Pyrolytic Carbon', *Encyclopedia of Biomaterials and Biomedical Engineering*, 1308–1319.

Nurdin N, François P, Mugnier Y, *et al.* (2003), 'Haemocompatibility evaluation of DLC- and SiC-coated surfaces', *European Cells Materials*, 5(6328), 17–26; discussion 26–28.

Okpalugo TIT, Ogwu AA, Maguire PD and McLaughlin JAD (2004), 'Platelet adhesion on silicon modified hydrogenated amorphous carbon films', *Biomaterials*, 25(2), 239–245.

Ong S-E, Zhang S, Du H, *et al.* (2007), 'Influence of silicon concentration on the haemocompatibility of amorphous carbon', *Biomaterials*, 28(28), 4033–4038.

Ozeki K, Nagashima I, Hirakuri K K and Masuzawa T (2010), 'Adsorptive properties of albumin, fibrinogen, and gamma-globulin on fluorinated diamond-like carbon films coated on PTFE', *Journal of Materials Science. Materials in Medicine*, 21(5), 1641–1648.

Robertson J (2002), 'Diamond-like amorphous carbon', *Materials Science and Engineering: R: Reports*, 37(4–6), 129–281.

Roy R K, Choi H W, Yi J W, *et al.* (2009), 'Hemocompatibility of surface-modified, silicon-incorporated, diamond-like carbon films', *Acta Biomaterialia*, 5(1), 249–256.

Roy RK and Lee K-R (2007), 'Biomedical Applications of Diamond-Like Carbon Coatings: A Review', *Journal of Biomedical Materials Research Part B: Appl Biomater*, 83B, 72–84.

Ruckenstein E and Gourisankar S V (1986), 'Preparation and characterization of thin film surface coatings for biological environments', *Biomaterials*, 7(6), 403–422.

Saito T, Hasebe T, Yohena S, *et al.* (2005), 'Antithrombogenicity of fluorinated diamond-like carbon films', *Diamond and Related Materials*, 14(3–7), 1116–1119.

Salahas A, Vrahatis A, Karabinos I, *et al.* (2007), 'Success, safety, and efficacy of implantation of diamond-like carbon-coated stents', *Angiology*, 58(2), 203–210.

Santavirta S (2003), 'Compatibility of the totally replaced hip – Reduction of wear by amorphous diamond coating', *Acta Orthopaedica Scandinavica Supplementum*, 74(310), 1–19.

De Scheerder I, Szilard M, Yanming H, *et al.* (2000), 'Evaluation of the biocompatibility of two new diamond-like stent coatings (Dylyn) in a porcine coronary stent model', *Journal of Invasive Cardiology*, 12(8), 389–394.

Shao W, Zhao Q, Abel E W and Bendavid A (2010), 'Influence of interaction energy between Si-doped diamond-like carbon films and bacteria on bacterial adhesion under flow conditions', *Journal of Biomedical Materials Research. Part A*, 93(1), 133–139.

Sheeja D, Tay B K, Lau S P and Nung L N (2001), 'Tribological characterisation of diamond-like carbon coatings on Co–Cr–Mo alloy for orthopaedic applications', *Surface and Coatings Technology*, 146–147(0), 410–416.

Sick P B, Gelbrich G, Kalnins U, *et al.* (2004), 'Comparison of early and late results of a Carbofilm-coated stent versus a pure high-grade stainless steel stent (the Carbostent-Trial)', *The American Journal of Cardiology*, 93(11), 1351–1356, A5.

Sin D-C, Kei H-L and Miao X (2009), 'Surface coatings for ventricular assist devices', *Expert Review of Medical Devices*, 6(1), 51–60.

Su X J, Zhao Q, Wang S and Bendavid A (2010), 'Modification of diamond-like carbon coatings with fluorine to reduce biofouling adhesion', *Surface and Coatings Technology*, 204(15), 2454–2458.

Sui J, Cai W, Liu Ailian, *et al.* (2006), 'Surface characterization and blood compatibility of diamond-like carbon (DLC) films on the NiTi alloys', *Materials Transactions*, 47(3), 691–693.

Tiainen V (2001), 'Amorphous carbon as a bio-mechanical coating – mechanical properties and biological applications', *Diamond and Related Materials*, 10, 153–160.

Tran H S, Puc M M, Hewitt C W, *et al.* (1999), 'Diamond-Like Carbon Coating and Plasma or Glow Discharge Treatment of Mechanical Heart Valves', *Journal of Investigative Surgery*, 12(3), 133–140.

Vallana F, Pasquino E, Rinaldi S, *et al.* (1993), 'Carbofilm™: Present and future applications in biomedical devices', *Ceramics International*, 19(3), 169–179.

Vinnichenko M, Gago R, Huang N, *et al.* (2004), 'Spectroscopic ellipsometry investigation of amorphous carbon films with different sp3 content: relation with protein adsorption', *Thin Solid Films*, 455–456, 530–534.

Wu Y, Simonovsky F I, Ratner B D and Horbett Thomas A (2005), 'The role of adsorbed fibrinogen in platelet adhesion to polyurethane surfaces: A comparison of surface hydrophobicity, protein adsorption, monoclonal antibody binding, and platelet adhesion', *Journal of Biomedical Materials Research Part A*, 74A(4), 722–738.

Yang P, Chen JY, Leng YX, *et al.* (2004), 'Effect of annealing on structure and biomedical properties of amorphous hydrogenated carbon films', *Surface and Coatings Technology*, 186(1–2), 125–130.

Yang P, Huang N, Leng YX, *et al.* (2006), 'Wettability and biocompatibility of nitrogen-doped hydrogenated amorphous carbon films: Effect of nitrogen', *Nuclear Instruments and Methods in Physics Research Section B*, 242(1–2), 22–25.

Young B, Lambrecht L, Cooper S and Mosher D (1982), 'Biomaterials, interfacial phenomena and applications', in Cooper SL and Peppas NA, *Biomaterials, interfacial phenomena and applications*, Washington DC, ACS, 317.

Yu L, Wang X, Wang X and Liu X (2000), 'Haemocompatibility of tetrahedral amorphous carbon films', *Surface and Coatings Technology*, 128–129, 484–488.

Zhao Q, Su X, Wang S, *et al.* (2009), 'Bacterial attachment and removal properties of silicon- and nitrogen-doped diamond-like carbon coatings', *Biofouling*, 25(5), 377–385.

Zolgharni M, Jones B J, Bulpett R, *et al.* (2008), 'Energy efficiency improvements in dry drilling with optimised diamond-like carbon coatings', *Diamond and Related Materials*, 17(7–10), 1733–1737.

Part II

Biomedical applications of diamond-based materials

5

Nanostructured diamond coatings for orthopaedic applications

S.A. CATLEDGE, V. THOMAS and Y.K. VOHRA,
University of Alabama at Birmingham, USA

DOI: 10.1533/9780857093516.2.105

Abstract: With increasing numbers of orthopaedic devices being implanted, greater emphasis is being placed on ceramic coating technology to reduce friction and wear in mating total joint replacement components, in order to improve implant function and increase device lifespan. In this chapter, we consider ultra-hard carbon coatings, with emphasis on nanostructured diamond, as alternative bearing surfaces for metallic components. Such coatings have great potential for use in biomedical implants as a result of their extreme hardness, wear resistance, low friction and biocompatibility. These ultra-hard carbon coatings can be deposited by several techniques resulting in a wide variety of structures and properties.

Key words: orthopaedic implant, nanostructured diamond coating, ultra-hard carbon, wear, biocompatibility.

5.1 Introduction

Orthopaedic surgery or orthopaedics is the branch of surgery concerned with conditions involving the musculoskeletal system. Orthopaedic surgeons use both surgical and non-surgical means to treat musculoskeletal trauma, sports injuries, degenerative diseases, infections, tumours and congenital disorders. Modern total hip replacement was pioneered by Sir John Charnley in the 1960s (Wroblewski, 2002). He found that joint surfaces could be replaced by metal or high density polyethylene implants cemented to the bone with methyl methacrylate bone cement. Since Charnley, there have been many improvements in the design of joint replacement (arthroplasty), including the development of uncemented arthroplasty techniques with the bone bonding directly to the implant. Recently, surface replacement of joints, especially the hip joint, has become more popular in younger and more active patients. This type of operation delays the need for the more traditional and less bone-conserving total hip replacement, but carries significant risks of early failure from fracture and bone death.

Despite all the innovations made with joint replacements over the years, wear of the bearing surfaces of components remains a substantial problem. Wear can lead to damage to surrounding bone and contribute to eventual failure of the implant. Use of alternative bearing surfaces has increased in recent years in an attempt to minimize wear debris of joint replacement components. These include ceramics and all-metal implants (as opposed to the more common metal-on-polyethylene). The polyethylene is traditionally of ultra-high molecular weight and can be modified in ways that may improve wear characteristics. Motivated by the extreme hardness of diamond and other ultra-hard carbon materials and the need for reducing wear in articulating implant devices, alternative bearing surfaces are actively being investigated. These technologies must undergo critical assessment in terms of their viability as being robust and more effective than the current state-of-the-art.

5.1.1 Limitations of current orthopaedic implant designs

Statistics from the American Academy of Orthopaedic Surgeons show that more than 418,000 total and partial knee replacements are performed each year, 15% of them on baby boomers; of the 328,000 total and partial hip replacements done, boomers are the recipients of more than 20%. According to a study presented at the 73rd annual meeting of the American Academy of Orthopaedic Surgery in Chicago (Kurtz *et al.*, 2006), the number of total knee replacements and total hip replacements performed in the USA will leap by 673% and 174%, respectively, by the year 2030. The new projections suggest that the number of revision surgeries will double by 2015 for total knee replacements, and that hip replacement revisions will double by 2026. Other joints, such as shoulders, elbows and temporomandibular joints are also routinely replaced. Despite improvements in surgical technique and in the designs of prostheses, revision rates do not seem to be declining over time. Revision surgery is much more complex a surgical procedure then the primary joint replacement. It is a longer, more complicated, technically demanding surgery, where optimal positioning and fixation of the prosthesis is a real challenge. With revision joint replacement surgery, the recovery is also longer, with more of a toll on the patient, and even a higher complication rate.

The apparent critical need to reduce the number of revision surgeries motivates a firm understanding of what causes initial implants to fail over time. A primary cause of failure is the generation of wear debris particles at the articulating surface that causes local pain and inflammation. Wear of articulating surfaces involving Co-Cr-Mo alloy-on-polyethylene (used in the majority of hip and knee arthroplasties) has been cited as a dominant factor limiting the long-term success of the implant (Amstutz *et al.*, 1992, Goldring *et al.*, 1983). An ongoing concern in conventional total joint replacement prostheses is osteolysis and aseptic loosening induced by wear debris originating from the interfaces of articulating components. Wear can lead to component loosening, deleterious biological responses, osteolysis (bone loss), mechanical instability, decreased joint mobility, increased pain and, ultimately, implant failure (Mercuri, 2000a). Large debris pieces are normally sequestered by fibrous tissue, whereas small debris is taken up by macrophages and multinucleated giant cells which may release cytokines that result in inflammation. This inflammation cascade damages surrounding bone, ultimately resulting in osteolysis. The inflammatory response also leads to the recruitment of activated osteoclasts at the bone–implant interface. This tissue death around the implant can eventually result in loosening and implant failure. One solution for this problem of osteolysis caused by wear debris is to develop harder materials for the articulating surfaces that are more wear resistant, which would reduce the number and size of debris particles generated. In early total joint arthroplasty systems, metal-on-metal articulating materials were selected. Cast cobalt alloy metal-on-metal components were used for temporomandibular arthroplasty and exhibited resistance to fretting and wear. Orthopaedic research (Amstutz and Grigoris, 1996, McKellop *et al.*, 1996, Medley *et al.*, 1996) has revealed that much less wear occurs with metal-on-metal hip prosthesis, up to 100 times less than that of polyethylene-on-metal. Unfortunately, there continue to be concerns associated with metal sensitivity and metallosis, the release of alloy constituents into the surrounding tissue. The term 'metallosis' has also been used to describe the intraoperative findings of gross metallic debris and blackening of periprosthetic tissue (McGovern and Moskal, 2002). Metal sensitivity, which affects approximately 10–15% of the general population, is much higher among patients with failed implants (Wagner and Wagner, 2000, Hallab *et al.*, 2001, Moran and Tourret, 2001).

The Food and Drug Administration (FDA) has acknowledged that recent data from orthopedic implant registries as well as peer-reviewed journal publications and presentations at scientific meetings suggests increases in potential safety issues associated with Metal-on-Metal (MoM) hip systems (FDA Gaithersburg, 2012). These safety issues include: (1) Local complications such as pseudotumors and aseptic lymphocytic vasculitis-associated lesions, (2) Early device failure and the need for revision surgery; and (3) Systemic complications from metal ion exposure. In addition, there have been recent concerns that the mechanical demands at the modular MoM total hip femoral junctions lead to enhanced wear and mechanically assisted corrosion at the head/stem junction (Fricka *et al.*, 2012). The MoM bearings include Total Hip Replacement (THR) systems that have been available in the United States (US) for decades, as well as MoM hip resurfacing devices that have been available in the US since 2006.

In 2011, the FDA received 12,137 adverse event reports associated with metal hip implants, compared with 6,332 associated with other types of hip implants, such as ceramic and plastic (Bloomberg, 2012). The DePuy ASR hip implants accounted for 74 percent of the incident reports received by the FDA. Emerging data on MoM hip systems have resulted in several actions by regulatory bodies across the world, including in the U.S. In May 2011, FDA issued orders for postmarket surveillance studies to each manufacturer of MoM THR systems requiring them to submit a study protocol to the FDA that addresses specific safety issues related to these devices. In the United Kingdom, the Medicines and Healthcare products and Regulatory Agency declared in February 2012 that patients with symptoms should have annual follow-up care for the rest of their lives rather than for five years. Also recommended were blood tests for metal levels and imaging tests of the joint and surrounding tissues. In a recent FDA Orthopedic and Rehabilitation Devices Panel discussion held in June 2012 (FDA Gaithersburg, 2012), a general consensus was that it should be left to an individual surgeon in discussion with his/her patient to choose the best technology.

In most commercial joint prostheses in use today, a polished metallic CoCrMo surface articulates with a much softer polyethylene surface. The rationale is that with this set-up, almost all of the debris generated will be the softer and relatively less toxic polyethylene debris. This approach effectively reduces the production of toxic metallic ions; however, even in ideal conditions, the wear rate of the polyethylene cup in a hip implant is expected to be 0.1–0.2 mm/year (National Institutes of Health, 1994). Dividing the thickness of the cup by this wear rate will give the maximum expected life, but there are many instances where scratches on the CoCrMo surface cause acceleration of this wear rate. Sources of scratches that commonly cause scratches on CoCrMo condyles originate from bone, bone cement, prosthetic coatings for bone ingrowth (especially titanium beads), wear and corrosion products from modular junctions, and metallic transfer from metal liner following a dislocation. When hard, third-body particles roughen the metal femoral component, it leads to scratches and increased abrasive wear of the softer poly counterface. Surfaces that are more resistant to abrasive scratching reduce the potential for abrasive wear. Now that implants are routinely reaching near the maximum life expectancy, requiring surgery to replace the polyethylene cup, a more permanent solution to minimize wear debris is needed.

The goal of minimizing polyethylene wear debris (or eliminating it altogether) has led to renewed interest in ceramic articulation components, and, with recent improvements in manufacturing and prosthetic designs, ceramic materials are performing much better than in their initial clinical uses in the 1970s. In addition to using metal-on-metal designs, (Lombardi *et al.*, 2004, Cuckler, 2005, Bal *et al.*, 2005), current trends in orthopaedic implant design involve developing ceramic surface components such as oxidized zirconium or nitrided titanium (Fig. 5.1). Titanium nitride (TiN) coatings on cp-Ti and Ti-6Al-4V alloy demonstrated reduced wear rates in hip simulator studies (Gutmanas and Gotman, 2004). TiN coatings deposited from cathodic arc physical vapour deposition techniques were shown to reduce fretting behaviour of untreated Ti-6Al-4V surfaces (Hendry and Pilliar, 2001). Oxidized zirconium, featuring a 3–5 μm thick diffused oxide layer on the surface of zirconium metal, has been associated with reduced wear rates when coupled with ultrahigh molecular weight (UHMW) polyethylene components (Good *et al.*, 2003, 2005). Short-term clinical success of oxidized zirconium in total knee arthroplasty has also been reported (Innocenti *et al.*, 2010). The rationale for this approach is that by employing materials with much greater hardness, the generation of wear debris can be minimized. Similarly, data of annual linear wear rates for several orthopaedic couplings show that volumetric wear for alumina–alumina couplings (0.002 mm/year) is much lower than

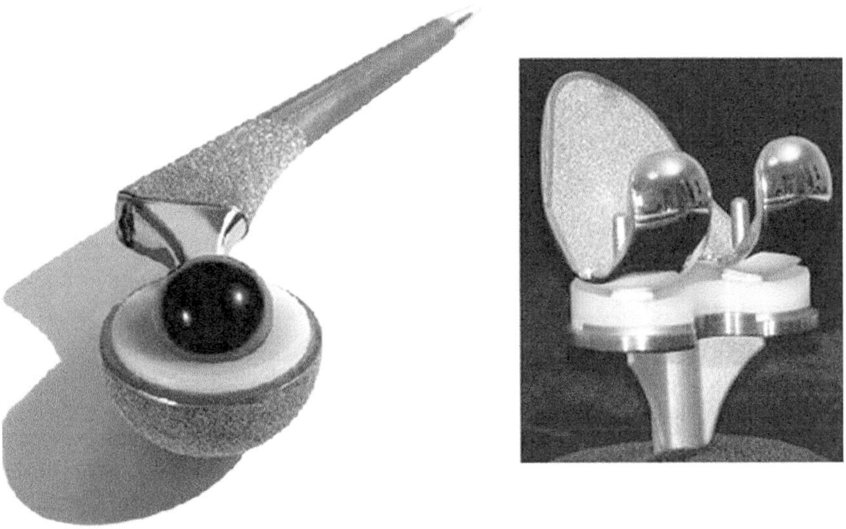

5.1 Examples of total hip and knee replacement devices used in industry. Both devices shown here have femoral head components with a ceramic surface layer (oxidized zirconium on left, titanium nitride on right). These devices also use a polyethylene liner.

for alumina–polyethylene (0.05–0.1 mm/year) or cobalt chrome–polyethylene (0.1–0.4 mm/year) couplings (www.wmt.com/ceramic/patients/weardata.asp). The benefits of ceramics for orthopaedic implant surfaces are becoming increasingly evident due to their outstanding mechanical and biocompatibility properties. There is also strong evidence showing that many nanostructured ceramics exhibit improved mechanical properties (such as hardness, ductility, and enhanced strain to failure) over their conventional larger-grained counterparts (Bohn *et al.*, 1991, Mayo *et al.*, 1990, 1992).

5.1.2 Joint resurfacing alternatives

Joint resurfacing may be considered an alternative to total joint arthroplasty, particularly in young active patients who would potentially outlive a total hip or knee prosthesis. Therefore, total hip resurfacing could be viewed as a time-buying procedure to delay the need for a total hip arthroplasty. For example, proposed advantages of total hip resurfacing compared to total hip arthroplasty include preservation of the femoral neck and femoral canal, thus facilitating revision or conversion to a total hip replacement, if required (Amstutz *et al.*, 2004, Beaule *et al.*, 2004). In May 2006 the FDA granted premarket application (PMA) approval to the metal-on-metal Birmingham Hip Resurfacing (BHR) System (Smith and Nephew, Inc.) for use in patients requiring primary hip arthroplasty for non-inflammatory or inflammatory arthritis. The BHR uses femoral and acetabular components made of high carbon cobalt–chromium alloy. Metal-on-metal total hip resurfacing with a fully FDA approved total hip resurfacing device may be considered medically necessary when the patient is likely to outlive a traditional prosthesis and would otherwise require a total hip replacement. The FDA lists several contraindications for total hip resurfacing. These contraindications include: bone stock inadequate to support the device, skeletal immaturity, vascular insufficiency, muscular atrophy, or neuromuscular disease severe enough to compromise implant stability or postoperative recovery, known moderate to severe renal insufficiency, severely overweight, known or suspected metal sensitivity, immunosuppressed or receiving high doses of corticosteroids.

Some outcomes have been reported with the BHR device suggesting medium to long-term durability. Treacy and colleagues reported that the 5-year survival of BHR arthroplasty in 144 patients was 98% overall (Treacy *et al.*, 2005). Shimmin and Back reviewed 3497 BHRs performed by 89 surgeons between April 1999 and April 2004 (Shimmin and Back, 2005). The authors reported that the incidence of femoral neck fracture was 1.46% (50 of 3497) and the mean time to fracture was 15.4 weeks. Glyn-Jones and colleagues evaluated the stability of BHR arthroplasties by radiographic analysis in 22 hips in 20 patients (Glyn-Jones *et al.*, 2004). At 24 months, migration of the head of the femoral component was not statistically significant (0.2 mm total three-dimensional). A substantial body of evidence shows that total hip resurfacing is associated with consistent and strong symptomatic and functional improvements comparable to those obtained with current total hip arthroplasty (THA) in patients less than 65 years old. The available evidence shows that the short-term symptomatic and functional health benefits of HR are at least as good as those of THA over midterm follow-up, with no substantial differences in revision rates, among patients younger than 65 years who are likely to outlive a traditional prosthesis. Also, inference from the available long-term evidence suggests that HR will be at least as beneficial as THA in patients who are likely to outlive a traditional prosthesis.

Despite the apparent benefits of joint resurfacing over total joint arthroplasty, a limitation of hip resurfacing is that the bearing is a cobalt–chrome alloy surface gliding against another cobalt–chrome surface. Although the wear rates of such metal-on-metal bearings are low, this technology has some potential concerns. Very rarely, a patient with a metal-on-metal bearing can develop a metal hypersensitivity reaction. Also, hip resurfacing is not recommended for women of child-bearing age and in patients with decreased kidney function. In both groups, it is speculated that the possible toxicity of metal particles could lead to future problems. With regards to long-term safety, literature summaries provided to the FDA demonstrated increased serum and urinary concentrations of metal ions postoperatively in patients, particularly after metal-on-metal procedures, although data show no conclusive evidence of significant detrimental effects (ASTM_ F732-00, 2003).

5.2 Ultra-hard carbon coatings

Highly crystalline chemical vapour deposition (CVD) diamond is often considered as a wear-resistant material for applications such as cutting tools. However, its extreme properties, including hardness close to 100 GPa, are not easily exploited due to its inherently brittle nature and high surface roughness. Conventional diamond films synthesized by the vapour phase exhibit columnar crystal growth; once cracks occur on the surface of the film, they tend to propagate through the columnar particles, leading to a decrease in film and interface toughness. A number of deposition techniques have been utilized to produce several variants of carbon structures, distinguished primarily by the nature of carbon bonding (sp^3 vs sp^2 hybridized) and the degree of order (crystalline vs amorphous), as well as by the degree to which hydrogen is incorporated into the structure. The sp^3 bonds can occur not only within crystals (i.e. with long-range order), but also within amorphous solids where the atoms are in a random arrangement. The bond types have a considerable influence on the material properties of carbon films. If the sp^2 type is predominant the film will be softer, if the sp^3 type is predominant the film will be harder. In addition to the various forms of purely amorphous carbon, designated as 'diamond-like carbon' (DLC), phase-pure 'nanocrystalline diamond' (NCD) with grain sizes of 30–100 nm and 'ultra-nanocrystalline diamond' (UNCD) (Shenderova and Gruen, 2006) with grain sizes as low as 3–5 nm have been developed for several applications. Yet another carbon structure has been associated with composite-like characteristics associated with nanocrystalline diamond grains embedded within an amorphous carbon matrix, designated as 'nanostructured diamond' (NSD) or 'ultra-smooth nanostructured diamond' (USND) (Konovalov *et al.*, 2006), depending on the size of diamond grains (as low as 5–6 nm). Of the various carbon structures reported, only DLC and NSD/USND coatings have been extensively investigated for wear-resistant articulating components in dental and orthopaedic devices.

5.2.1 Diamond-like carbon (DLC) coatings for orthopaedic implants

DLC is a purely amorphous carbon material with varying amounts of sp^3 bonding and has been investigated for use in medical applications as a result of its excellent wear properties and biocompatibility (Roy and Lee, 2007, Narayan, 2005). Hydrogen-containing amorphous carbon (a-C:H), amorphous carbon without hydrogen (a-C) and pure sp^3-hybridized amorphous carbon (ta-C) are typical forms, each with potentially different mechanical properties. Vickers hardness for a-C and a-C:H are typically between 1500 and 3500 HV and up to ~40% sp^3, whereas tetrahedral amorphous carbon (ta-C) can have 4000–9000HV with 80–85% sp^3. Raman spectroscopy has been a valuable tool in characterizing these coatings for predicting structure, optical and mechanical properties (Ferrari and Robertson, 1999, Tamor and Vassell, 1994). Traditionally, the largest inherent problem with DLC coatings has been issues of residual stress; higher sp^3 contents lead to a harder coating but at the expense of higher compressive stress (Morshed *et al.*, 2003, Schwan, 1997). The internal compressive stress in DLC coatings can be as high as 10 GPa, which dramatically limits coating thickness. Such stresses can create unstable interfaces (i.e. adhesion and/or cohesion issues) and the film may become prone to delamination. It has been shown that for the case of ultra-hard ta-C coatings thermal annealing at ~650°C can dramatically reduce the large compressive stress to near zero without substantial change in sp^3 bonding (Grierson *et al.*, 2010, Friedmann *et al.*, 1997).

Although DLC in its various forms is widely studied, issues regarding instability of the coating caused by high levels of residual stress and poor adhesion in aqueous environments remain of concern. For a thorough review of DLC coatings for biomedical applications, the reader is referred to the comprehensive work by Roy and Lee (Roy and Lee, 2007).

5.2.2 Nanostructured diamond coatings for orthopaedic implants

Another potential coating system to address the issues associated with wear and metal ion release in orthopaedic and dental implants is that of ultra-smooth nanostructured diamond (NSD and USND) coatings. These have been developed for metal implant surfaces including titanium and cobalt-based alloys using microwave plasma CVD (Catledge *et al.*, 2011, Catledge and Vohra, 1999, Chowdhury *et al.*, 2008). The NSD coatings could prove to be more resistant to scratching by third body wear particles, such as bone cement, due to the high hardness (56–80 GPa) and low surface roughness (rms value <10 nm) of the coatings (Papo *et al.*, 2004, Konovalov *et al.*, 2006, Chowdhury, 2006, Catledge *et al.*, 2002). They have been characterized as a mixture of sp^3 and sp^2 bonded carbon, with nanometre sized diamond particles embedded in an amorphous carbon matrix. They combine high hardness, low surface roughness, and excellent fracture toughness and adhesion, especially to titanium alloys.

The inherent challenges in successfully coating NSD onto a metal substrate by CVD methods have been largely overcome for titanium and Ti-6Al-4V alloy substrates. By nature of the ultra-hard, yet somewhat compliant NSD coating and the strong interfacial carbide that naturally forms during deposition onto titanium surfaces, coating adhesion and tribological properties are excellent (Hill *et al.*, 2008, Catledge and Vohra 2004, Catledge, 1995, Booth *et al.*, 2011). A more difficult challenge faces NSD coating of cobalt–chromium (CoCr) alloys that are so widely used as wear bearings in the orthopaedic industry. The high cobalt content of this alloy acts as a catalyst for graphite that inevitably forms as an interfacial layer (Lawson *et al.*, 2005). Such is the case for other transition metals of iron or nickel that have such high solubility for carbon. The formation of interfacial graphitic carbon and the lack of strongly bonded interfacial carbides is believed to be responsible for the poor coating quality and adhesion to this material. However, recently it was shown (Catledge *et al.*, 2011) that use of oxygen in the feedgas can promote early formation of chromium oxides that act as an effective diffusion barrier to cobalt and therefore minimize interfacial graphite. These chromium oxides combined with chromium carbides that form at elevated substrate temperature are believed to be important interfacial phases that have led to improved adhesion of NSD coatings on CoCr orthopaedic alloys.

Nanostructured diamond on cobalt–chromium substrates

Cobalt–chromium alloys are widely used as the bearing surfaces in orthopaedic implants such as needed in total hip and knee replacement surgeries, because of their superior mechanical properties and resistance to corrosion and biodegradation (Black, 1992). Wear of articulating surfaces involving CoCr alloy-on-polyethylene (used in the majority of hip and knee arthroplasties) has been cited as a dominant factor limiting the long-term success of the implant (Amstutz *et al.*, 1992, Goldring *et al.*, 1983). Diamond coatings have been considered for these alloys in order to reduce the problems associated with wear and metal ion release, thereby increasing the lifetime of the implant in the body. Smooth NSD coatings would be expected to reduce friction and wear, which are the primary sources of failure in current orthopaedic implant devices. In addition, the diamond coating may act to prevent or slow the release of potentially toxic heavy metal ions into surrounding tissue from the alloy itself (Kobayashi *et al.*, 2007, Ohgoe *et al.*, 2006). However, CVD diamond deposition onto transition metals such as nickel and cobalt which have partially filled d-electron shells is made difficult because of the catalytic formation of graphite (Lettington and Steeds, 1994, Davis, 1993, Chen and Narayan, 1993) during initial stages of growth. These transition metals have high carbon diffusivity and do not form stable carbides, making nucleation of the diamond phase difficult. Once a graphitic layer is formed, the adhesion of a subsequently formed diamond layer is very weak. Several attempts have been made to improve diamond nucleation and adhesion using interlayers (Godbole *et al.*, 1999, Wei *et al.*, 2009, Polini *et al.*, 2007, Zuo *et al.*, 2003) to act as a buffer to limit carbon exposure to the substrate, by using laser irradiation to partially melt the substrate surface and react molten metal with carbon (Narayan *et al.*, 1991), or by using $C+$ ion implantation (Lee *et al.*, 1992). These approaches often involve an extra processing step and have yielded limited success.

One particularly promising method of CVD diamond deposition developed by Godbole *et al.* (Godbole *et al.*, 1999) used a composite approach by sequential deposition of aluminium nitride with diamond followed by titanium carbide with diamond, as shown schematically in Fig. 5.2. The titanium carbide component, although found to be a very stable and effective barrier to the diffusion of cobalt, was not useful as a stand-alone buffer layer due to excessive thermally induced stress with consequent film cracking. However, the composite consists of

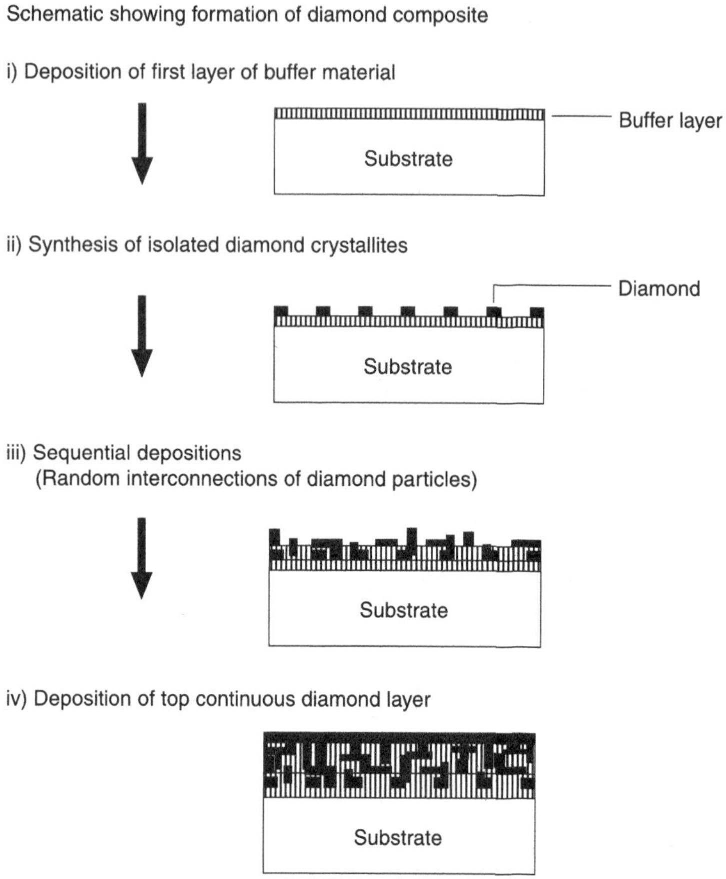

5.2 Schematic showing different stages of the formation of diamond composites for deposition on cobalt-chromium substrate. Reprinted from *Materials Science and Engineering B*, 58, Godbole, V. P., Narayan, R., Xu, Z., Narayan, J. and Sankar, J., Diamond films and composites on cobalt-chromium alloys, 254, Copyright (1999), with permission from Elsevier.

randomly interconnected micron sized diamond crystallites, which are primarily surrounded by buffer material (AlN or TiC), whereas the contact area between neighbouring diamond crystallites is minimum. The presence of such a discontinuous morphology of diamond crystallites renders more toughness and also leads to compensation of stresses in localized regions (local stress management) and thus reduces bulging and subsequent delamination effects. Although the surface of the diamond coating is not nanostructured and therefore appears rough and faceted on a micron-scale, the method demonstrates the potential for reducing graphite formation and subsequent coating delamination that is so problematic for this alloy.

In light of the need for a single-step CVD process resulting in improved adhesion of ultra-hard and smooth NSD coatings on CoCr alloy, Catledge *et al.* report the use of oxygen in a feedgas mixture containing hydrogen along with high methane content (up to 15 vol%). It has been shown that one of the key roles of oxygen atoms in CVD diamond film growth is the sp^2-sp^3 conversion of C-C bonds on the surface (Dementjev and Petukhov, 1998). However, its influence on interfacial structure/composition and diffusion of Co for growth of hard carbon films on CoCr substrates is not well studied. It was demonstrated that when oxygen is added to the H_2/CH_4 feedgas mixture for growth of NSD on CoCr alloy, the deleterious interaction of cobalt with carbon can be minimized through formation of an interfacial chromium oxide layer that effectively acts as a diffusion barrier to cobalt. Figure 5.3 shows the dramatic influence that oxygen has during the diamond nucleation and initial growth stages (before the coating has a chance to fully coalesce) through analysis of X-ray photoelectron spectroscopy (XPS) survey scans of the incomplete coatings, grown with and without use of oxygen. The most striking observation from these spectra is the absence of surface cobalt and molybdenum when oxygen is used in the feedgas. However, surface chromium is present and, as expected, a more intense oxygen peak is detected when oxygen

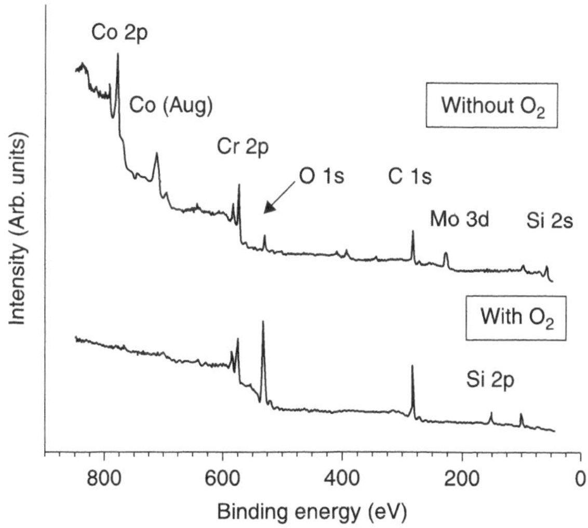

5.3 XPS survey spectra after nucleation of nanostructured diamond films grown on CoCrMo with and without oxygen at T_{sub} = 915°C. When oxygen is used, no cobalt or molybdenum is detected on the surface, although chromium is still present. Reprinted with kind permission from Springer Science + Business Media: *Journal of Materials Science: Materials in Medicine*, Improved adhesion of ultra-hard carbon films on cobalt-chromium orthopaedic implant alloy, 22, 2011, Catledge, S. A., Vaid, R., Diggins, P. T., Weimer, J. J., Koopman, M. and Vohra, Y. K., Figure Number 6.

feedgas is used. The Co/Cr and Co/C atomic ratios drop two orders of magnitude when oxygen is used and, as expected, the O/Cr and O/Co increase dramatically. High resolution spectra for Co 2p and Cr 2p, shown in Fig. 5.4, demonstrate the nature of bonding with oxygen for these metals in the early terminated films. Whereas no cobalt was detected when oxygen was used, without the use of oxygen Co 2p spectra show a primary component of elemental cobalt with some bonding as cobalt oxide and cobalt hydroxide. The Cr 2p spectra also show a primarily elemental chromium component when oxygen is not used, along with chromium oxide. However, when oxygen is used, the chromium forms an oxide with essentially no elemental chromium remaining.

It was found that NSD coatings grown with oxygen on CoCrMo at substrate temperature in the range of 915–970°C show excellent adhesion, whereas those grown at lower temperatures or without oxygen delaminate. Despite the expected increase of thermally induced stress at the elevated temperature, improved adhesion of these coatings is attributed to a combined effect: higher interfacial chromium carbide content (observed at higher temperature) and reduced cobalt migration into the growing film (observed when oxygen is used). In contrast, the films grown at lower temperature (even in the presence of oxygen) show the presence of carbon nanotubes (Fig. 5.5) at the interface side of delaminated films, indicative of cobalt interaction with carbon. One might suggest that an interfacial carbide layer may itself be sufficient to act as a diffusion barrier to elemental cobalt. However, substantial graphitic soot is formed and adhesion is poor when oxygen is not used, even at the higher temperatures. Therefore, oxygen plays an important role in achieving soot-free, adhered diamond films on CoCrMo, particularly for the substrate temperature range of 915–970°C. Overall, these results provide hope for successful coating of CoCrMo orthopaedic implant materials for improved joint performance and lifetime. Artificial joints involving diamond-on-diamond articulation may be a viable option leading to fewer and less invasive surgeries while maintaining high performance of the joint.

Nanostructured diamond on titanium substrates

CVD diamond on titanium and the biomedical alloy Ti-6Al-4V has been explored by numerous researchers (Scardi *et al.*, 1997, Perry, 1993, Ager and Drory, 1993, Askari *et al.*, 2008, Azevedo *et al.*, 2005, Baek *et al.*, 2003, Buccioni *et al.*, 1999, Fu *et al.*, 2003, Terranova, 1996). Issues deemed to be particularly important in this system include the potential hydrogen embrittlement of titanium, the large thermally induced residual stress in the diamond coating, relative amounts of interfacial titanium carbide, titanium hydride, and titanium oxide phases, and plastic flow of the substrate. Despite large residual stress in CVD diamond coatings on titanium substrates, as much as 7–8 GPa, the coating adhesion can be quite good, in large part because of the strongly bonded interfacial titanium

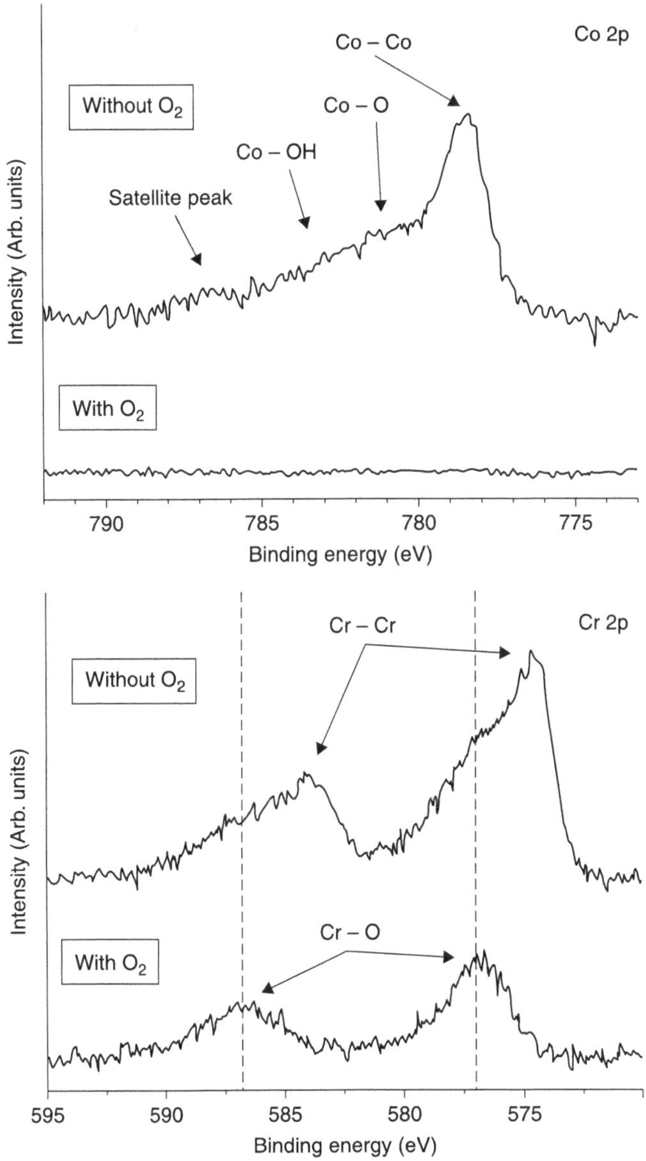

5.4 High resolution XPS spectra for Co 2p and Cr 2p after nucleation of nanostructured diamond films grown on CoCrMo with and without oxygen at T_{sub} = 915°C. When oxygen is not used, chromium is detected primarily in elemental form, whereas it is primarily bonded with oxygen when oxygen is used in the feedgas. Reprinted with kind permission from Springer Science + Business Media: *Journal of Materials Science: Materials in Medicine*, Improved adhesion of ultra-hard carbon films on cobalt-chromium orthopaedic implant alloy, 22, 2011, Catledge, S. A, Vaid, R., Diggins, P. T., Weimer, J. J., Koopman, M. and Vohra, Y. K., Figure Number 7.

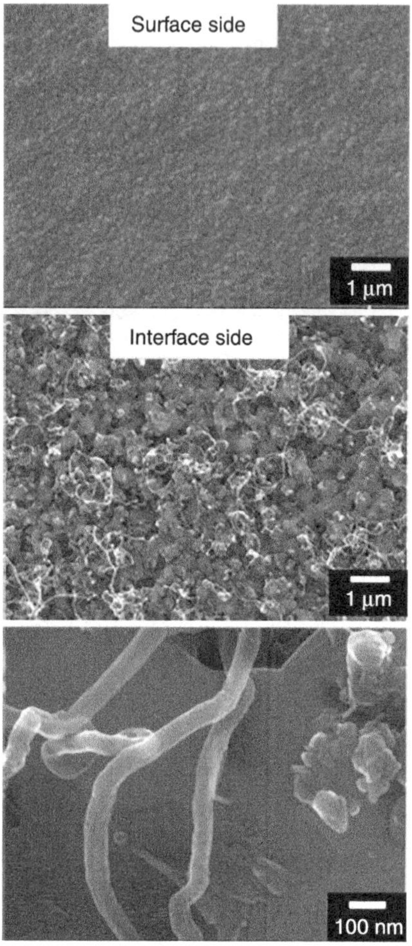

5.5 SEM images showing surface (top) and interface (middle and bottom) morphology from a delaminated nanostructured diamond film grown on CoCrMo with oxygen at a low substrate temperature (825°C). Carbon nanotubes are observed to develop at the interface. Reprinted with kind permission from Springer Science + Business Media: *Journal of Materials Science: Materials in Medicine*, Improved adhesion of ultra-hard carbon films on cobalt-chromium orthopaedic implant alloy, 22, 2011, Catledge, S. A, Vaid, R., Diggins, P. T., Weimer, J. J., Koopman, M. and Vohra, Y. K., Figure Number 5.

carbide (Drory and Hutchinson, 1994, Vandenbulcke, 1998). Stress relaxation is influenced by tensile stress in the substrate (to offset compressive stress in the coating and interface), the thickness of the interfacial carbide and the nature of the diamond film itself.

The present authors have extensive experience in the deposition of NSD on Ti-6Al-4V alloy and have demonstrated exceptional coating adhesion while maintaining very low surface roughness and ultra-high hardness. Well-adherent NSD coatings on Ti-6Al-4V substrates synthesized by microwave plasma CVD with feedgas consisting of high methane (15 vol%), hydrogen and nitrogen have been previously established (Toprani *et al.*, 2000, Catledge, 1999). Based on these deposition conditions, the coatings feature low surface roughness (14–30 nm) and high hardness (70–90 GPa). Additionally, USND coatings synthesized with helium-rich plasmas were shown to further reduce grain size (5–6 nm) and surface roughness (9–10 nm), while maintaining high hardness in the range of 56–72 GPa (Chowdhury *et al.*, 2006). These coatings may be described as a mixture of sp^3 and sp^2 bonded carbon, with nanometre sized diamond particles embedded in an amorphous carbon matrix.

Conventional micro-crystalline diamond films contain large micron size facets and are too rough to be used for implant components requiring low friction and minimal wear during articulation. The addition of N_2 into the feedgas mixture (Jin, 1994) results in substantial changes in film morphology, structure and mechanical properties, and can lead to NSD as shown in Fig. 5.6 (Catledge, 1998, 1999, Chowdhury *et al.*, 2008). *In situ* plasma diagnostics involving optical emission spectroscopy (OES) as well as thermodynamic equilibrium calculations to model the gas phase composition, revealed that the CN radical concentration in the plasma was an important parameter involved in the transformation from rough microcrystalline to smooth NSD films (Corvin, 2002). The NSD coating fracture toughness was also found to improve as a result of the addition of N_2 to the feedgas (Toprani *et al.*, 2000). Upon bulk indentation with a Rockwell indenter, films were observed to undergo significant plastic deformation without hard elastic-to-brittle fracture occurring. Strain energy could be released through stable circumferential microcracks emanating from near the edges of the indent craters, but without film spallation.

Although bare titanium and Ti-6Al-4V alloy is not considered appropriate in articulating biomedical implants because of its poor wear characteristics, NSD coating of these materials may be a viable solution as long as coating adhesion is not a concern. The high hardness, low surface roughness, excellent adhesion and resilience of these coatings should be considered when searching for alternative bearing surfaces in total joint replacements.

Diamond on steel substrates

CVD deposition of diamond onto substrates comprising primarily transition elements cobalt, iron or nickel is inherently difficult because of the propensity of these elements to act as a catalyst for graphite formation (Lettington and Steeds, 1994, Davis, 1993, Chen and Narayan, 1993) during initial stages of growth. An additional hurdle for diamond deposition on steel is the large mismatch in thermal coefficients of expansion (1×10^{-6}/°C for diamond and 17×10^{-6}/°C for stainless steel, at room temperature). This leads to residual stresses present in the diamond

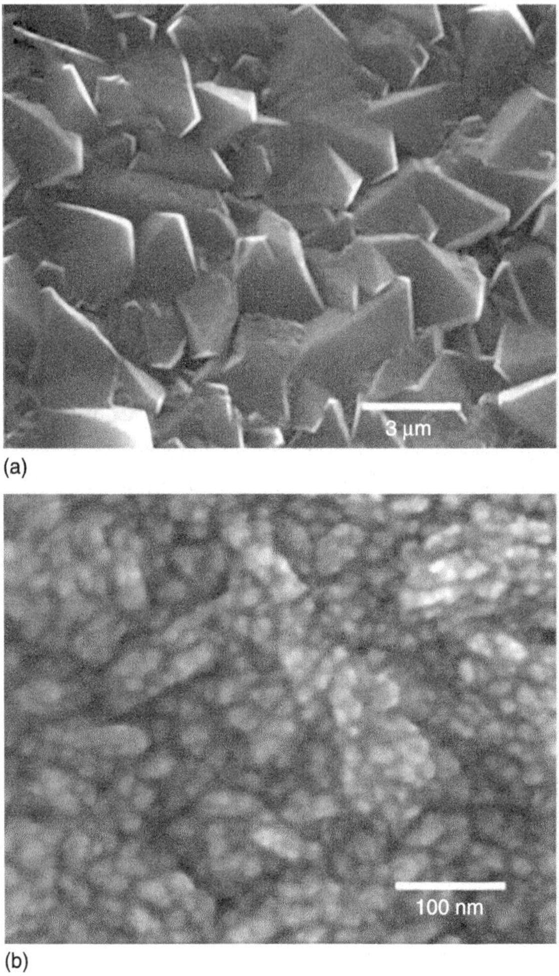

5.6 SEM images showing CVD diamond films grown (a) without N_2 and (b) with N_2 feedgas addition to a $H_2 + CH_4$ plasma consisting of 15% vol CH_4. Note the difference in scale bars.

film upon cooling from the high deposition temperatures, leading to poor adhesion. Therefore, in addition to lower substrate temperature during deposition, manipulation of interfacial chemistry is often used to improve adhesion of diamond coatings on steel. The most common method to attempt to overcome the hindrances for diamond deposition on ferrous substrates is through the use of an intermediate layer or system of layers. Choice of the intermediate layer should be based on its ability to act as a diffusion barrier to carbon, and to allow strongly bonded metal carbides and/or other interfacial reaction layers, ideally without sharp discrete interfacial boundaries that may act as regions of stress concentration.

Many different intermediate layers or layer systems have been tried over the years, including the nitrides of chromium and titanium with mixed reports in achieving adhered diamond films for both systems (Fayer *et al.*, 1995, Buijnsters *et al.*, 2002, Negrea and Vermesan, 2000, Lorenz, 1995). Buijnsters *et al.* used arc-plated CrN interlayers for coating diamond onto austenitic AISI-type 316 stainless steel as well as high speed steel. The use of the CrN interlayer was found not to result in a continuous diamond film on the stainless steel, but good quality adherent coatings did form on the high speed steel for substrate temperature as low as 650°C. Polini *et al.* (Polini *et al.*, 2006) demonstrated that well-adherent diamond films can be grown on high speed steels using a TiC interlayer deposited by the physical vapour deposition (PVD) arc technique. Their results showed that diamond films deposited on rough TiC interlayers exhibited a wide distribution of stress values and that very large compressive stress (as much as 10 GPa) could be accommodated without delamination.

The use of a pack bording process to create a thick boride case on ferritic tool and austenitic stainless steel resulted in the formation of FeB and/or Fe_2B phases believed to have a strong influence on the adherence of the diamond films (Buijnsters *et al.*, 2003). In particular, the presence of FeB on the surface of the borided steels resulted in very high thermal stresses and consequent delamination of the diamond films on both ferritic tool and austenitic stainless steels. The boron-rich FeB phase was deemed to be not desirable, as it is more brittle and the large difference in expansion coefficients between the FeB and Fe_2B phases leads to crack formation at the FeB/Fe_2B interface. However, on the borided tool and stainless steels without the FeB phase (but with Fe_2B), continuous and adherent diamond films with very low residual stress were obtained. Preliminary findings (Ballinger and Catledge, 2011) reveal improved adhesion of NSD coatings on 440C stainless steel ball bearings using a plasma surface modification process to create iron and chromium boride interfacial layers. The NSD coatings were found to adhere much better on the plasma-borided ball bearings when compared to bearings that instead had a titanium nitride interfacial layer. Overall, these results suggest that with appropriate interfacial structure and chemistry, well-adhered diamond coatings may be possible on a variety of steels, despite the large driving force for delamination from graphitic carbon and from thermal expansion mismatch.

5.3 Wear measurements for ceramic-based orthopaedic implants

Fully dense ceramics, alumina and zirconia, are used in total joint replacements specifically for the purpose of providing more wear resistant bearing surfaces. Because of their hardness, ceramics can be polished to a very smooth finish and remain relatively scratch resistant while in use as a bearing surface. The most significant disadvantage of ceramics is their brittle nature, making them susceptible to fracture. Improvements in metallurgy have sparked renewed interest of metal-on-metal bearings, and similarly, improvements in ceramic quality have led to increased interest in ceramic bearings. Over the long term, alumina-on-polyethylene bearings for hip replacement show reduced wear rates over those typically seen with metal-on-polyethylene bearings, with an associated decrease in osteolysis (Wright *et al.*, 2009). However, the use of zirconia as a bearing surface against polyethylene has not proven as successful clinically as alumina-on-polyethylene bearings. In comparing alumina-, zirconia-, and metal-on-conventional polyethylene bearings in total hip patients, the highest wear rate occurs in the zirconia group. Zirconia, which is as wear resistant as alumina, tends to change its crystalline structure to a form that is less tough and more prone to wear. In general, alumina-on-alumina joints have shown very low wear rates clinically, although the results are design dependent. Recent reports also show excellent wear resistance in young patients, with no measurable wear and no evidence of osteolysis even beyond a decade of follow-up (Wright *et al.*, 2009). Furthermore, very few implant fractures have been observed, even in this high demand patient population, providing support for the improved mechanical properties of alumina. Oxidized zirconium is used for femoral heads in hip replacement and the femoral component in knee replacement, and initial results look promising. However, longer term studies will be needed to prove that the improved bearing properties of oxidized zirconium lead to longer lasting implants.

5.3.1 Wear of DLC coatings for orthopaedic implants

A review of ceramic coatings for orthopaedic implants shows that the significant research effort devoted to develop TiN and DLC coatings for orthopaedic bearings by many research groups worldwide has not led to widespread clinical applications (Piconi *et al.*, 2004). The laboratory tests on DLC coatings often show conflicting and controversial results on the improvements in wear in comparison to CoCr alloy. A comparison of these results shows that care must be taken with regard to the source of DLC, methane being superior to acetylene, and above all to the smoothness of the substrate. When conditions are favourable, the tests indicate that DLC coatings have the potential to provide the lowest wear rates of ultrahigh molecular weight polyethylene (UHMWPE), perhaps half that against alumina, without the risks associated with fracture of ceramic components. However, better control of the high internal stresses in these coatings may be needed in order to avoid issues with coating spallation and detachment.

With regard to application involving orthopaedic materials, hard DLC coatings have been deposited on CoCr and magnesia-stabilized zirconia substrates, with enhanced scratch resistance on the latter substrate due to its better resistance to plastic deformation (Roy *et al.*, 2009). DLC-coated titanium alloy femoral heads performed well in hip simulator tests (Affatato *et al.*, 2000) but fared poorly in clinical use (Taeger *et al.*, 2003). DLC-coated CoCr alloy femoral heads were undamaged in aggressive wear tests employing third-body bone cement particles (Santavirta *et al.*, 1999), but hip simulator tests using bovine serum as a lubricant have not shown reduced polyethylene wear compared to non-coated CoCr heads (Saikko *et al.*, 2001, Galvin *et al.*, 2007). Wear tests aimed to evaluate DLC as a coating for tibial trays of knee prostheses (Jones *et al.*, 2001) measured 3.5 increase in wear of UHMWPE pins sliding against DLC-coated vs. cast CoCr alloy plates, leading the authors to remark on the unsuitability of DLC coating for the intended application. Also the results of biaxial hip simulator tests were controversial: similar wear of UHMWPE cups against CoCr DLC-coated and uncoated heads was reported (Saikko *et al.*, 2001), both values higher than the wear of the same cups against alumina heads, whereas other authors (Affatato *et al.*, 2000) measured wear rates of UHMWPE cups similar for alumina and DLC-coated heads, both higher than CoCr coupled to the same cups. In pin-on-disk tests against PMMA pins (Mishra and Davidson, 1992), DLC-coated Ti6Al4V disks performed worse than wrought CoCrMo alloy raising doubts about coating resistance to third-body wear. In comparison, several reports involving DLC are very encouraging. An original bearing couple DLC-on-DLC was tested in a simplified hip simulator and in pin-on-disk wear tests with satisfactory results (Lappalainen *et al.*, 1998). In a National Science Foundation (NSF)-funded study, Xu and Pruitt (Xu and Pruitt, 1999) examined DLC coatings on Ti–6Al–4V alloy against UHMWPE in pin-on-disk tests in water. The DLC was prepared by the plasma source method described above. The rate of PE wear was reduced by a factor of 3–4, compared with uncoated alloy. For amorphous diamond coatings deposited by pulsed plasma arc techniques, the wear rates determined in a commercial hip simulator for 15 million walking cycles (corresponding to about 15 years of clinical use) in serum lubrication were even 1 000 000 times lower than the clinical values for conventional total hip replacements (THRs) (polyethylene–metal or metal–metal pairs) (Lappalainen *et al.*, 2003). Clearly, the variability of reports for the effectiveness of DLC in orthopaedic wear couples must be treated with caution, and may be explained, at least in part, by differences in coating roughness and test procedure (Dearnaley and Arps, 2005).

5.3.2 Wear of nanostructured diamond coatings for orthopaedic implants

NSD coatings have been tested to a much lesser extent than DLC coatings. The NSD coatings could prove to be more resistant to scratching by third-body wear particles, such as bone cement, due to the high hardness of the coatings (56–72 GPa) (Papo *et al.*, 2004). In one study (Hill *et al.*, 2008), NSD coatings were deposited onto Ti6Al4V by microwave plasma-assisted chemical vapour deposition (MPCVD), with both hydrogen-rich, NSD-(H), and helium-rich, NSD-(He), feedgas mixtures. Pin-on-disk wear testing was performed in serum lubrication with an OrthoPOD® wear tester to evaluate the wear of polyethylene against the NSD coatings and CoCr. The average wear factor calculated for polyethylene-on-CoCr, $5.7 \pm 0.8 \times 10^{-7}$ mm^3/Nm, falls within the range determined from retrieval studies of total replacement hip joints, $9.0 \times 10^{-8} - 7.2 \times 10^{-6}$ mm^3/Nm (Atkinson *et al.*, 1985). As shown in Fig. 5.7, no statistically significant difference in wear factor was found between polyethylene against NSD-(H), NSD-(He) and CoCr. However, polyethylene experienced lower wear against nine of the 12 NSD samples compared to CoCr, despite NSD exhibiting higher roughness and higher coefficient of friction against polyethylene. Scanning electron microscopy (SEM) images of the worn pins revealed multiple protuberances of polyethylene rising above the surface in polyethylene-on-CoCr, and a single, large, elevated protuberance in polyethylene-on-NSD. These protuberances were thought to be areas of high wear resistance. It was concluded that as a counterface to polyethylene, NSD coatings gave comparable wear with CoCr, with several NSD samples giving lower wear. Although pin-on-disk wear testing is a valid screening tool for candidate materials, similar results may not be observed *in vivo*. Although the present wear results for the polyethylene-on-CoCr were consistent with those found in the literature, simulator studies are required to further evaluate the NSD coatings. To examine the resistance of NSD to this third-body damage, bone cement particles should be added to future wear tests of polyethylene-on-NSD. Investigation into

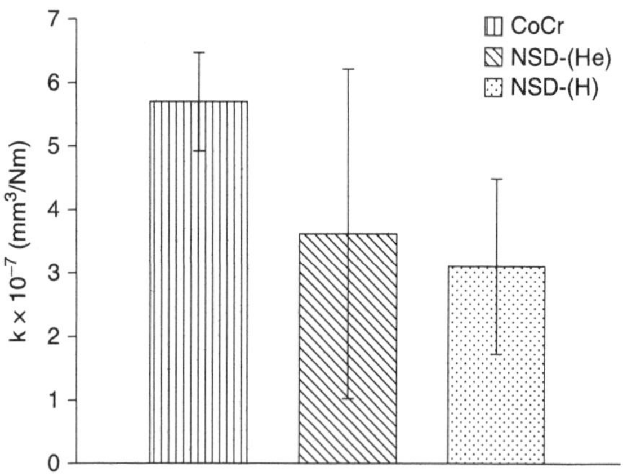

5.7 Average wear factor for polyethylene on CoCr, NSD-(He) and NSD-(H). Error bars represent one standard deviation. Reprinted with permission from *Journal of Biomedical Materials Research B: Applied Biomaterials*, Preliminary tribological evaluation of nanostructured diamond coatings against ultra-high molecular weight polyethylene, 85, 2008, Hill, M. R., Catledge, S. A, Konovalov, V., Clem, W. C., Chowdhury, S. A, Etheridge, B. S., Stanishevsky, A, Lemons, J. E., Vohra, Y. K. and Eberhardt, A W., Copyright © 2007 Wiley Periodicals, Inc.

the role of protein concentration and on the formation of the polyethylene surface features may provide further insight into the wear mechanisms.

5.4 Mesenchymal stem cells derived from bone marrow and their interactions with nanostructured diamond surfaces

Clinical success of diamond coated orthopaedic implants that required to be anchored in surrounding bone tissue requires biointegration resulting from the growth of bone-forming osteogenic cells onto the surface *in vivo*. Therefore, orthopaedic materials designed for bone implantation are tested *in vitro* on cell cultures and then *in vivo* on animals to evaluate their efficacy for cell growth and subsequent bone formation. The anchorage-dependent cells studied on these materials typically adhere with spreading across tens of micrometres (Stevens and George, 2005). Under *in vitro* conditions, usually, the materials or surfaces are allowed to interact with either established cell lines or primary cells derived from laboratory animals. Examples of animal cell lines often used for bone-implant screening as well as for bone-tissue engineering include osteoblast-like UMR-106 cells, mouse bone marrow MBA-15 cells and mouse progenitor MC3T3-E1 cells (having a fibroblast-like phenotype capable of differentiating into osteoblasts in appropriate culture environments (Kanazawa *et al.*, 2007)). Human bone-derived cell lines (derived from osteosarcoma) include osteoblast-like cells CPC-2, TE-85, MG-63, SaOS-2 and U-2OS. Although these cell lines generally retain the most important markers of osteogenic cell differentiation, such as the activity of alkaline phosphatase and production of osteocalcin (Zhao *et al.*, 2007, Amaral *et al.*, 2008, Rudnik *et al.*, 2008, Kalbacova *et al.*, 2009, Vandrovcova and Bakacova, 2011), as a result of tumour origin, they may sometimes lose their markers of differentiation compared to primary low-passaged cells (Tan and Saltzman, 2004).

Primary cells of animal and human origin used to interact with materials for bone implants or scaffolds for bone regeneration include differentiated osteoblasts, such as osteoblasts from neonatal rat calvaria (Webster *et al.*, 2000a,b, de-Oliveiera and Nanci, 2004, de-Oliveira *et al.*, 2007), human osteoblasts (hOB) obtained from surgical bone specimens (Anselme and Bigerelle, 2005) and also stem cells, such as mesenchymal stem cells derived from the bone marrow (Clem *et al.*, 2008, Kilpadi *et al.*, 2004, Jose *et al.*, 2010) or embryonic stem cells (Bedi *et al.*, 2009). Adhesion, growth and differentiation of osteoblasts on the surface of materials developed for bone implants were reviewed recently by Vandrovcova and Bacakova *et al* (Vandrovcova and Bakacova, 2011). Multipotent mesenchymal stem cells (MSC), which can rapidly proliferate in response to injury (Caplan, 2005) and differentiate into a variety of functional cells including bone forming osteoblasts, have attracted much attention in orthopaedic research (Deans and Moseley, 2000). As MSCs differentiate into a committed cell type, they lose their ability for rapid proliferation (Bruder *et al.*, 1994). For this reason, it is the MSCs, rather than osteoblasts, that are primarily recruited for early stage bone healing (Okumura *et al.*, 1997). The process of bone deposition on the surface of a biomaterial is thought to be dependent on cell attachment and proliferation of MSCs on the material surface, followed by osteoblastic differentiation, and finally, production of a mineralized matrix. Attachment of MSCs occurs primarily via integrin receptors, which recognize specific sequences on extracellular matrix (ECM) proteins. Integrins are composed of an α-subunit and a β-subunit, which together recognize specific peptide-domains on collagen, laminin, fibronectin, vitronectin, fibrinogen, osteopontin, sialoprotein and others which mediate the cell adhesion on artificial implant materials. As blood contains large amounts of fibronectin, vitronectin and fibrinogen, spontaneous adsorption of these proteins onto the surface of materials with a geometrical conformation favouring good contact between their specific bioactive sites (e.g. RGDs) and cell-integrins can increase biomaterial capacity for cell attachment. As integrins attach to ECM proteins, they activate intracellular cascade events that regulate cell spreading, proliferation, migration and differentiation (Giancotti, 1999). It has been recently reported that MSC attachment to adhesive proteins, such as fibronectin, occurs by different mechanisms than those in attachment of cell lines (Kilpadi *et al.*, 2004, Vohra *et al.*, 2008). For example, MG-63 and Saos-2 cell attachment to fibronectin is mediated by both α5- and αv-containing integrin heterodimers, whereas only αv-containing integrins are used by MSCs in fibronectin adhesion. Additionally, MSCs have higher levels of α2-integrin subunits than either MG-63 or Saos-2 cells (Vohra *et al.*, 2008).

CVD diamond surfaces are biocompatible, according to Tang *et al.* (Tang *et al.*, 1995), who were among the first to report the biocompatibility of CVD diamond, comparable with titanium and stainless steel. Since then, NSD surfaces or films produced by CVD technique have been repeatedly shown to be an excellent non-cytotoxic material for cell adhesion and growth (Fig. 5.8) in biotechnological applications (Bacakova *et al.*, 2008, Rezek *et al.*, 2011). Many recent studies, using a variety of cell types such as osteoblasts (Amaral *et al.*, 2008, Kalbacova *et al.*, 2009, Yang *et al.*, 2009a), fibroblasts (Amaral *et al.*, 2009), epithelial cells (Lechleitner *et al.*, 2008), endothelial cells (Grousova *et al.*, 2008), bone marrow derived MSCs (Clem *et al.*, 2008) and neural cells (Chen *et al.*, 2009), have focused to understand and control the cell responses on NSD by varying the CVD process parameters to obtain nanocrystallinity, grain size and roughness and also post-surface treatments to obtain different surface chemistry, wettability, and surface functional groups and surface change and conductivity. General findings from these studies so far are that NSD surfaces enhance the growth of osteogenic cells including mesenchymal stem cells and that control of cell adhesion, proliferation and subsequent bone formation can be achieved by altering NSD surface properties as a result of the correlation between the surface properties and the adsorbed endogeneous proteins that regulate the cell behaviour (Clem *et al.*, 2008, Kanazawa *et al.*, 2007, Kloss *et al.*, 2008b).

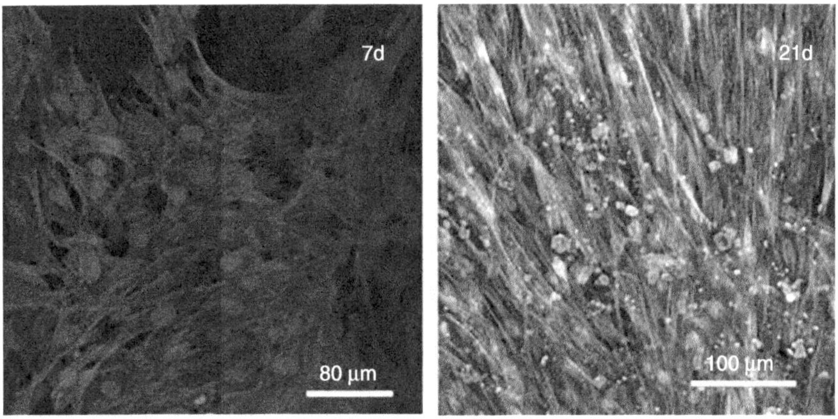

(a) (b)

5.8 CLSM observation of human bone marrow osteoblastic cells cultured on NCD films at days 7 (a) and 21 (b) (calcein, phalloidin and propidium iodide labelling). Reprinted with permission from *Journal of Biomedical Materials Research*, Nanocrystalline diamond: *In vitro* biocompatibility assessment by MG 63 and human bone marrow cells cultures, 87A, 2008, Amaral, M., Dias, A G., Gomes, P. S., Lopes, M. A., Silva, R. F. and Santos, J. D. Copyright © 2008 Wiley Periodicals, Inc.

5.4.1 Effect of nanotopology and nanoroughness

It is well documented that cells respond differently to nanostructured compared with conventional classic material topographies in terms of cell adhesion, proliferation and function (Kalbacova *et al.*, 2009, Webster *et al.*, 2000a, Catledge *et al.*, 2002, Grausova *et al.*, 2011). Many features of nanofibre or nanophase or nanostructured materials with irregularities less than 100 nm mimic or simulate the nanoscaled architecture of native ECM, irregularities of biomacromolecules such as folding, branching etc., and size of ECM parts of cell adhesion receptors (Thomas *et al.*, 2006). Regarding the major bone constituents, hydroxyapatite (the major mineral component) is between 2 and 5 nm in width and 50 nm in length; Type I collagen (the major protein component of bone tissue) is 300 nm in length, 0.5 nm in width and has a periodic bandwidth of 67 nm (Thomas *et al.*, 2006, Kaplan *et al.*, 1994). The osteogenic cells interact with surfaces with a large degree of nanometric-scale morphological features. Surface roughening treatments have been performed on the anchoring region of an implant in order to generate interlocking with bone for stabilization. Webster's research group has published several reports demonstrating increased adhesion of osteoblasts on nanophase ceramics as well as polymer-ceramics nanocomposites (Webster and Smith, 2005, Kay *et al.*, 2002, Webster and Ejiofor, 2004, Palin *et al.*, 2005, Balasundaram *et al.*, 2006). Studies on primary rat calvarial osteoblast cultured on nanophase titania (grain size 20–56 nm), alumina (grain sizes 20–67nm) and conventional much rougher titania and alumina (grain sizes 2120 nm and 177 nm) demonstrated increased attachment of osteoblast on nanophase ceramics (Webster *et al.*, 1990). Human osteoblast like MG63 cells cultured on titania (Ra = 40 nm) also induced larger cell-spreading and higher cell numbers (viability) than surface with higher roughness (Ra = 100–170 nm) (Vandrovcova *et al.*, 2010). Enhanced cell performance on nanophase materials was attributed to the higher number of surface atoms, surface defects and grain boundaries (Webster, 2004), which in turn have been shown to influence initial protein adsorption in terms of concentration, conformation and bioactivity, the factors that trigger and control cell adhesion and proliferation (Webster *et al.*, 2000a,b).

Regarding the NSD coating, which is a nanocrystalline material, composed of agglomerated nanocrystals embedded in amorphous carbon matrix having topographical features (roughness and grain size) in nanoscale, the same nanofeatures can be extrapolated from nanophase ceramics. The quantitative increase in the total length of grain boundaries and total number of pores between surface particles of NSD provide very high surface area-to-volume ratio compared with micron-structured diamond surfaces. Therefore, cell culture on NSD grains exposes cells to an increased number of grain boundaries favouring a positive cell behaviour. Among nanocrystalline diamond surfaces created with identical grain size (200 nm), but with nano-roughness (RMS=20 nm), nano/micro-roughness (RMS=270 nm) and micro-roughness (RMS=500 nm), the nano-rough surface of 20 nm provided the best results for the initial adhesion of SaOS-2 cells, for metabolic activity, for osteogenic differentiation and biomineralization (Kalbacova *et al.*, 2009). However, in an early study, Bacakova *et al.* (2007) reported that the best osteoblast proliferation could be on diamond with combined micro- and nano-structured features compared to NCD and polystyrene (PS) plates. A search for the optimum roughness for a better bone fixation on diamond surface concluded that nanocrystalline diamond (ND) with grain sizes <100 nm and roughness <20 nm promoted osteoblast functions, that could be due to its similarity to the topography of a real bone surface (Kalbacova *et al.*, 2009), whereas microcrystalline diamond (MD) with larger grain sizes (200 nm to 2 μm) prohibited these osteoblast functions (Yang *et al.*, 2009b).

5.4.2 Effect of terminal functional groups and surface wettability

CVD deposited NSD is usually hydrogen terminated, which makes the surface hydrophobic with contact angles of 85–95° range (Clem *et al.*, 2008, Lechleitner *et al.*, 2008, Yang *et al.*, 2009b). Inducing oxygen terminal-functionalities on as-deposited NSD could render the surface highly hydrophilic with a contact angle as low as 2° (Clem *et al.*, 2008). Oxygen plasma treatment was expected to enhance cell adhesion on nanodiamond films and several studies have confirmed this rationale (Kalbacova *et al.*, 2009, Lechleitner *et al.*, 2008, Kloss *et al.*, 2008b).

However, depending on the phenotype characteristics of cells used for the NSD interaction studies, mixed reports are found in literature. In a study, Lechleitner *et al.* (Lechleitner *et al.*, 2008) reported that hydrogen-terminated NCD (hydrophobic) inhibited renal epithelial cell (HK-2 cell line) attachment but oxygen-terminated NCD (hydrophilic) improved HK-2 cell attachment and proliferation compared to borosilicate glass. According to the authors, this selective inhibition could be due to the lack of functional polar groups or interaction sites which prevent adherent cells from setting on the surface whether nanostructured or not. Hydrophilic O-terminated NCD on the other hand, appears to offer a multitude of interaction sites for polar and ionic components of the cell culture medium and subsequently favour the attachment of cells. Immobilization of BMP-2 on O-terminated nanocrystalline diamond followed by *in vitro* studies using primary human mesenchymal stromal cells and subsequent bone formation *in vivo* by implanting into sheep calvaria confirmed this fact (Kloss *et al.*, 2008b).

Our studies (Clem *et al.*, 2008) performed on the mesenchymal cell cultures on the surface of USND (RMS=5 nm) with terminal functional group such as H-terminal hydrophobic USND, F-terminated hydrophobic USND and O-terminated hydrophilic USND, revealed that MSC adhesion and proliferation favoured on H-terminated NSD but not on F-terminated or O-terminated NSD (Fig. 5.9). At shorter time (1 hour), numerous cells had adhered to the H-terminated samples and the cells had adopted a well-spread morphology, with pseudopodia extending randomly along the biomaterial surface (Fig. 5.10). In contrast, no cells attached to the F-terminated samples and a limited number of very rounded cells were observed on O-terminated NCD (Clem *et al.*, 2008). At longer culture times, both O-terminated or F-terminated USND surfaces have been found to fully inhibit cell adhesion, whereas the H-terminated USND surfaces consistently supported adhesion and spreading of MSCs up to 14 days wherein a confluent layer had covered the surface, indicating that the MSCs were proliferating (Fig. 5.11).

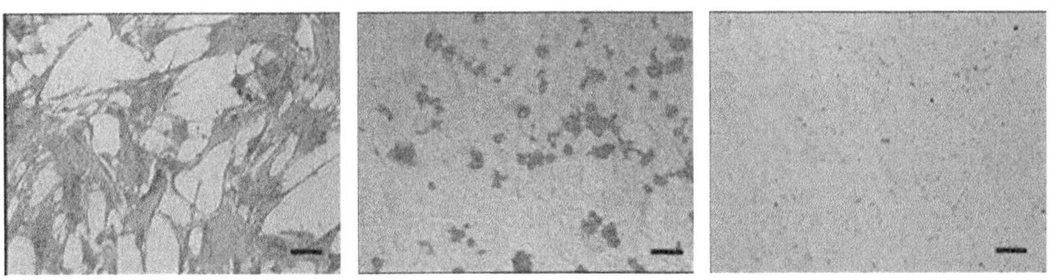

(a) (b) (c)

5.9 Reflected light microscopy images demonstrating the morphology of MSCs cultured in serum-free DMEM for 1 hour on (a) H-terminated USND, (b) O-terminated USND and (c) F-terminated USND. The cells readily attach to the H-terminated surface, whereas adhesion is very weak to the O-terminated or F-terminated surfaces. Scale bar = 100 μm. Clem *et al. Biomaterials* 29 (2008) 3461–3468 © Elsevier 2008.

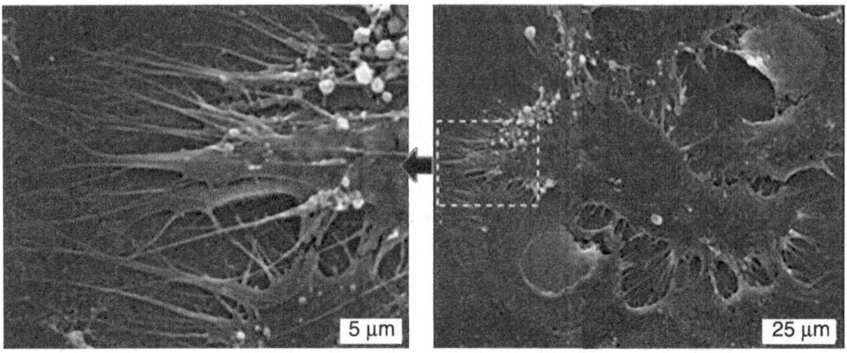

5.10 SEM images of MSCs cultured for 24 hours on H-terminated USND. The image on the left shows a higher magnification of the area indicated in the right image. The cells adopt a spread morphology and extend many pseudopodia along the surface. Reprinted with permission from Clem *et al. Biomaterials* 29 (2008) 3461–3468 © Elsevier 2008.

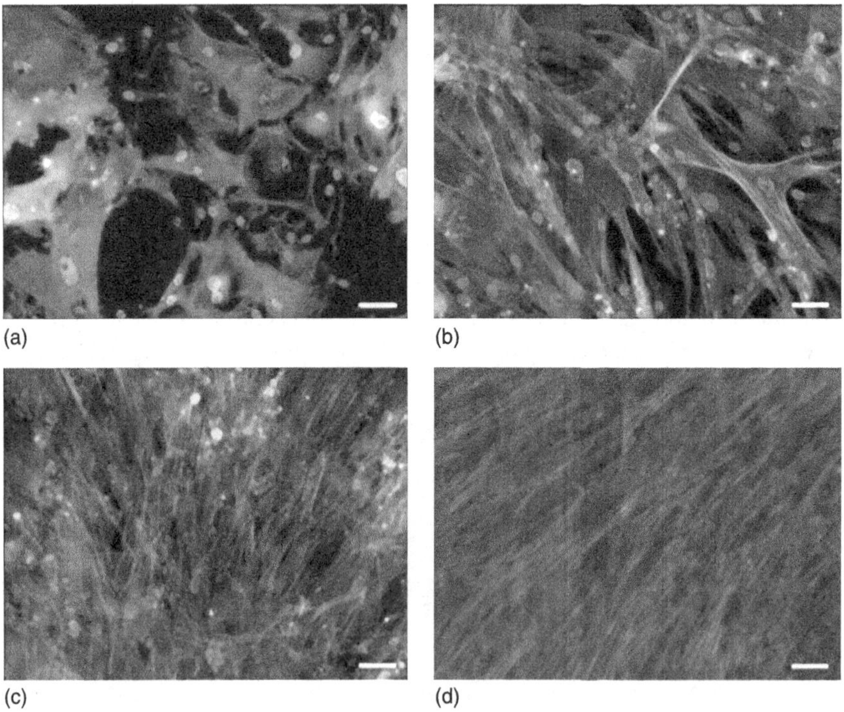

5.11 Fluorescent images showing morphology of MSCs cultured for up to 2 weeks on H-terminated USND coatings. The cells were cultured on a USND surface for (a) 3 hours, (b) 24 hours, (c) 7 days, and (d) 14 days. MSCs readily attach, spread, and eventually form a confluent layer on this surface. Scale bar = 50 µm. Reprinted with permission from Clem *et al. Biomaterials* 29 (2008) 3461–3468 © Elsevier 2008.

The mechanism underlying the high degree of MSC adhesion to H-terminated, but not F- or O-terminated USND is not clear yet. It is known that cell adhesion is optimum on moderately hydrophilic surfaces. Highly hydrophilic substrates bind the cell adhesion mediating proteins with relatively weak forces (Bacakova *et al.*, 2008), which can lead to the detachment of these proteins at a longer culture time. Another possibility may relate to the intrinsic surface conductive properties of H-terminated surfaces. The opposite cell material behaviour of two H-terminated nanodiamond surfaces with more less similar contact angles (86° and 90°) indicates that surface wettability alone is inadequate to explain the cell responses on NSD and that the role of other surface properties (such as surface atoms ratio, grain size etc.) on the regulation of cells needs to be considered. Yang *et al.* (Yang *et al.*, 2009a) have also compared the osteoblast cell functions on H-terminated nanocrystalline diamond (NCD) with grain sizes between 30 and 100 nm and submicron grain size 100 and 600 nm (SMCD) having similar wettability (92–98° contact angles). Osteoblastic short-term functions (such as adhesion and proliferation) and long-term functions (ALP activity, collagen synthesis and extra cellular calcium deposition) were found to be enhanced significantly on relatively smooth NCD (RMS roughness =~20 nm) than on SMCD with rough diamond surface (RMS=60 nm). SEM imaging (Fig. 5.12) of the osteoblast filopodia protrusions on NCD and SMCD revealed that filopodia on NCD spread randomly, indicating a greater number of focal contact sites on surface via optimal protein interactions, whereas many filopodia converged on minimal site on SMCD, indicating only a few protein binding sites on the surface (Yang *et al.*, 2009a). It is asserted that two adhesive sites with proper receptors on adjacent grains with a separation greater than 73 nm might limit osteoblast spreading and subsequent proliferation, as reported by Arnold *et al.* (Arnold *et al.*, 2004). However, it is noteworthy that hydrophobic H-terminated NCD exhibited favourable long-term osteoblast functions comparable or better than those of hydrophilic Bioglass (contact angle ~38°) and silicon surface (contact angle ~32°) as observed in Fig. 5.13 (Yang *et al.*, 2009a). In a recent study Pareta *et al.* (Pareta *et al.*, 2010) showed that among the H_2, O_2 and NH_3^- plasma treated NCD, enhanced osteoblast adhesion was observed on NH_3^- plasma treated NCD. Further systematic studies might be useful to elucidate the extent to which both surface chemistry and wettability play a role in cell adhesion and growth in the case of mesenchymal stem cells.

5.4.3 Effect of electric conductivity of surface

Electric properties (electric charge, potential and conductivity) have been reported to favour positively on the cell performance even without additional electrical stimulation in the case of neural cells, cardiac myoblasts and bone cells also. H-terminated CVD diamond surface posses p-type surface conductivity and show negative electron affinity (Pakes *et al.*, 2007). The p-type electrical conductivity of NCD films can be further improved by boron doping (Gajewski *et al.*, 2009). Only a couple of studies reported the influence of boron doped NCD films on the

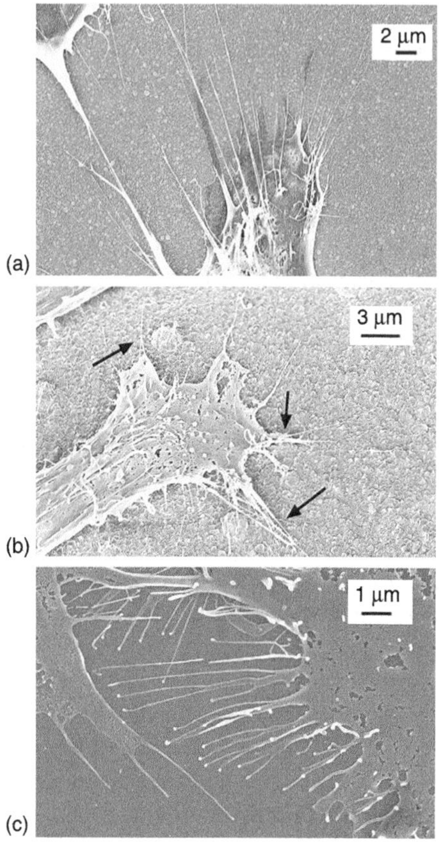

5.12 Osteoblast filopodia extensions on NCO (a), SMCD (b) and Si (c) after 48h of culture. The arrows in (b) indicate filopodia extensions converging to some spots on the diamond surfaces. Osteoblast seeding density was 10000 cells/cm^2. Reprinted from *Biomaterials, 30,* The impact of diamond nanocrystallinity on osteoblast functions, 3463, Yang, L., Sheldon, B. W. and Webster, T. J., Copyright (2009), with permission from Elsevier.

adhesion, growth, differentiation and functions of osteoblasts (Grausova *et al.*, 2011, Kopecek *et al.*, 2008). Human osteoblast-like MG 63 cells cultured on NCD with varying concentrations of boron (133, 1000 and 6700 ppm) indicated that the highest number of cells were obtained on NCD with low and medium boron concentrations (Grausova *et al.*, 2011). However, NCD films with the highest boron concentration (6700 ppm) indicated signs of increased cell matrix adhesion (manifested by the highest concentration of focal adhesion protein vinculin and increased adsorption of collagen I) and also osteogenic differentiation (suggested by a higher concentration of osteocalcin and ALP). The relatively low proliferation activity of cells on the samples of highest boron concentration was attributed, in

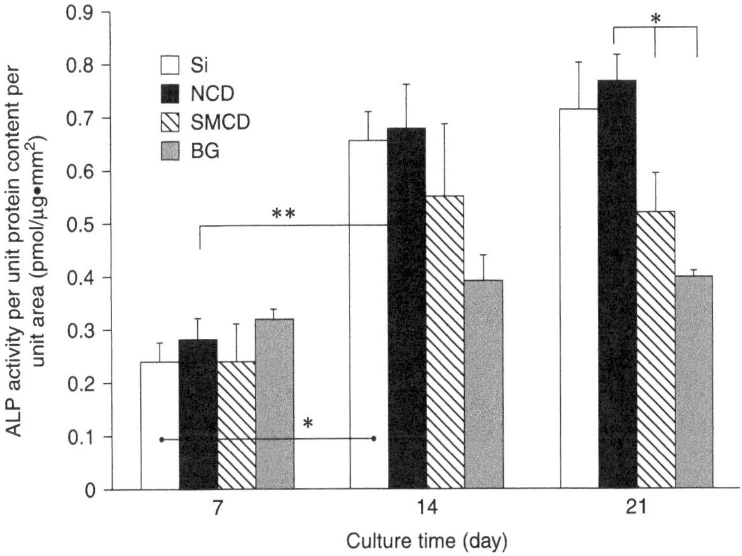

5.13 Alkaline phosphatase (ALP) activity of osteoblasts on NCD, SMCD, Si and borosilicate glass (BG) after 7, 14 and 21 days. Data were expressed as mean ± standard deviation of the mean (n = 9). *$p < 0.01$ and **$p < 0.05$. Osteoblast seeding density was 100000 cells/cm^2. Reprinted from *Biomaterials, 30,* The impact of diamond nanocrystallinity on osteoblast functions, 3463, Yang, L., Sheldon, B. W. and Webster, T. J., Copyright (2009), with permission from Elsevier.

part, to the higher amount of sp^2 bonded carbon (graphite or amorphous carbon) and to the relatively higher hydrophilicity of the surface (water contact angle = 13°) (Grausova *et al.*, 2011). Although not well understood, these studies support the fact that p-type electric conductivity influences the cell attachment, growth and differentiation on the NSD surface.

5.4.4 Effect of orthopaedic substrate chemistry

A comparative study (Clem *et al.*, 2008) of MSC attachment and growth to H-terminated USND coated surface and known orthopaedic implant surfaces such as CoCrMo and Ti-6Al-4V revealed that USND supported greater cell adhesion than CoCrMo, although less than Ti-6Al-4V (Fig. 5.14). Subsequent quantification of cell proliferation by MTT assay at 3–7 days indicated that MSCs exhibited a similar degree of proliferation on USND and Ti-6Al-4V (Fig. 5.15). A recent study by Pareta *et al.* (Pareta *et al.*, 2010) revealed similar levels of osteoblast adhesion on H-terminated NCD-coated titanium and uncoated titanium with an osteoblast adhesion efficiency between 30% and 40% after 4 hours of culture. In contrast, reduced cell number on CoCrMo may reflect a slower rate of proliferation, reduced cell survival on CoCrMo or both (Clem *et al.*, 2008). Attachment and

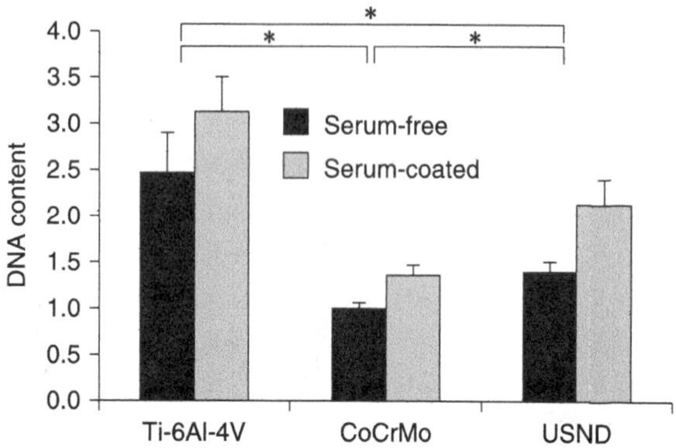

5.14 Quantitative analysis of MSC adhesion to H-terminated USND, Ti-6Al-4V and CoCrMo. Prior to cell seeding, the surfaces were either pre-coated with serum (FBS) or left uncoated. Cells were cultured for 90 minutes, followed by mechanical agitation to remove loosely bound MSCs. Remaining attached cells were quantified by assay for DNA content. Adhesion of MSCs to USND was found to be intermediate between that of Ti-6Al-4V and CoCrMo, in both serum-free conditions and in the presence of serum. * denotes $p < 0.05$. Reprinted with permission from Clem *et al.*, *Biomaterials* 29 (2008) 3461–3468 © Elsevier 2008.

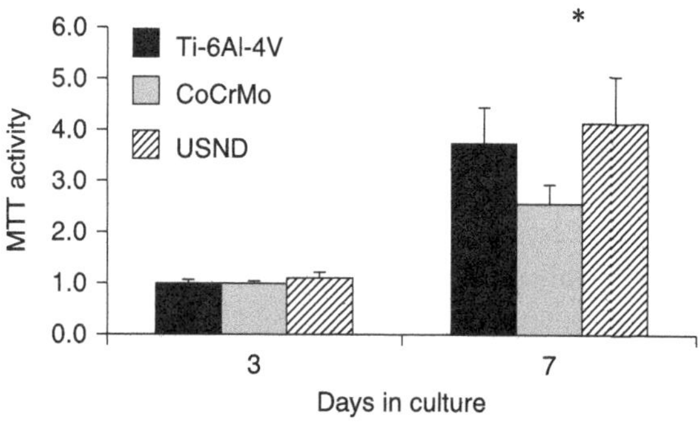

5.15 Proliferation assay to assess potential long-term effects of exposure to USND on cell behaviour. A small number of MSCs were seeded onto H-terminated USND, Ti-6Al-4V, or CoCrMo and cultured for up to **one** week. The number of viable cells was quantified at days 3 and 7 by an MTT assay. Cell proliferation on USND was not significantly different from Ti-6Al-4V, but was greater than that observed for cells grown on CoCrMo. * denotes $p < 0.05$. Reprinted with permission from Clem *et al.*, *Biomaterials* 29 (2008) 3461–3468 © Elsevier 2008.

proliferation of MSCs to the surface of the biomaterial are critical steps in the osseointegration of an implant. Cellular response to biomaterials depends initially on the interaction of adhesion receptors with proteins adsorbed to the surface. Adsorbed proteins can be detected on biomaterials within a second of exposure to the blood, and a monolayer of adsorbed proteins forms in seconds to minutes (Raffaini and Ganazzoli, 2007). Fibronectin, vitronectin and fibrinogen are pro-adhesive proteins that are recognized by various cellular integrins and platelet receptors, and play an important role in the initial recruitment of cells to the implant surface. Surface properties (surface energy, charge, chemistry, topography and wettability) influence greatly the protein adsorption and subsequent confirmation. Ideally, the proteins should adsorb in a confirmation that allows for the pro-adhesive motifs, such as RGD, to be accessible by MSC or osteoblastic integrins.

Ultimately, firm fixation of an orthopaedic implant depends on deposition of mineralized matrix directly on the surface of the implant by osteoblasts. For osseointegration of an implant, the implant surface should not only support the attachment and proliferation of MSCs, but also favour the differentiation of stem cells along an osteoblastic lineage (bone forming cells). Our studies (Clem *et al.*, 2008) by quantification of calcium content for the MSC cultured on H-terminated NCD surface, cobalt chrome and titanium alloy (under osteogenic condition, OS+) showed that similar amounts of mineralized matrix were deposited by the cells onto USND and cobalt chrome, whereas a slight increase in mineral deposition was observed for titanium alloy (Fig. 5.16). Processes of osteoblastic differentiation and matrix mineralization occurring readily on USND coatings is an indicator for osseointegration necessary for anchoring regions of bone implants.

5.5 Macrophage cell interactions to diamond wear debris

As mentioned previously, wearing of joint-implants and the generation of wear-debris particles can lead to mechanical instability, decreased joint mobility, increased pain, deleterious biological responses, osteolysis and ultimately component loosening and implant failure (Mercuri, 2000b, Maloney and Smith, 1995, Bauer, 2002, Wang *et al.*, 2004, Archibeck *et al.*, 2001, Purdue *et al.*, 2007, Aspenberg, 1996). Macrophages are the primary scavengers of wear debris particles and their response appears to depend on the nature, size and concentration of particles accumulated. Large debris pieces are normally sequestered by fibrous tissue, whereas small debris is phagocytosed by macrophages and multinucleated giant cells. Phagocytic cells engulf wear debris and become activated, releasing pro-inflammatory cytokines, degradative enzymes and other factors that stimulate osteoclasts (Ingham and Fisher, 2005, Glant *et al.*, 1993, Merkel *et al.*, 1999) at the bone implant interface and the bone resorption around the implant.

Regarding NSD-coated implants; the brittleness/delamination of a thin diamond coating may lead to the formation wear debris of nanodiamonds from diamond-

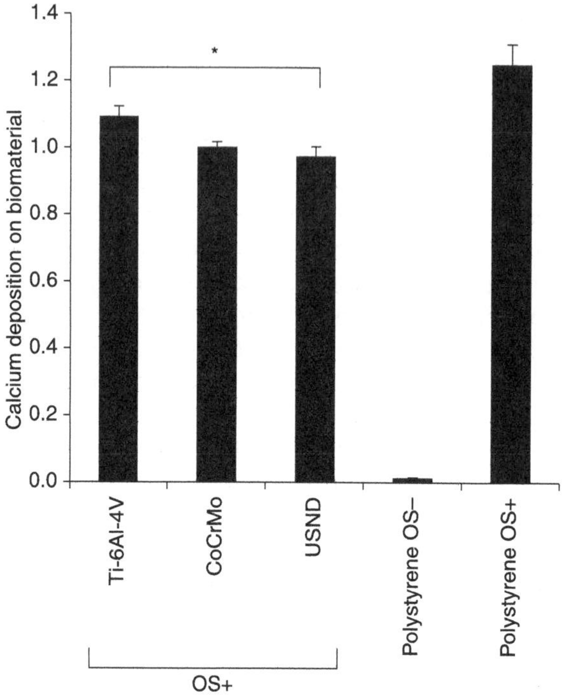

5.16 Analysis of mineralized matrix deposited on H-terminated USND, Ti-6Al-4V and CoCrMo. Osteoblastic differentiation of MSCs adherent to the metal substrates was induced by culture for four weeks in an osteogenic medium (OSp). The cells were allowed to deposit mineral on the biomaterial surfaces, and then the calcium content was quantified at week 4. Cells were also cultured on tissue culture plastic in osteogenic media (OSp, positive control) or in normal growth media (OS negative control). Slightly more mineral was deposited on Ti-6Al-4V than USND, but the difference in mineral deposition between USND and CoCrMo surfaces was not significant. * denotes $p < 0.05$. Reprinted with permission from Clem *et. al.*, *Biomaterials* 29 (2008) 3461–3468 © Elsevier 2008.

on-diamond and diamond-on-polyethylene couples. In a hip simulator study (Lappalainen *et al.*, 2003), diamond–diamond couples have shown a huge reduction in wear debris volume ($<10^{-4}$ mm^3/year), compared to first-generation CoCrMo–CoCrMo couples (1–5 mm^3/year) and to couples using polyethylene (50–100 mm^3/year). The reduced wear volume and particle size expected for diamond articulation is a major advantage over conventional orthopaedic bearings. Similarly the average particle size of debris produced from a diamond-on-diamond and diamond couple is expected to be considerably smaller than polyethylene debris due to its superior hardness, smoothness and wear-resistant properties. However, a very low wear volume itself is not the only key factor governing the long-term clinical outcome of a total joint replacement. The number, size or morphology and biological response to any wear particles released are also important. In addition, there exists considerable discussion over the possible distribution of these smaller nanoparticles in the body, and their biological effects on cells and tissues. A few studies have reported the cytocompatibility of detonation nanodiamond particles (2–10 nm) from a standpoint of cell viability using MTT assay and ATP production or reactive oxygen species (ROS) measurement with different cell types, including macrophages (Schrand *et al.*, 2007, Huang *et al.*, 2008). A variety of cells of other phenotypes, such as neuroblastoma cells, keratinocytes, macrophages and pheochromocytoma P12 cells, in cultures on NCD films or exposed to diamond nanoparticle suspensions (concentration of 5–100 mg/mL of the culture media), also retained their typical morphology, metabolic activity and viability (Schrand *et al.*, 2007). Moreover, diamond nanoparticles were found to generate no significant amount of ROS (Schrand *et al.*, 2007). In cultures of HeLa cells, micro sized diamond crystals (diameter approximately 1 μg/mL, concentration ≥1 μm/mL) caused considerable stress to the cells and attenuated their growth and viability, whereas nanodiamond crystals (diameter ~2 nm) showed no harmful effects in comparable concentrations (Fucikova *et al.*, 2009).

Activated macrophages generally release inflammatory cytokines and chemokines including bone-resorbing factors such as tumour necrosis factor α (TNFα), interleukin (IL-6 and IL1), inducible nitric oxide synthetase (iNOs) etc., in response to increasing concentration of the wear debris (for a recent review, see Goodman and Ma, 2010). Huang *et al.* have reported no significant variation in the *m*RNA levels for TNFα, IL-6 and iNOS genes due to the exposure of detonation nanodiamond particles (2–8 nm) at a relatively low concentration of 30 μg/mL (Huang *et al.*, 2008). In an objective to evaluate systematically the effect of size (6–500 nm) of synthetic nanodiamond particles as potential wear debris from diamond on diamond couples on cell toxicity, apoptosis and pro-inflammatory cytokine gene expression, we have recently cultured RAW 264.7 macrophage cells in a medium containing free-floating diamond particles (10–200 μg/mL) (Thomas *et al.*, 2012). Figure 5.17 illustrates that cells both with and without the addition of ND solutions grew healthily, with no noticeable cell morphology difference. However, more elongated cells can be seen in PBS and in wells of low concentration particles (20 μg/mL) than wells of 70 μg/mL where they displayed a rounded morphology whether they had consumed particles or not. A reduction of relative mRNA levels was found for genes such as TNF-α, IL-1β, Cxcl2, Ccl2, VEGF and PDGF with the introduction of nanodiamonds (50 μg/mL) in culture medium (Thomas *et al.*, 2012). But, apoptosis and necrosis (downstream events in response to cytotoxic stimuli) showed reduction in cell viability with a pronounced effect with smaller particles (6 and 60 nm). This data were in agreement with the results obtained in BrdU assay by measuring the cells that are actively replicating their DNA (Thomas *et al.*, 2012). This could be due to the increased number of

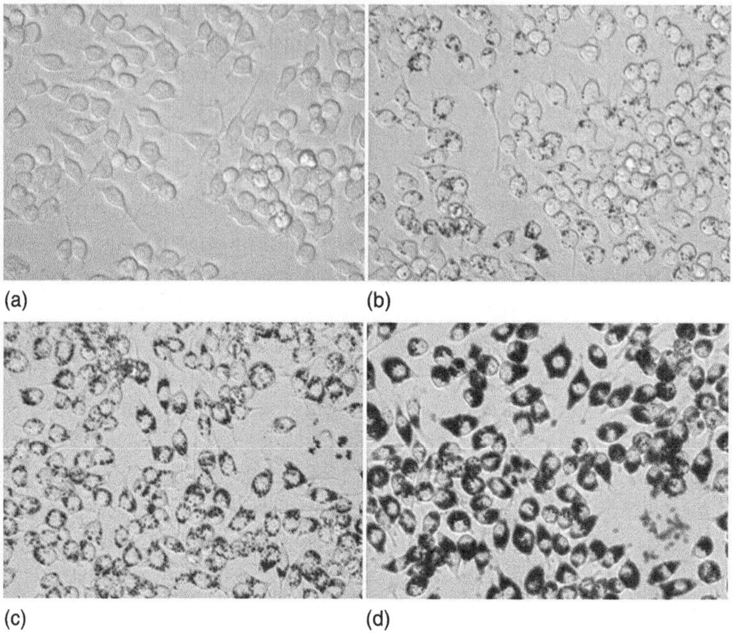

5.17 Optical micrographs (400×) of free-floating nanodiamond particles (2–10 nm) of varying concentrations cultured with macrophage cells for 24 hours; macrophage cells without diamond particles (a) and cells with diamond particles of 10 μg/mL (b),100 μg/mL (c), and 200 μg/mL (d).

particles with the size reduction at a constant concentration (50 μg/mL) and huge surface area of nanoparticles when size is reduced to 100 nm and below. A comparable *in vitro* study using stainless steel particles with the RAW 264.7 cell line reported upregulation of both TNF-α and IL-1β with a significant number of late apoptotic cells (Bailey *et al.*, 2005).

The translational potential of the NSD-coated implants is in a large way determined by their biocompatibility and bio-performance (wear resistance of articulating surface and osteointegration of the rest). Failure or loosening of joint replacement components is often multifactorial (Revel, 2008). Among them, an important factor is wear debris and its response to macrophage mediated osteolysis, which can potentially occur in any implant system regardless of implant design or fixation mode. For this reason, the reduction of wear debris should be a primary goal of orthopaedic research. Although NSD coating can improve the smoothness and wear characteristics of metallic components of total hip replacements and increase their longevity, *in vivo* response of macrophage cells to the possible nanodiamond wear debris and the fate of phagocytosed nanodiamond (nanotoxicology) are not well understood and future translational research must be focused on these aspects.

5.6 *In vivo* evaluation of nanostructured diamond surfaces

Although the biocompatibility of DLC coatings has been well established through numerous studies (for a comprehensive review, see Dearnaley and Arps, 2005), a thorough *in vivo* evaluation of NSD coatings is lacking. Work by Kloss *et al.* (Kloss *et al.*, 2008a) demonstrated that coating of endosseous implants with nanocrystalline diamond allows stable functionalization by means of physisorption with BMP-2. Strong physisorption was shown to be directly related to the unique properties of NCD, and BMP-2 in its active form interacted strongly when NCD was oxygen-terminated. Implant surfaces refined in such a manner yielded enhanced osseointegration *in vivo*, when inserted into sheep calvaria.

In another study, initial *in vivo* biocompatibility profiles showed evidence that bone integration with NSD may be comparable with Ti-6Al-4V, observed from staining of bone on the diamond surface. In this study (Lemons *et al.*, 2003), the distal femoral and proximal tibial bone regions of four New Zealand white rabbits were aseptically implanted with 8 mm diameter by 2 mm thick discs (one side alloy, one side NSD-coated). Specimens were followed clinically and radiographically and examined macroscopically during euthanization at times to 8 weeks. Non-decalcified transversely oriented twin sections (five per disc) were prepared with an Exakt system; specimens were stained and examined by optical microscopy. All specimens showed trabecular and compact bone directly associated with the alloy (Ti-6AI-4V) and diamond surfaces (biointegration), with no foreign body reactions and no abnormal characteristics within the marrow-bone spaces. It was concluded that the NSD coatings were similar macro- and microscopically to titanium alloy with respect to general and histological biocompatibility. The results, shown in Fig. 5.18, were consistent throughout the retrieved samples, indicating that NSD appears to be biocompatible and can perform well in applications where bone integration is needed.

5.7 Future trends

From a clinical perspective, the superior wear characteristics of NSD on metal prostheses may allow for a hard-on-hard approach of implant design providing a less invasive surgical procedure. In the current market the industry standard for orthopaedic and dental total joint replacement involves articulation of UHMWPE against a cobalt-chromium alloy. The UHMWPE component requires considerable thickness to stand up to the articular loads. In the case of the temporomandibular joint, for example, a hard-on-hard device (metal-on-metal device with NSD coatings on articular surfaces) engineered to be of sufficient rigidity to allow for a thin design of the fossa and condyle would allow for significant advantages: 1) allow for more minimally invasive surgery through a single incision; 2) allow for a more nature articulating position; 3) maintain normal structures such as the

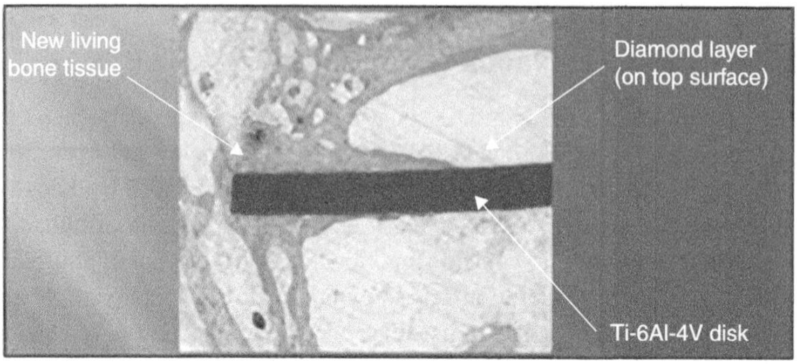

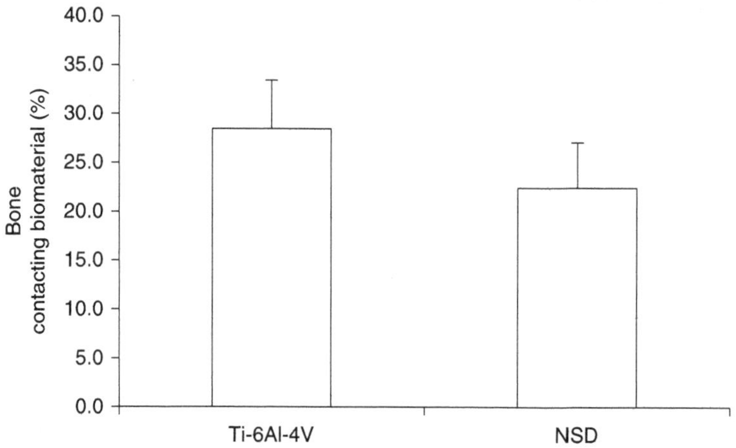

5.18 Results of *in vivo* studies for NSD-coated Ti-6Al-4V disc implanted into the leg bone of New Zealand white rabbits showing comparable bone coverage against uncoated Ti-6Al-4V control (top) and showing excellent biocompatibility (bottom).

condyle and muscle attachments, maintaining normal muscle function; 4) the smaller design of the prosthesis with smaller surface area could result in a lower risk of infection; and 5) salvage procedures, if necessary, would be simpler to perform due to more native tissue being left in place.

Localized and 'on-demand' or prolonged drug delivery is also a priority for clinical research in implant devices. Electrochemical anodization of titanium has been used to create a layer of ordered titania nanotubes (inner diameters less than 100 nm), which mimic the size and pattern of components of natural bone. Anodized titanium possessing nanotubular structures may be ideal drug storage matrices to locally deliver a wide range of drugs after implantation. Possible candidates for drugs to be delivered from nanotubular anodized titanium include those to fight infection, decrease inflammation and promote bone cell functions. The on-demand release of drugs could be triggered by local sonication near the implant site.

Infusion of orthopaedic and dental materials with therapeutics, including antioxidants and antimicrobials is gaining more widespread acceptance in the marketplace. For example, the polyethylene used in orthopaedic devices has recently undergone new technology by infusion of vitamin E, a naturally occurring antioxidant that can stabilize the free radicals that would otherwise lead to polyethylene oxidation and accelerated wear. Carbon-based nanomaterials also have potential as drug-carriers or free-radical scavengers. Fullerenes, for example, are believed to be extremely efficient antioxidants and are being investigated for biological applications. Fullerene-C_{60} is a non-toxic antioxidant 100–1000 times more active than vitamin E. Although C_{60} itself is not at all water soluble, many highly water soluble fullerene derivatives have now been prepared. Ultimately, it seems, nanoscale science and engineering for medical device development is relying more and more on the integration of structure, mechanical and biochemical functionality in its design. In this way, we hope to provide implant devices that are inherently less intrusive, longer lasting and more effective in fighting disease and infection.

5.8 Acknowledgements

The authors acknowledge support by Award Number R01AR056665 from the National Institute of Arthritis and Musculoskeletal and Skin Diseases. The content is solely the responsibility of the authors and does not necessarily represent the official views of the National Institute of Arthritis and Musculoskeletal and Skin Diseases or the National Institutes of Health.

5.9 References

Affatato, S., Frigo, M. and Toni, A. (2000) An in vitro investigation of diamond-like carbon as a femoral head coating. *J Biomed Mater Res*, 53, 221–226.

Ager, J. W., III and Drory, M. D. (1993) Quantitative measurement of residual biaxial stress by Raman spectroscopy in diamond grown on a Ti alloy by chemical vapor deposition. *Physical Review B*, 48, 2601–2607.

Amaral, M., Fdias, A. G., Gomes, P. S., *et al.* (2008) Nanocrystalline diamond: In vitro biocompatibility assessment by MG 63 and human bone marrow cells cultures. *J Biomed Mater Res A*, 87, 91–99.

Amaral, M., Gomes, P. S., Lopes, M. A., *et al.* (2009) Cytotoxicity evaluation of nanocrystalline diamond coatings by fibroblast cell cultures. *Acta Biomater*, 5, 775–763.

American Academy of Orthopaedic Surgeons. 2006 [cited; Available from: <http://www.aaos.org/>.

Amstutz, H. C., Beaule, P. E., Dorey, F. J., *et al.* (2004) Metal-on-metal hybrid surface arthroplasty: two to six-year follow-up study. *J Bone Joint Surg Am*, 86-A, 28–39.

Amstutz, H. C., Campbell, P., Kossovsky, N. and Clarke, I. C. (1992) Mechanism and clinical significance of wear debris-induced osteolysis. *Clin Orthop Relat Res*, 7–18.

Amstutz, H. C. and Grigoris, P. (1996) Metal on metal bearings in hip arthroplasty. *Clin Orthop Relat Res*, S11–34.

Anselme, K. and Bigerelle, M. (2005) Topography effects of pure titanium substrates on human osteoblast long-term adhesion. *Acta Biomater*, 1, 211–222.

Archibeck, M. J., Jacobs, J. J., Roebuck, K. A. and Glant, T. T. (2001) The basic science of periprosthetic osteolysis. *Instr Course Lect*, 50, 185–195.

Arnold, M., Calvacanti-Adam, E. A., Glass, R., *et al.* (2004) Activation of integrin function by nanopatterned adhesive interface. *Chem Phys Chem*, 5, 383–388.

Askari, S. J., Chen, G. C. and Lu, F. X. (2008) Growth of polycrystalline and nanocrystalline diamond films on pure titanium by microwave plasma assisted CVD process. *Materials Research Bulletin*, 43, 1086–1092.

Aspenberg, P. (1996) Benign response to particles of diamond and SiC: bone chamber studies of new joint replacement coating materials in rabbits. *Biomaterials*, 17, 807.

ASTM_F732–00 (2003) *Standard test method for wear testing of polymeric materials used in total joint prostheses*. Philadelphia, PA.

Atkinson, J. R., Dowson, D., Isaac, J. H. and Wroblewski, B. M. (1985) Laboratory wear tests and clinical observations of the penetration of femoral heads into acetabular cups in total replacement hip joints: III: The measurement of internal volume changes in explanted Charnley sockets after 2–16 years in vivo and the determination of wear factors. *Wear*, 104, 225–244.

Azevedo, A. F., Corat, E. J., Ferreira, N. G. and Trava-Airoldi, V. J. (2005) Wettability and corrosion tests of diamond films grown on Ti6Al4V alloy. *Surface and Coatings Technology*, 194, 271–275.

Bacakova, I., Grausova, L., Vacik, J., *et al.* (2007) Improved adhesion and growth of human osteoblast-like MG63 cells on biomaterials modified with carbon nanoparticles. *Diamond and Related Materials*, 16, 2133–2140.

Bacakova, L., Grausova, L., Vandrovcova, M., *et al.* (2008) Carbon nanoparticles as substrates for cell adhesion and growth. In Lombardi, S. L. (Ed.) *Nanoparticles: New Research*. New York, Nova Science Publishers Inc, Hauppauge.

Baek, S., Mihec, D. and Metson, J. (2003) Interfacial Properties Between CVD Diamond and Titanium. *International Journal of Modern Physics B*, 17, 1127–1133.

Bailey, L. O., Lippiatt, S., Biancanello, F. S., *et al.* (2005) The quantification of cellular viability and inflammatory response to stainless steel alloys. *Biomaterials*, 26, 5296–5302.

Bal Bs, A. T., Garino J.P., Toni A. and Hendricks K. J. (2005) Ceramic-on-ceramic versus ceramic-on-polyethylene bearings in total hip arthroplasty: Results of a multicenter prospective randomized study and update of modern ceramic total hip trials in the United States. *Hip International*, 15, 129–135.

Balasundaram, G., Sato, M. and Webster, T. J. (2006) Using hydroxyapatite nanoparticles and decreased crystallinity to promote osteoblast adhesion similar to functionalizing with RGD. *Biomaterials*, 27, 2798–2805.

Ballinger, J. and Catledge, S. A. (2011) Adhered nanostructured diamond coatings on plasma borided stainless steel, unpublished results.

Bauer, T. W. (2002) Particles and periimplant bone resorption. *Clin Orthop Relat Res*, 405, 138–143.

Beaule, P. E., Amstutz, H. C., Le Duff, M. and Dorey, F. (2004) Surface arthroplasty for osteonecrosis of the hip: hemiresurfacing versus metal-on-metal hybrid resurfacing. *J Arthroplasty*, 19, 54–58.

Bedi, R. S., Beving, D. E., Zanello, L. P. and Yan, Y. (2009) Biocompatibility of corrosion-resistant zeolite coatings for titanium alloy biomedical implants. *Acta Biomater*, 5, 3265–3271.

Black, J. (1992) *Biological Performance of Materials: fundamentals of bio-compatibility*, New York, Marcel Dekker.

bloomberg.com/news/2012-06-21/hip-implant-concerns-reached-16-800-in-a-decade-fda-says.html

Bohn, R., Haubold, R., Birringer, R. and Gleiter, H. (1991) Nanocrystalline intermetallic compounds. An approach to ductility. *Scripta Metall Mater*, 25, 811.

Booth, L., Catledge, S. A., Nolen, D., Thompson, R. G. and Vohra, Y. K. (2011) Synthesis and Characterization of Multilayered Diamond Coatings for Biomedical Implants. *Materials (Basel)*, 4, 857–867.

Bruder, S. P., Fink, D. J. and Caplan, A. I. (1994) Mesenchymal stem cells in bone development, bone repair, and skeletal regeneration therapy. *J Cell Biochem*, 56, 283–294.

Buccioni, E., Braca, E., Kenny, J. M. and Terranova, M. L. (1999) Processing-structure-adhesion relationship in CVD diamond films on titanium substrates. *Diamond and Related Materials*, 8, 17–24.

Buijnsters, J. G., Shankar, P., Fleischer, W., *et al.* (2002) CVD diamond deposition on steel using arc-plated chromium nitride interlayers. *Diamond and Related Materials*, 11, 536–544.

Buijnsters, J. G., Shankar, P., Gopalakrishnan, P., *et al.* (2003) Diffusion-modified boride interlayers for chemical vapour deposition of low-residual-stress diamond films on steel substrates. *Thin Solid Films*, 426, 85–93.

Caplan, A. I. (2005) Review: Mesenchymal Stem Cells: Cell-Based Reconstructive Therapy in Orthopedics. *Tissue Engineering*, 11, 1198–1211.

Catledge, S. (1998) High density plasma processing of nanostructured diamond films on metals. *J Appl Phys*, 84, 6469.

Catledge, S. (1999) Effect of nitrogen addition on the microstructure and mechanical properties of diamond films grown using high-methane concentrations. *J Appl Phys*, 86, 698.

Catledge, S. and Vohra, Y. (1999) Effect of nitrogen addition on the microstructure and mechanical properties of diamond films grown using high-methane concentrations. *J Appl Phys*, 86, 698.

Catledge, S. A., Fries, M. D., Vohra, Y. K., *et al.* (2002) Nanostructured ceramics for biomedical implants. *J Nanosci Nanotechnol*, 2, 293–312.

Catledge, S. A., Vaid, R., Diggins, P. T., *et al.* (2011) Improved adhesion of ultra-hard carbon films on cobalt-chromium orthopaedic implant alloy. *J Mater Sci Mater Med*, 22, 307–316.

Catledge, S. A. and Vohra, Y. K. (1995) High Density Plasma Processing of Diamond Films on Titanium: Residual Stress and Adhesion Measurements. *J Appl Phys*, 78, 7053.

Catledge, S. A., Frees, M. and Vohra, Y. K. (2004) Nanostructured Surface Modifications for Biomedical Implants. In Nalwa, H. S. (Ed.) *Encyclopedia of Nanoscience and Nanotechnology*. American Scientific Publishers.

Chen, X. and Narayan, J. (1993) Effect of the chemical nature of transition-metal substrates on chemical-vapor deposition of diamond. *J Appl Phys*, 74, 4168–4173.

Chen, Y. C., Lee, D. C., Hsiao, C. Y., *et al.* (2009) The effect of ultra nanocrystalline diamond films on the proliferation and differentiation of neural stem cells. *Biomaterials*, 30, 3428–3435.

Chowdhury, S., Borham, J., Catledge, S. A., *et al.* (2008) Synthesis and Mechanical Wear Studies of Ultra Smooth Nanostructured Diamond (USND) Coatings Deposited by Microwave Plasma Chemical Vapor Deposition with He/H(2)/CH(4)/N(2) Mixtures. *Diamond Related Materials*, 17, 419–427.

Chowdhury, S., Hillman, D. A., Catledge, S. A., *et al.* (2006) Synthesis of ultrasmooth nanostructured diamond films by microwave plasma chemical vapor deposition using a He/H2/CH4/N2 gas mixture. *Journal of Material Research*, 21, 2675–2682.

Clem, W. C., Chowdhury, S., Catledge, S. A., *et al.* (2008) Mesenchymal stem cell interaction with ultra-smooth nanostructured diamond for wear-resistant orthopaedic implants. *Biomaterials*, 29, 3461–3468.

Corvin, R. (2002) Gas-phase thermodynamic models of nitrogen-induced nanocrystallinity in chemical vapor-deposited diamond. *Appl Phys Lett*, 80, 2550.

Cuckler, J. M. (2005) The rationale for metal-on-metal total hip arthroplasty. *Clin Orthop Relat Res*, 441, 132–136.

Davis, R. F. (1993) *Diamond Films and Coatings*, New Jersey, Noyes Publications.

De-Oliveiera, P. T. and Nanci, A. (2004) Nanotexturing of titanium-based surfaces upregulates expression of bone sialoprotein and osteopontin by cultured osteogenic cells. *Biomaterials*, 25, 403–413.

De-Oliveira, P. T., Zalzal, S. F., Beloti, M. M., *et al.* (2007) Enhancement of in vitro osteogenesis on titanium by chemically produced nanotopography. *J Biomed Mater Res A*, 80, 554–564.

Deans, R. J. and Moseley, A. B. (2000) Mesenchymal stem cells: Biology and potential clinical uses. *Experimental Hematology*, 28, 875–884.

Dearnaley, G. and Arps, J. H. (2005) Biomedical applications of diamond-like carbon (DLC) coatings: A review. *Surface and Coatings Technology*, 200, 2518–2524.

Dementjev, A. P. and Petukhov, M. N. (1998) The role of oxygen atoms in sp2-sp3 conversion on the growing surface of carbon film. In Gielisse, P. J., Ivanov-Omskii, V. I., Popovici, G. and Prelas, M. (Eds.) *Diamond and Diamond-Like Film Applications*. Lancaster, PA, Technomic Publishing Company, Inc.

Drory, M. D. and Hutchinson, J. W. (1994) Diamond Coating of Titanium Alloys. *Science*, 263, 1753–1755.

Fayer, A., Glozman, O. and Hoffman, A. (1995) *Deposition of continuous and well adhering diamond films on steel*, AIP.

FDA Gaithersburg, Maryland Executive Summary Memorandum: *Metal-on-metal hip implant systems* (Prepared for the June 27–28, 2012 Meeting of the Orthopaedic and Rehabilitation Devices Advisory Panel)

Ferrari, A. and Robertson, J. (1999) Raman Signature of Bonding and Disorder in Carbons. *MRS Proceedings*, 593, 299.

Fricka, K. B., Ho, H., Peace, W. J. and Engh, Jr, C. A. (2012) Metal-on-metal local tissue reaction is associated with corrosion of the head taper junction. *J Arthroplasty*, 27, 26–31.e21

Friedmann, T. A., Sullivan, J. P., Knapp, J. A., *et al.* (1997) *Thick stress-free amorphous-tetrahedral carbon films with hardness near that of diamond*, AIP.

Fu, Y., Du, H. and Sun, C. Q. (2003) Interfacial structure, residual stress and adhesion of diamond coatings deposited on titanium. *Thin Solid Films*, 424, 107–114.

Fucikova, A., Valenta, J., Pelant, I. and Brezina, V. (2009) Novel use of silicon nanocrystals and nanodiamonds in biology. *Chem Pap*, 63, 704–708.

Galvin, A.L., Tipper, I.L., Jennings, L.M., *et al.* (2007) Wear and biological activity of highly crosslinked polyethylene in the hip under low serum protein concentrations. *Proceedings of the Institution of Mechanical Engineers. Part H, Engineering in Medicine.*

Gajewski, W., Achatz, P., Williams, O. A., *et al.* (2009) Electronic and optical properties of boron-doped nanocrystalline diamond films. *Phys Rev B*, 79, 045206.

Giancotti, F. G. (1999) Integrin Signaling. *Science*, 285, 1028–1033.

Glant, T. T., Jacobs, J. J., Molna, R. G., *et al.* (1993) Bone resorption activity of particulate-stimulated macrophages. *J Bone Miner Res*, 8, 1071–1079.

Glyn-Jones, S., Gill, H. S., Mclardy-Smith, P. and Murray, D. W. (2004) Roentgen stereophotogrammetric analysis of the Birmingham hip resurfacing arthroplasty. A two-year study. *J Bone Joint Surg Br*, 86, 172–176.

Godbole, V. P., Narayan, R., Xu, Z., Narayan, J. and Sankar, J. (1999) Diamond films and composites on cobalt-chromium alloys. *Materials Science and Engineering B*, 58, 251–257.

Goldring, S. R., Schiller, A. L., Roelke, M., *et al.* (1983) The synovial-like membrane at the bone-cement interface in loose total hip replacements and its proposed role in bone lysis. *J Bone Joint Surg Am*, 65, 575–584.

Good, V., Ries, M., Barrack, R. L., *et al.* (2003) Reduced wear with oxidized zirconium femoral heads. *J Bone Joint Surg Am*, 85A, 105–110.

Good, V., Widding, K., Hunter, G. and Heuer, D. (2005) Oxidized zirconium: a potentially longer lasting hip implant. *Materials and Design*, 26, 618–622.

Goodman, S. B. and Ma, T. (2010) Cellular chemotaxis induced by wear particles from joint replacements. *Biomaterials*, 31, 5045–5050.

Grausova, L., Kromka, A., Burdikova, Z., *et al.* (2011) Enhanced growth and osteoblastic differentiation of human osteoblast-like cells on boron doped nanocrystalline diamond thin films. *PLos ONE,* 6, e20943. doi:10.1371/journal.pone.0020943.

Grierson, D. S., Sumant, A. V., Konicek, A. R., *et al.* (2010) *Thermal stability and rehybridization of carbon bonding in tetrahedral amorphous carbon*, AIP.

Grousova, L., Kromka, A., Bacakova, L., *et al.* (2008) Bone and vascular endothelial cells in cultures on nanocrystalline diamond films. *Diamond Relat Mater*, 17, 1405–1409.

Gutmanas, E. Y. and Gotman, I. (2004) PIRAC Ti nitride coated Ti-6Al-4V head against UHMWPE acetabular cup-hip wear simulator study. *Journal of Materials Science-Materials in Medicine*, 15, 327–330.

Hallab, N., Merritt, K. and Jacobs, J. J. (2001) Metal sensitivity in patients with orthopaedic implants. *J Bone Joint Surg Am*, 83-A, 428–436.

Hendry, J. A. and Pilliar, R. M. (2001) The fretting corrosion resistance of PVD surface-modified orthopedic implant alloys. *Journal of Biomedical Materials Research*, 58, 156–166.

Hill, M. R., Catledge, S. A., Konovalov, V., *et al.* (2008) Preliminary tribological evaluation of nanostructured diamond coatings against ultra-high molecular weight polyethylene. *J Biomed Mater Res B Appl Biomater*, 85, 140–8.

Huang, H., Pierstorff, E., Osawa, E. and Ho, D. (2008) Protein-Mediated Assembly of Nanodiamond Hydrogels into a Biocompatible and Biofunctional Multilayer Nanofilm. *ACS Nano*, 2, 203–212.

Ingham, E. and Fisher, J. (2005) The role of macrophages in osteolysis of total joint replacement. *Biomaterials*, 26, 1271–86.

Innocenti, M., Civinini, R., Carulli, C., *et al.* (2010) The 5-year Results of an Oxidized Zirconium Femoral Component for TKA. *Clinical Orthopaedics and Related Research*, 468, 1258–1263.

Jin, S. (1994) Effect of nitrogen on the growth of diamond films. *Appl Phys Lett*, 65, 403.

Jones, V. C., Barton, D. C., Auger, D. D. *et al.* (2001) Simulation of tibial counterface wear in mobile bearing knees with uncoated and ADLC coated surfaces. *Biomed Mater Eng*, 11, 105–115.

Jose, M. V., Thomas, V., Xu, Y., *et al.* (2010) Multifunctional aligned nanofibrous nanocomposite scaffolds of PLGA/Collagen/HA for bone tissue engineering. *Macromol Biosci*, 10, 433–444.

Kalbacova, M., Rezek, B., Baresova, V., *et al.* (2009) Nanoscale topography of nanocrystalline diamonds promotes differentiation of osteoblasts. *Acta Biomater*, 5, 3076–3085.

Kanazawa, I., Yamaguchi, T., Yano, S., *et al.* (2007) Adiponectin and AMP kinase activator stimulate proliferation, differentiation, and mineralization of osteoblastic MC3T3-E1 cells. *BMC Cell Biology*, 8, 51.

Kaplan, F. S., Hayes, W. C., Keaveny, T. M., *et al.* (1994) Form and function of bone. In: Simon S.P., (Ed.) *Orthopedic Basic Science.* Columbus, OH, American Academy of Orthopedic Surgeons.

Kay, S., Thapa, A., Haberstroh, K. M. and Webster, T. J. (2002) Nanostructured polymer/nanophase ceramic composites enhance osteoblast and chondrocyte adhesion. *Tissue Eng*, 8, 753–761.

Kilpadi, K. L., Sawyer, A. A., Prince, C. W., *et al.* (2004) Primary human marrow stromal cells and Saos-2 osteosarcoma cells use different mechanisms to adhere to hydroxylapatite. *J Biomed Mater Res A*, 68, 273–285.

Kloss, F. R., Gassner, R., Preiner, J., *et al.* (2008a) The role of oxygen termination of nanocrystalline diamond on immobilisation of BMP-2 and subsequent bone formation. *Biomaterials*, 29, 2433–2442.

Kloss, F. R., Gassner, R., Preiner, J., *et al.* (2008b) The role of oxygen termination of nanocrystalline diamond on immobilization of BMP-2 and subsequent bone formation. *Biomaterials*, 29, 2433–2442.

Kobayashi, S., Ohgoe, Y., Ozeki, K., *et al.* (2007) Dissolution effect and cytotoxicity of diamond-like carbon coatings on orthodontic archwires. *J Mater Sci Mater Med*, 18, 2263–2268.

Konovalov, V. V., Melo, A., Catledge, S. A., *et al.* (2006) Ultra-smooth nanostructured diamond films deposited from He/H2/CH4/N2 microwave plasmas. *J Nanosci Nanotechnol*, 6, 258–261.

Kopecek, M., Bacakova, L., Vacik, J., *et al.* (2008) Improved adhesion, growth and maturation of human bone-derived cells on nanocrystalline diamond films. *Phys Stat Sol (a)*, 205, 2146–2153.

Kurtz S., Lau E., Mowat F., *et al.* (2006) *The future burden of hip and knee revisions: U.S. projections from 2005 to 2030.* Paper presented at: 73rd Annual Meeting of the American Academy of Orthopaedic Surgeons: Chicago, IL.

Lappalainen, R., Anttila, A., and Heinonen, H. (1998) Diamond coated total hip replacements. *Clin Orthop Relat Res*, 118–127.

Lappalainen, R., Selenius, M., Anttila, A., *et al.* (2003) Reduction of wear in total hip replacement prostheses by amorphous diamond coatings. *Journal of Biomedical Materials Research Part B: Applied Biomaterials*, 66B, 410–413.

Lawson, T. R., Catledge, S. A. and Vohra, Y. K. (2005) Nanostructured Diamond Coated CoCrMo Alloys for Use in Biomedical Implants. *Key Engineering Materials*, 284–286, 1015.

Lechleitner, T., Klauser, F., Seppi, T., *et al.* (2008) The surface properties of nanocrystalline diamond and nanoparticulate diamond powder and their suitability as cell growth support surfaces. *Biomaterials*, 29, 4275–4284.

Lee, S.-T., Chen, S., Agostinelli, J., *et al.* (1992) Laser processing of carbon-implanted Cu, Ni, and Co crystals – An attempt to grow diamond films. *Applied Physics Letters*, 60, 2213–2215.

Lemons, J., Louis, P. J., Beck, P., *et al.* (2003) Biocompatibility of Nanostructured Diamond Surfaces for TMJ Articulation. *32nd Annual Meeting and Exhibition of the AADR*. San Antonio, TX.

Lettington, A. and Steeds, J. W. (1994) *Thin Film Diamond*. New York, Chapman and Hall, London.

Lombardi, A. V., Jr., Mallory, T. H., Cuckler, J. M., *et al.* (2004) Mid-term results of a polyethylene-free metal-on-metal articulation. *J Arthroplasty*, 19, 42–47.

Lorenz, H. P. (1995) Investigation of TiN as an interlayer for diamond deposition on steel. *Diamond and Related Materials*, 4, 1088–1092.

Maloney, W. J. and Smith, R. L. (1995) Periprosthetic osteolysis in total hip arthroplasty: The role of particulate wear debris. *J Bone Joint Surg Am*, 77, 1448–1461.

Mayo, M., Siegel, R. W., Liao, Y. X. and Nix, W. D. (1992) Nanoindentation of nanocrystalline ZnO. *Journal of Materials Research*, 7, 973.

Mayo, M., Siegel, R. W., Narayanasamy, A. and Nix, W. D. (1990) Mechanical properties of TiO_2 as determined by nanoindentation. 5, 1073.

McGovern, T. F. and Moskal, J. T. (2002) Radiographic evaluation of periprosthetic metallosis after total knee arthroplasty. *J South Orthop Assoc*, 11, 18–24.

McKellop, H., Park, S. H., Chiesa, R., *et al.* (1996) In vivo wear of three types of metal on metal hip prostheses during two decades of use. *Clin Orthop Relat Res*, S128–140.

Medley, J. B., Chan, F. W., Krygier, J. J. and Bobyn, J. D. (1996) Comparison of alloys and designs in a hip simulator study of metal on metal implants. *Clin Orthop Relat Res*, S148–159.

Mercuri, L. G. (2000a) The TMJ Concepts patient fitted Total Temporomandibular Joint Reconstruction Prosthesis in Total Temporomandibular Joint Reconstruction. *Oral and Maxillofacial Surgery Clinics of North America*, 12, 73–91.

Mercuri, L. G. (2000b) The TMJ Concepts patient fitted Total Temporomandibular Joint Reconstruction Prosthesis in Total Temporomandibular Joint Reconstruction. *Oral and Maxillofacial Surgery Clinics of North America*, 12, 73–91.

Merkel, K. D., Erdmann, J. M., Mchugh, K. P., *et al.* (1999) Tumor necrosis factor-a mediates orthopedic implant osteolysis. *Am J Pathol*, 154, 203–210.

Mishra, A. and Davidson, J. (1992) Abrasion Resistance of candidate coatings for orthopedic articulating surfaces. In Doherty, P., *et al.* (Ed.) *Advances in Biomaterials*. Amsterdam, NL, Elsevier Science publ.

Moran, C. G. and Tourret, L. J. (2001) Recent Advances: Orthopaedics. *BMJ*, 322, 902–905.

Morshed, M. M., McNamara, B. P., Cameron, D. C. and Hashmi, M. S. J. (2003) Effect of surface treatment on the adhesion of DLC film on 316L stainless steel. *Surface and Coatings Technology*, 163–164, 541–545.

Narayan, J., Godbole, V. P. and White, C. W. (1991) Laser Method for Synthesis and Processing of Continuous Diamond Films on Nondiamond Substrates. *Science*, 252, 416–418.

Narayan, R. J. (2005) Nanostructured diamondlike carbon thin films for medical applications. *Materials Science and Engineering: C*, 25, 405–416.

National Institutes of Health (1994) Total Hip Replacement. NIH Consensus Statement Online 12(5):1–31.

Negrea, G. and Vermesan, G. (2000) Investigations Of Diamond Layers Growth On Steel. *Journal of Optoelectronics and Advanced Materials*, 2, 698–703.

Ohgoe, Y., Kobayashi, S., Ozeki, K., *et al.* (2006) Reduction effect of nickel ion release on a diamond-like carbon film coated onto an orthodontic archwire *Thin solid films,* 497, 218–222.

Okumura, M., Ohgushi, H., Dohi, Y., *et al.* (1997) Osteoblastic phenotype expression on the surface of hydroxyapatite ceramics. *J Biomed Mater Res A*, 37, 122–129.

Pakes, C. I., Hoxley, D., Rubanov, S., *et al.* (2007) Work function of hydrogen terminated diamond surfaces under ion impact. *Surf Sci*, 601, 5732–5735.

Palin, E., Liu, H. and Webster, T. J. (2005) Mimicking the nanofeatures of bone increases bone-forming cell adhesion and proliferation. *Nanotechnology*, 16, 1828–1835.

Papo, M. J., Catledge, S. A., Vohra, Y. K. and Machado, C. (2004) Mechanical wear behavior of nanocrystalline and multilayer diamond coatings on temporomandibular joint implants. *J Mater Sci Mater Med*, 15, 773–777.

Pareta, R., Yang, L., Kothari, A., *et al.* (2010) Tailoring nanocrystalline diamond coated on titanium for osteoblast adhesion. *J Biomed Mater Res A*, 95, 129–136.

Perry, S. (1993) Interface characterization of chemically vapor deposited diamond on titanium and Ti-6Al-4V. *J Appl Phys*, 74, 7542.

Piconi, C., Maccauro, G., Muratori, F., *et al.* (2004) Ceramic Coatings in Metal-PE Joints: Where Are We Now? *Bioceramics in Joint Arthroplasty*, Steinkopff.

Polini, R., Mantini, F. P., Braic, M., *et al.* (2007) Effects of Ti- and Zr-based interlayer coatings on hot-filament chemical vapor deposition of diamond on high-speed steel. *Journal of Materials Engineering and Performance*, 15, 201–207.

Polini, R., Mattei, G., Valle, R. and Casadei, F. (2006) Raman spectroscopy characterization of diamond films on steel substrates with titanium carbide arc-plated interlayer. *Thin Solid Films*, 515, 1011–1016.

Purdue, P. E., Koulouvaris, P., Potter, H. G., *et al.* (2007) The cellular and molecular biology of periprosthetic osteolysis. *Clin Orthop Relat Res*, 454, 251–261.

Raffaini, G. and Ganazzoli, F. (2007) Sequential adsorption of proteins and the surface modification of biomaterials: a molecular dynamics study. *Journal of Materials Science: Materials in Medicine*, 18, 309–316.

Revel, P. A. (2008) The combined role of wear particles, macrophages and lymphocytes in the loosening of total joint prostheses. *J Roy Soc Interface*, 5, 1263.

Rezek, B., Kratka, M., Ukraintsev, E., *et al.* (2011) Diamond as functional material for bioelectronics and biotechnology. In: Serra P.A., (Ed.) *Biosensors for Health, Environment and Biosecurity Intech.* Open Access Publisher.

Roy, R. K. and Lee, K. R. (2007) Biomedical applications of diamond-like carbon coatings: a review. *J Biomed Mater Res B Appl Biomater*, 83, 72–84.

Roy, M. E., Whiteside, L. A., *et al.* (2009) Diamond-like carbon coatings enhance scratch resistance of bearing surfaces for use in joint arthroplasty: Hard substrates outperform soft. *Journal of Biomedical Materials Research Part B: Applied Biomaterials* 89B(2), 527–535.

Rudnik, V., Sanyal, A., Syed, F. A., *et al.* (2008) Loss of ERE binding activity by estrogen receptor-alpha alters basal and estrogen-stimulated bone-related gene expression by osteoblastic cells. *J Cell Biochem*, 103, 896–907.

Saikko, V., Ahlroos, T., Calonius, O. and Keranen, J. (2001) Wear simulation of total hip prostheses with polyethylene against CoCr, alumina and diamond-like carbon. *Biomaterials*, 22, 1507–1514.

Santavirta, S. S., Lappalainen, R., *et al.* (1999). The Counterface, Surface Smoothness, Tolerances, and Coatings in Total Joint Prostheses. *Clinical Orthopaedics and Related Research*, 369, 92–102.

Scardi, P., Leoni, M., Cappuccio, G., et al. (1997) Residual stress in polycrystalline diamond/Ti-6Al-4V systems. *Diamond and Related Materials*, 6, 807–811.

Schrand, A. M., Huang, H., Cataleya, C., *et al.* (2007) Are diamond nanoparticles cytotoxic? *J Phy Chem B*, 111, 2–7.

Schwan, J. (1997) Stress-induced formation of high-density amorphous carbon thin films. *J Appl Phys*, 82, 6024.

Shenderova, O. A. and Gruen, D. M. (2006) *Ultrananocrystalline Diamond: Synthesis, Properties, and Applications*. Norwich/US, William Andrew Publishing.

Shimmin, A. J. and Back, D. (2005) Femoral neck fractures following Birmingham hip resurfacing: a national review of 50 cases. *J Bone Joint Surg Br*, 87, 463–464.

Stevens, M. M. and George, J. H. (2005) Exploring and engineering the cells surface interface. *Science*, 310, 1135–1138.

Taeger, G., Podleska, L. E., *et al.* (2003). Comparison of Diamond-Like-Carbon and Alumina-Oxide articulating with Polyethylene in Total Hip Arthroplasty. *Materialwissenschaft und Werkstofftechnik*, 34(12), 1094–1100.

Tamor, M. A. and Vassell, W. C. (1994) *Raman fingerprinting of amorphous carbon films*, AIP.

Tan, J. and Saltzman, W. M. (2004) Biomaterials with hierarchically defined micro- and nanoscale structure. *Biomaterials*, 25, 3593–3601.

Tang, L., Tsai, C., Gerberich, W. W., Kruckeberg, L. and Kania, D. R. (1995) Biocompatibility of chemical vapour-deposited diamond. *Biomaterials*, 16, 483–488.

Terranova, M. (1996) Structural investigation of the titanium/diamond film interface. *J Appl Phys*, 80, 3552.

Thomas, V., Dean, D. R. and Vohra, Y. K. (2006) Nanostructured biomaterials in regenerative medicine. *Curr Nanosci*, 2, 155–177.

Thomas, V., Halloran, B., Catledge, S. A., *et al.* (2012) In vitro studies on the effect of particle-size on the macrophage cells responses to potential nanodiamond wear debris-particles. *Acta Biomaterialia*, 8(5), 1939–1947.

Toprani, N., Catledge, S. A., Vohra, Y. K. and Thompson, R. (2000) Interfacial adhesion and toughness of nanostructured diamond coatings. *Journal of Materials Research*, 15, 1052–1055.

Treacy, R. B., McBryde, C. W. and Pynsent, P. B. (2005) Birmingham hip resurfacing arthroplasty. A minimum follow-up of five years. *J Bone Joint Surg Br*, 87, 167–170.

Vandenbulcke, L. (1998) Two-step process for improved diamond deposition on titanium alloys at moderate temperature. *Appl Phys Lett*, 72, 501.

Vandrovcova, M. and Bakacova, L. (2011) Adhesion, growth and differentiation of osteoblasts on surface modified materials developed for bone implants. *Physiol Res*, 60, 403–417.

Vandrovcova, M., Hanus, J., Kylian, O., *et al.* (2010) Effect of different surface nanoroughness of TiO2 films on the growth of MG63 cells. *Abstracts 2nd International Conference on Cellular and Molecular Bioengineering (ICCMB2)*. Singapore.

Vohra, S., Hennessy, K. M., Sawyer, A. A., *et al.* (2008) Comparison of mesenchymal stem cell and osteosarcoma cell adhesion to hydroxyapatite. *J Mater Sci Mater Med*, 19, 3567–3574.

Wagner, M. and Wagner, H. (2000) Medium-term results of a modern metal-on-metal system in total hip replacement. *Clin Orthop Relat Res*, 123–133.

Wang, M. L., Sharkey, P. F. and Tuan, R. S. (2004) Particle bioreactivity and wear mediated osteolysis. *J Arthroplasty*, 19, 1028–1038.

Webster, T. J. (2004) Proteins: Structure and interactions patterns to solid surfaces. In: Schwarz Ja, C. C., Putyera K, (Eds.) *Encyclopedia of Nanoscience and Nanotechnology*. New York, Marcel Dekker.

Webster, T. J. and Ejiofor, J. U. (2004) Increased osteoblast adhesion on nanophase metals: Ti, Ti6A14V, and CoCrMo. *Biomaterials*, 25, 4731–4739.

Webster, T. J., Ergun, C., Doremus, R. H., *et al.* (2000a) Specific proteins mediate enhanced osteoblast adhesion on nanophase ceramics. *J Biomed Mater Res A*, 51, 475–483.

Webster, T. J., Ergun, C., Doremus, R. H., *et al.* (2000b) Enhanced functions of osteoblasts on nanophase ceramics. *Biomaterials*, 21, 1803–1810.

Webster, T. J., Siegal, R. W. and Bizios, R. (1990) Osteoblast adhesion on nanophase ceramics. *Biomaterials*, 20, 1221–1227.

Webster, T. J. and Smith, T. A. (2005) Increased osteoblast function on PLGA composites containing nanophase titania. *J Biomed Mater Res A*, 74, 677–686.

Wei, Q., Yu, Z., Ma, L. and Yin, D. (2009) Enhanced Nucleation and Smoothness of Nanocrystalline Diamond Films via W-C Gradient Interlayer. *International Journal of Modern Physics B*, 23, 1676–1682.

Wright, T., Sculco, T. P., Su, E. P., *et al.* (2009) Joint Replacement: Implant Bearing Surface Materials. New York.

Wroblewski, B. M. (2002) Professor Sir John Charnley (1911–1982). *Rheumatology (Oxford)*, 41, 824–825.

Xu, T. and Pruitt, L. (1999) Diamond-like carbon coatings for orthopaedic applications: an evaluation of tribological performance. *Journal of Materials Science: Materials in Medicine*, 10, 83–90.

Yang, L., Sheldon, B. W. and Webster, T. J. (2009a) The impact of diamond nanocrystallinity on osteoblast functions. *Biomaterials*, 30, 3458–3465.

Yang, L., Sheldon, B. W. and Webster, T. J. (2009b) Orthopedic diamond coating: control of surface properties and their impact on osteoblast adhesion and proliferation. *J Biomed Mater Res A*, 91, 548–556.

Zhao, G., Raines, A. L., Wieland, M., *et al.* (2007) Requirement for both micron- and submicron scale structure for synergistic responses of osteoblasts to substrate surface energy and topography. *Biomaterials*, 28, 2821–2829.

Zuo, D., Li, X. F., Wang, M., *et al.* (2003) Adhesion improvement of CVD diamond film by introducing an electro-deposited interlayer. *J Mat Proc Technol*, 138, 455.

6
Ultrananocrystalline diamond (UNCD) films for ophthalmological applications

O. AUCIELLO and P. GURMAN, Argonne National Laboratory, USA, A. BERRA, Universidad Nacional de Buenos Aires, Argentina, M. SARAVIA, Hospital Austral, Argentina and R. ZYSLER, Centro Atómico Bariloche, Argentina

DOI: 10.1533/9780857093516.2.151

Abstract: This chapter discusses the integration of physiology, new biomaterials and micro and nanofabrication technologies, which enable the development of new devices implantable in the human eye for diagnosis, monitoring, and/or therapeutic treatment of vision. The chapter focuses on the science and technology of biomaterials for three main applications: to restore sight to people blinded by genetically induced degeneration of retina photoreceptors; for draining aqueous humour from the eyes of people with glaucoma condition; and a novel method for retina detachment therapy.

Key words: ultrananocrystalline diamond (UNCD), coating, biocompatible, encapsulation, microchip, vision restoration, retinitis pigmentosa, glaucoma valve, superparamagnetic, nanoparticles, retina reattachment.

6.1 Introduction

A new paradigm in biomaterials is emerging, enabling a new generation of implantable biomedical devices to treat a broad range of human diseases. The integration of physiology, new biomaterials and micro and nanofabrication technologies are enabling the development of new devices implantable in the human body for diagnosis, monitoring, and/or therapeutic treatment of vision, hearing, and motion, degraded or lost either through genetically induced degenerative conditions or through traumatic events. This chapter focuses on the science and technology of biomaterials for three main applications as described in three sections, namely:

1. Section 6.2: focuses on the synthesis and properties of a novel bioinert/biocompatible ultrananocrystalline diamond (UNCD) film as a coating for encapsulation of an implantable microchip, as a key component of an artificial retina to restore sight to people blinded by genetically induced degeneration of retina photoreceptors.
2. Section 6.3: focuses on the development of a low temperature growth process for UNCD films for encapsulation of valves or novel devices implantable in

the eye for draining saline solution from the eyes of people with glaucoma condition.

3. Section 6.4: focuses on a novel method for retina detachment therapy based on superparamagnetic nanoparticles injected into the eye and a magnet coated with UNCD film on the outside wall of the eye to produce a magnetic field to attract the particles to press a detached retina back against the inner eye wall to treat retina detachment.

6.2 The use of ultrananocrystalline diamond (UNCD) films as coatings in the restoration of sight in people blinded by degenerated photoreceptors

Age-related macular degeneration (AMD) is an eye disease primarily affecting the central vision regions in people aged 60 years and older.[1] According to the Macular Degeneration Research Fund, a case of AMD is diagnosed in the USA every 3 minutes.

6.2.1 Background on blindness due to genetically induced degeneration of photoreceptors

Each year, 1.2 million of the estimated 12 million people with AMD in the USA will suffer severe vision loss. Patients with AMD have dark areas in their central area vision (Fig. 6.1(a)) caused by fluid leakage or bleeding in the macula, the center of the retina in the back of the eye that is responsible for the central vision, providing the ability to read, drive, and perform other activities that require fine, sharp, straight-ahead vision.

Injury to the macula can impair the ability to see straight ahead clearly and sometimes make it difficult to read, drive, or perform other daily activities that require fine central vision. As people read, light is focused onto the macula where millions of cells capture the incoming light and transduce it into nerve electrical signals that travel to the brain, which process the electrical signals into complex patterns that will become the visual percept known as 'image'.

There are two types of AMD, i.e. the dry and the far more frequent wet type. An early symptom of wet AMD is revealed by the fact that straight lines appear wavy when seen by the person with AMD. This happens because the newly formed blood vessels leak fluid under the macula. The fluid raises the macula from its normal place at the back of the eye and distorts vision. Another sign that a person may have wet AMD is rapid loss of central vision. Dry AMD, on the other hand, results in a much slower loss of central vision. For both dry and wet AMD, the person may also notice a blind spot. The brain initially may compensate for these dark patches. Early cellular dysfunction (photoreceptors death) or spotting in the macula may go undetected until the disease is in advanced stages. If any of these changes in vision are noticed, an ophthalmologist should be consulted without delay.

Retinitis pigmentosa (RP) is the most common inherited cause of blindness in people between the ages of 20 and 60 years worldwide. Around 500 000 people in the USA suffer some level of visual impairment from RP, and, of those, 20 000 are totally blind. RP is a degenerative disease of the retina that results in genetically induced death of photoreceptors (i.e. cone cells, responsible for the color vision, and rod cells, responsible for night or dim light vision). Vision loss is gradual and may result in diminished or lost peripheral vision (tubular vision, Fig. 6.1(b)) all the way up to blindness when all photoreceptors die.

RP may be inherited in a number of different ways: as an autosomal dominant, autosomal recessive, or X-linked recessive trait or as a mitochondrial disorder. More than 30 different genes have been linked to RP.

6.2.2 Synthesis and characterization of UNCD films as coating for encapsulation of silicon microchip for artificial retina

Implantable medical devices are being used to address a growing number of medical problems. This rapidly growing field integrates physiology and micro and nanofabrication technology to produce implantable systems for diagnosis and monitoring, therapeutic treatment, and functional restoration. One example of these applications is the artificial retinal implant for restoring lost vision due to genetically induced degeneration of retina photoreceptors,[1,2] as is the case for RP and AMD. In 2002, the U. S. Department of Energy (DOE) set up the Artificial Retina Research Project with the goal of designing and fabricating an artificial retina to restore sight to people suffering from RP or AMD. The artificial retina includes the following critical components: 1) a microchip implantable on the retina at the ganglion cell layer level, 2) peripheral components also implantable in the eye (e.g. coil for coupling the RF signal carrying the image from an external

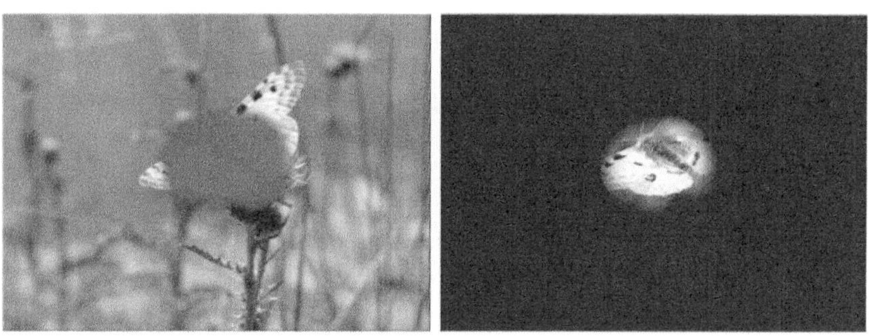

(a) (b)

6.1 (a) Picture showing the vision of a person with age-related macular degeneration. (b) Picture showing the so-called tubular vision for a person with advanced retinitis pigmentosa.

charge coupled device (CCD) camera into the microchip, and electrode array to transfer electrical pulses from the microchip into the ganglion cells); 3) a CCD camera, similar to those used in portable computers for people to communicate through systems such as Skype, allowing people to see each other on the computer screen; 4) a power source to provide power to the microchip.

The artificial retina helps to restore limited vision to people who have gone blind as a result of advanced RP and AMD. It enables them to read, have unaided mobility, and recognize faces.[1] The basic principle of the retinal implant under development by the DOE consortium is to translate the visual information captured by an external CCD camera, mounted on glasses, into a pattern of electrical stimulation pulses that are applied directly to the ganglion cells for transmission to the brain to restore image formation.[1,2] Clinical trials of a prototype retinal prosthesis show that completely blind individuals interpret this stimulus as a visual sensation,[1,2] and with the current prototype of 240 biocompatible platinum electrodes in a polymer matrix, they read letters of about 5 mm high, recognize objects, and find doors and windows following the light coming through them. The current microchip is implanted outside the eye and connected to an array of Pt electrodes on a polymer matrix on the ganglion cells, via an array of thin Pt wires encapsulated in polymer and penetrating through the eye wall. In order to improve on this device, it will be necessary to develop an implantable microelectronic system that can stimulate the retina at hundreds of individual locations in the same way a display uses hundreds of pixels to create an image.[1,2]

Packaging the retina microchip is a significant technical challenge, as the package must simultaneously protect the chip from corrosive eye fluids, protect the eye from the chip materials, and allow the circuit to interface with the retina through microelectrodes. The surface of this retina microchip will be exposed to the physiological environment of the eye for many years. Therefore, the permanently implanted microchip must fulfill special requirements in terms of biocompatability and bioinertness, that is, no adverse reaction induced to the surrounding retina tissue that may influence its physiological function and no electrochemical reaction with the physiological environment that might evolve gas (e.g. oxygen or hydrogen) and lead to chemical attack of the microchip surface affecting its functionality. The microchip used in the artificial retinal implant of the DOE consortium and most other implantable electronic medical devices uses Si as the structural and functional material. However, Si is soluble in human fluids over long time.[1,2] Therefore, hermetic coatings with good biocompatibility and bioinertness are critically needed for encapsulation of bioimplantable devices.

Coating materials currently being evaluated for encapsulating artificial retinal prototype implants include SiO_2,[2] SiN_x,[2] SiC,[2,3] and polyimide.[2,4] However, dissolution and decay of SiO_2 passivation layer has been found for some retinal implants when implanted in animals for up to six months.[5] SiN_x coatings often exhibit structural defects (pin holes) and degenerations, which could not protect the encapsulated micro-photodiode. Polyimide and other polymers are cheap and flexible, but tend to absorb significant quantities of water, which in turn leads to electrical leakage after some time.

Diamond is being considered as 'the biomaterial of the 21st century', and diamond films are strong candidates for protective coatings on bioimplants or as the bioimplant itself, because of their exceptional mechanical properties, chemical inertness, and biocompatibility.[6] However, the high substrate temperatures (>700°C) typically required for growing microcrystalline or nanocrystalline diamond using conventional deposition techniques with hydrogen-rich plasmas,[6] limit the selection range of the substrate materials. In particular, for implants that use silicon microchips based on complementary metal oxide semiconductor (CMOS) technology, the deposition/processing of the hermetic diamond coating should be within a thermal budget of ≥400°C. Also, large grain size and low nucleation density for microcrystalline diamond coatings make it difficult to achieve conformal deposition on complicated features, so hermetic sealing is unobtainable. The solution to this problem has been provided by a new diamond thin film technology developed and patented at Argonne National Laboratory in the form of UNCD thin films. These films are synthesized using microwave plasma chemical vapor deposition with argon-rich Ar/CH_4 plasma chemistries. UNCD consists of diamond grains 3–5 nm in size and atomically abrupt grain boundaries, which consist of carbon atoms in a mixture of sp^3 (diamond) and sp^2 (graphitic) bonding, and intermediates.[6] This unique nanostructure results in a very smooth as-deposited surface roughness of about 5–8 nm (rms), and also excellent mechanical properties and chemical inertness. In addition, a very important distinction between the UNCD and the conventional diamond deposition process is that UNCD can be grown at 400°C with growth rates similar to those observed for high temperature growth.[6] Furthermore, the capability to covalently functionalize the surface of UNCD makes it amenable to the specific physiological environment and makes it more biocompatible.[6] The combination of all these properties makes UNCD a strong, reliable candidate for application as a hermetic coating for the protection of the artificial retinal microchip and other implantable medical devices.

UNCD films grown using a $CH_4/Ar/H_2$ gas mixture with 1% added hydrogen (2.5% total H_2 content in the plasma) exhibit an extremely smooth surface (Fig. 6.2(a)), which enables production of a high density layer for encapsulation of the Si microchip (Fig. 6.2(b)) to be implanted inside the eye. Laboratory experiments, measuring the leakage current flowing from the Si microchip through the UNCD encapsulating layer in a saline solution, simulating the eye environment, showed that UNCD coatings exhibit leakage currents of $\sim 7\times10^{-7}$ A/cm^2 (Fig. 6.2(c)).[6,7] This leakage is borderline to what is required by agencies like the FDA in the USA for approval of functionality of a microchip inside the eye. Therefore, more recent work at Argonne has focused on growing an Al_2O_3

encapsulation layer on the Si microchip, followed by an interface layer on top of the Al_2O_3 layer, and finally the external UNCD top layer to be in contact with the eye saline. The UNCD/Al_2O_3 heterostructure encapsulating coating can yield the high electrical insulation with low leakage current in eye saline, provided by the Al_2O_3 layer (Fig. 6.3), and the external UNCD layer in contact with the eye saline provides resistance to chemical attack and inhibits cell and protein attachment on the implant surface (Fig 6.2(d–g)).

Long term (~6 months) *in vivo* tests, involving implantation, of UNCD-coated Si chips in rabbit eyes, demonstrated that UNCD is hermetic (Fig. 6.1(b)), bioinert and biostable (Fig. 6.2(d–f)), further proven by chemical analysis via X-ray photoelectron spectroscopy (Fig. 6.2(g)). These results provide preliminary validation of using low temperature UNCD as a hermetic coating for the artificial retina microchip and other biomedical chip implants. Further work is ongoing to

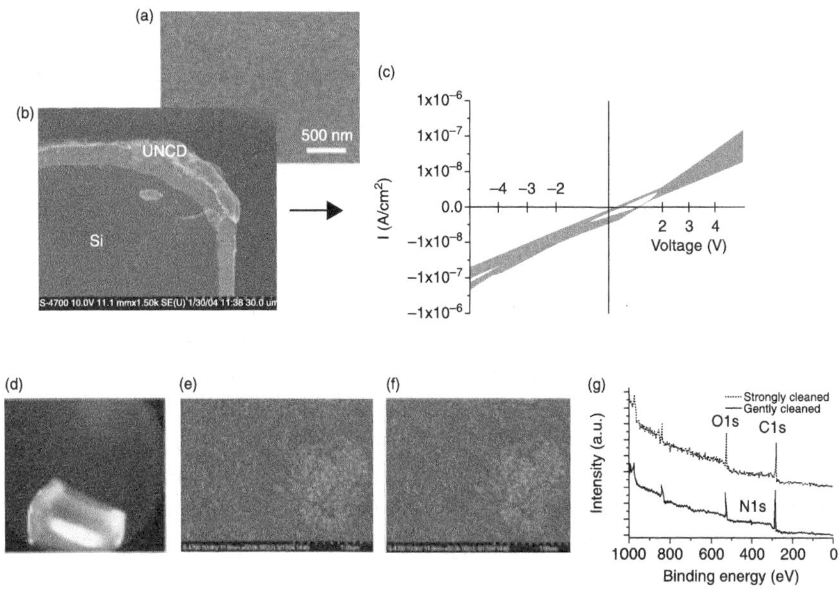

6.2 (a) Surface nanomorphology of UNCD film grown with 1% H_2 in the Ar/CH_4 mixture (2–5 nm grain size). (b) Cross-section SEM picture showing UNCD coating encapsulating a Si chip. (c) Leakage current vs. voltage in saline solution to test performance of UNCD encapsulating coating in the eye saline environment. (d) *In vivo* picture of UNCD-coated Si chip implanted in rabbit eye for six months; SEM pictures of UNCD coating before implantation (e) and after six month implantation in rabbit eye (f); and (g) XPS analysis of UNCD surface after six months implantation in rabbit eye, showing no adsorption of biomolecules on the surface of UNCD. Reprinted from *Diamond and Related Materials*, 19 (2010) 699. O. Auciello and A.V. Sumant, Copyright (2001), with permission from Elsevier Publishers.

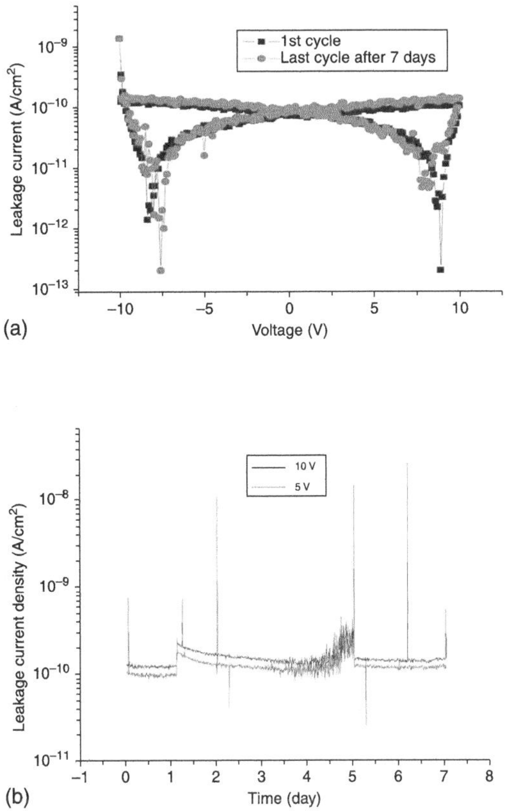

6.3 Leakage current for an Al_2O_3 microchip encapsulating layer measured in saline solution. (a) Cycle test for leakage current density vs. voltage from –10 V to +10 V with steps of 0.5 V; (b) nA/cm^2 leakage current for an Al_2O_3 (2 μm thick)-coated Si chip.

overcome the remaining technical barriers to fully integrate UNCD coatings into future generations of retinal prostheses and eventually other microchip implants.

6.3 The use of UNCD films in the treatment of glaucoma

Glaucoma is an eye condition characterized by increased intra-ocular pressure (IOP) (pressure within the eye) either through increased production or decreased outflow of fluid, called aqueous humour, in the eye anterior chamber (Fig. 6.4(a),(c)). Normally, the aqueous humour flows out of the eye through a mesh-like channel. If this channel becomes blocked, fluid builds up, causing glaucoma. The direct cause of this blockage is unknown, but doctors do know that it is most often inherited, meaning it is passed from parents to children.

6.3.1 Background on glaucoma condition

Less common causes of glaucoma include a blunt or chemical injury to the eye, severe eye infection, blockage of blood vessels in the eye, inflammatory conditions of the eye, and occasionally eye surgery to correct another condition. Glaucoma usually occurs in both eyes, but it may involve each eye to a different extent.

The increased IOP may result in optic nerve damage (Fig. 6.4(b)), permanently damaging vision in the affected eye(s), as the optic nerve carries to the brain the pattern of electrical pulses with encoded images generated from the ganglion cells as a result of the transduction of light based images into electrical pulses by the photoreceptors. The nerve damage involves loss of retinal ganglion cells in a characteristic pattern. Glaucoma can be divided into two main categories, 'open angle' and 'closed angle' glaucoma. Closed angle glaucoma can appear suddenly and is often painful, such that visual loss can progress quickly, but the discomfort often leads patients to seek medical attention before permanent damage occurs. Open angle, chronic glaucoma tends to progress at a slower rate and patients may not notice they have lost vision until the disease has progressed significantly. Once lost, the damaged visual field cannot be recovered. Worldwide, it is the second leading cause of blindness after cataracts. It is also the leading cause of blindness among African Americans in the USA. Glaucoma affects one in 200 people aged 50 and younger, and one in 10 over the age of 80. If the condition is detected early enough, it is possible to arrest the development or slow the progression with medical and surgical means.

Glaucoma is often, but not always, associated with increased pressure of the fluid in the eye (aqueous humour). The term 'ocular hypertension' is used for cases having constantly raised IOP without any associated optic nerve damage. 'Normal' or 'low tension glaucoma' is used for the typical visual field defects associated with a normal or low IOP. There are many different subtypes of glaucoma, but they can all be considered a type of optic neuropathy. Raised IOP is a significant risk factor for developing glaucoma (above 21 mmHg or 2.8 kPa). One person may develop nerve damage at a relatively low pressure, whereas another person may have high eye pressure for years and yet never develop damage.

Increased resistance to outflow of aqueous humour may occur due to an abnormal or clogged trabecular meshwork or obliteration of the meshwork due to injury or disease of the iris. However, increased IOP is neither sufficient nor necessary for development of primary open angle glaucoma, although it is a major risk factor. Uncontrolled glaucoma typically leads to visual field loss and ultimately to blindness. The mechanism whereby the IOP is naturally controlled is described below.

The aqueous humour is secreted into the posterior chamber by the ciliary body (Fig. 6.4(c)), specifically the non-pigmented epithelium of the ciliary body, from where it flows through the narrow cleft between the front of the lens and the back of

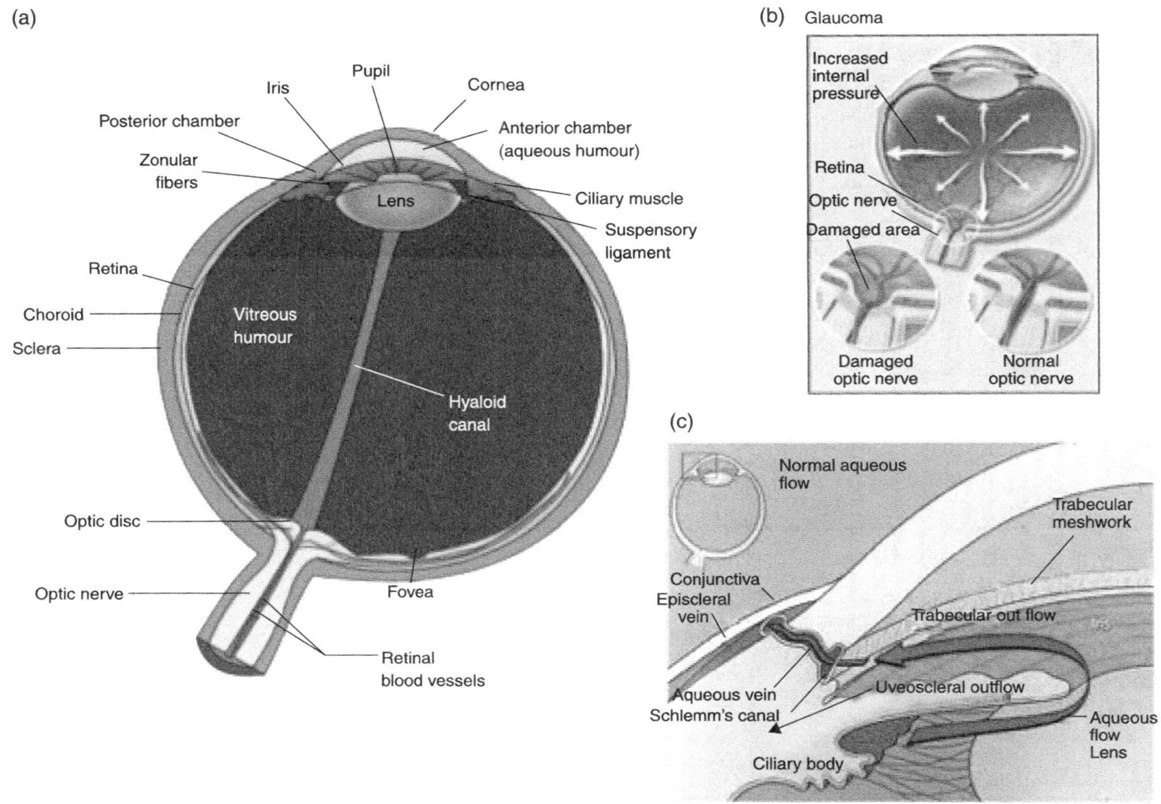

6.4 (a) Schematic of human eye, showing components that play critical roles in the glaucoma condition. (b) Schematic showing how high IOP produces damage in the optic nerve, which can lead to blindness. (c) Schematic showing detail of how the aqueous humour flows to control IOP.

the iris, to escape through the pupil into the anterior chamber, and then to drain out of the eye via the trabecular meshwork. From the trabecular meshwork, the aqueous humour is drained into the Schlemms's canal in one of two ways: directly, via the aqueous vein to the episcleral vein, or indirectly, via collector channels to the episcleral vein by the intrascleral plexus and eventually into the veins of the orbit.

The processes involved in the control of aqueous humor flow include:

1. Filtration; i.e. as blood flows in the capillaries of the ciliary body, it is filtered by the endothelial cells of the capillaries. The resulting plasma is then re-filtered by the pigmented and non-pigmented ciliary epithelial cells and is secreted into the posterior chamber before travelling between the lens and iris into the anterior chamber of the eye as aqueous humour.
2. The Diamond-Bossert model indicates that active fluid transport occurring in the non-pigmented ciliary epithelial cells induces small osmotic pressure gradients in between the cells. A higher concentration of solutes in the proximal part of the intercellular space generates a flow of water. The concentration diminishes from the proximal part to the distal part, releasing the liquid into the posterior chamber.
3. The ciliary cells continually produce aqueous humour, and this rate of production must be balanced by an equal rate of aqueous humour drainage. Small variations in the production or outflow of aqueous humour have a large influence on the IOP. The drainage route for aqueous humour flow is first through the posterior chamber, then the narrow space between the posterior iris and the anterior lens (contributes to small resistance) (Fig. 6.4(a)), through the pupil to enter the anterior chamber (Fig. 6.4(a)). From there, the aqueous humour exits the eye through the trabecular meshwork into the Schelmm's canal (a channel at the limbus, i.e. the joining point of the cornea and sclera, which encircles the cornea) (Fig. 6.4(c)). The fluid flows through 25–30 collector canals into the episcleral veins. The greatest resistance to aqueous flow is provided by the trabecular meshwork, and this is where most of the aqueous outflow occurs. The internal wall of the canal is very delicate and allows the fluid to filter due to high pressure of the fluid within the eye. The uveoscleral drainage provides a secondary route for aqueous flow, which does not affect the IOP, and enables the flow of the eye's fluid to a lesser extent than through the trabecular meshwork. The fluid is normally 15 mm (0.6 inch) Hg above atmospheric pressure, so when a syringe is injected the fluid flows easily. If the fluid is leaking, due to collapse and wilting of the cornea, the hardness of the normal eye is therefore corroborated.

In conclusion, the most important factor in treating glaucoma is early detection of the disease. Most patients will be treated with eye drops to control eye pressure. Laser treatment and surgery are also options for certain cases. In other cases, glaucoma is treated via implantation of valves in the sclera (Fig. 6.5) to drain the eye fluid in a controlled manner,[8] as done by the natural trabecular tubes.

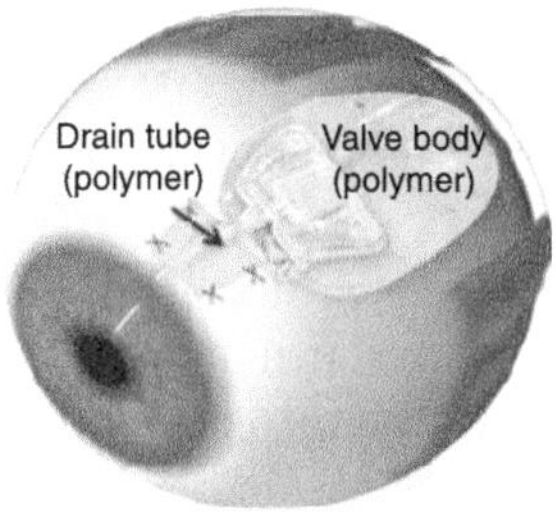

6.5 Schematic of human eye showing implantation of a fluid drain valve to treat glaucoma. Note that there is need for two incisions: one for inserting the relatively large (1.7 × 1 cm) body of the valve, and the second for insertion of the drain tube.

6.3.2 UNCD films as hermetic bioinert/biocompatible coatings for glaucoma valves

Current glaucoma valves in the market face several problems. The valves are made mainly of polymers and are rather large (~1.7 × 1 cm), and the implant surgery requires two incisions, one to insert the body of the valve in the sclera (Fig. 6.5) and the other to insert the polymer tube inside the eye to drain the fluid (Fig. 6.5). An important and so far unsolved problem with current glaucoma valves (as with most implantable devices) is the host reaction against the implant that occurs immediately after implantation (seconds to minutes), where a protein layer adheres to the device. As a consequence of protein adhesion and within the first eight hours, inflammatory cells such as macrophages are recruited by chemical signals to the implant site where they become activated and secrete growth factors that stimulate fibroblast cells responsible for collagen production that will be part of the fibrous capsule around the implant which will appear within a few days. After a few weeks, a complete fibrotic reaction known as a foreign body reaction will occur, isolating the implant from the rest of the body. This fibrous capsule could have deleterious effects on medical implants, such as impairing sensor performance or diffusion of drugs in drug delivery devices. To overcome this issue, several approaches have been investigated. Initial *in vivo* experiments were performed in collaboration between scientists at Argonne National Laboratory and the University of Buenos Aires-Argentina, and a surgeon at the Hospital Austral in Pilar, Buenos Aires, Argentina. These aimed to demonstrate the effectiveness of a UNCD coating in avoiding fibrotic capsule development around glaucoma silicone valves that could jeopardize the performance of the valve by impairing the drainage of the humour, as the fibrotic tissue could block the drainage tube of the valve which would demand the valve replacement. Using animal trial protocols approved by ANMAT (Argentine Agency equivalent to the FDA in the USA), the experiments involved the implantation of two glaucoma valves. Each rabbit had one valve coated with a UNCD film implanted into one eye and one uncoated valve implanted into the other eye, in order to avoid any difference related to the use of different animals in the same experiment (see Fig. 6.6(a) and (b)).

Coating the polymer of a glaucoma valve with a UNCD film, using the growth process described in Section 6.2, resulted in practical elimination of fibrosis after several months of implantation (see Fig. 6.6(b)), whereas extensive fibrotic tissue was observed around the uncoated glaucoma valve only 24 hours after implantation (see Fig. 6.6(a)).

The practical elimination of fibrosis on the surface of the UNCD-coated glaucoma valve is attributed to the fact that the surface of UNCD films is extremely hydrophobic (no water adhesion), due to the hydrogen termination of the surface of the as-deposited UNCD films, as demonstrated by extensive experiments by the Argonne research group.[6,7]

UNCD films can, in principle, be grown on high temperature polymers because the unique growth process developed to produce UNCD films (see Section 6.2) enables growth of diamond films at temperatures in the range 350–400°C. However, this temperature range is still relatively high for growth of UNCD films on the surface of polymers, and may result in embrittlement (loss of flexibility of the polymer). Therefore, further work, currently under way is necessary to try to reduce the growth of the UNCD films to temperatures below 300°C. In this sense, research currently under way at Argonne is focused on developing a new process called bias enhanced nucleation/bias enhanced growth (BEN-BEG) of UNCD films. This process requires an electrically conductive substrate to apply a negative voltage on the surface of the substrate, to establish an electric field between the

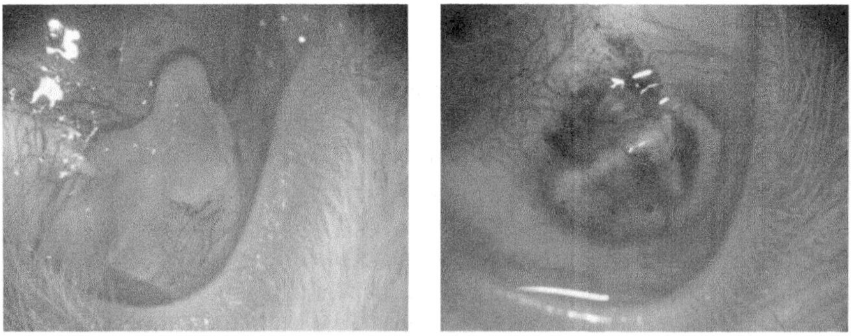

(a) (b)

6.6 (a) Optical picture of glaucoma valve only after 24 hours implantation into rabbit eye (notice the extensive fibrosis around the implant surface). (b) Glaucoma valve coated with a UNCD film after about four months implantation in the second eye of the same rabbit for which the uncoated valve was implanted (note that the glaucoma valve is clear, without fibrosis).

positively charged plasma boundary, from the Ar/CH_4 plasma used to grow the UNCD films, and the substrate. The electric field accelerates C^+ ions from the plasma towards the surface of the substrate, resulting in energies high enough (~100–300 eV) for the C^+ ions to get subplanted underneath the surface of the substrate, leading to the nucleation of a layer that induces the growth of UNCD films (read Chen *et al.*, 2008[9] and Zhong *et al.*, 2009[10] for a detailed description of the BEN-BEG process to produce UNCD films). As the polymers are generally electrical insulators, it is necessary to grow a very thin layer (~10–20 nm only) of an electrically conductive material that can form carbide layers on C atom implantation (e.g. tungsten or titanium).[9,10] The W or Ti layers are grown using magnetron sputter-deposition or atomic layer deposition.[9,10] The energy provided to the C^+ ions by the electrical bias on the substrate surface enables the motion of the C atoms landed on the surface at much lower temperatures than when no bias is applied, to establish the chemical bonds characteristic of diamond.[9,10]

It is expected that coating of polymers with UNCD films will enable not only more biocompatible glaucoma valves, but also other implantable biomedical devices made of polymers.

6.3.3 Novel UNCD-coated grid as new glaucoma treatment device

The glaucoma valves are relatively large and require two surgical incisions as indicated in Fig. 6.5. Therefore the Argonne-University of Buenos Aires-Hospital Austral group is developing an alternative approach involving implantation of a small grid (~3 mm in diameter) featuring hundreds to thousands of small holes formed by the boundaries of the very thin wires used to fabricate the grid. It is expected the large number of holes present in the grid will provide a very efficient drainage of the eye fluid. The grid is coated with an UNCD film to make it bioinert and biocompatible, and is implanted in the trabecular region, where the clogged natural trabecular tubes are located, in order to replace them as the drainage device. Initial experiments were performed using grids of copper (Cu) to demonstrate the power of the UNCD film as a bioinert/biocompatible coating. Copper elicits unacceptable toxicity on the eye, and if the UNCD coating was not hermetic, eye fluid would permeate though it, and the eye would recognize the presence of Cu underneath the UNCD film and eject the grid from the eye. Figure 6.7(a) shows a Cu grid implanted in the trabecular region of one rabbit eye, using a new surgical technique developed by Dr M. Saravia (Hospital Austral). The animal clinical trials were conducted in the animal facility of Dr A. Berra in the University of Buenos Aires under protocols approved by ANMAT (the Argentinian Agency equivalent to the FDA in the USA). Figure 6.7(a) shows a schematic of the new surgical procedure for implantation of the UNCD-coated drain grid in the trabecular region of the eye. Figure 6.7(b) shows an optical picture of the UNCD-coated Cu grid in one of the rabbit eyes (no rejection at all

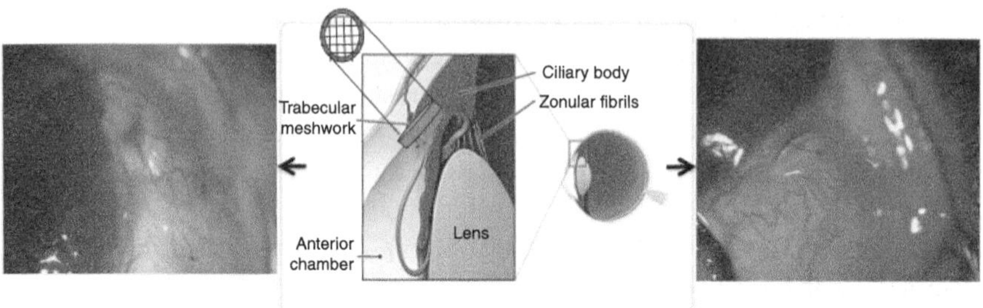

(b) (a) (c)

6.7 (a) Schematic of the new eye fluid drain device based on a UNCD-coated grid with hundreds to thousands of holes, for efficient drainage, implanted in the trabecular region, via a new surgical procedure developed by Dr M. Saravia. (b) Optical picture of a UNCD-coated Cu grid implanted in the trabecular region of one rabbit eye, showing no rejection after several months of implantation. (c) Optical picture of a Cu grid implanted in the second eye of the same rabbit.

after several months of implantation due to the excellent protection provided by the hermetic/bioinert/biocompatible UNCD film). Figure 6.7(b) shows a Cu grid without coating implanted on the second eye of the same rabbit. The figure shows the grid being rejected by the rabbit eye in only about 24 hours.

This initial work described above shows a new promising drain device technology and surgical procedure for treating glaucoma with a much less invasive approach due both to the much smaller device and simpler surgical procedure. The base material to be used for the grids on which the bioinert/biocompatible UNCD coating will be deposited will be a biocompatible metal such as Ti. UNCD films grow very well on Ti, and provide even better performance than Ti from the wear and bioinertness point of view, when implanted in the human body. Work is now in progress to optimize the new glaucoma device as described above.

6.4 Integrated magnet/superparamagnetic nanoparticles interacting system for new treatment of retina detachment

The retina is a thin, transparent and light-sensitive tissue located in the back of the eye. A detached retina has become disconnected from the other tissues of the eye.

6.4.1 Background on physiology of the retina

The retina is a thin, transparent and light-sensitive tissue located in the back of the eye. The cornea allows light to enter into the eye, and the lens focuses the light onto the retina, exiting the photoreceptors on the retina layer in contact with the inner eye wall. The photoreceptors act as a transducer, changing the light signals into electrical pulses that excite the bipolar cells (the layer next to the photoreceptors layer), which amplify the pulses and inject them into the ganglion cells (the most external layer of the retina), the axons of which form the optic nerve that carries the electrical pulses to the brain, where the information is processed to create the visual percept commonly known as 'image'.

6.4.2 Background on retina detachment

The retina that has become disconnected from the other tissue of the eye is a detached retina. According to the extensive literature (see for example MedicineNet.com[11]), two-thirds of the inside of the eye are filled with a clear vitreous gel. If this gel becomes disconnected from the retina it can cause the retina to tear. A torn retina can allow the vitreous gel to collect in front of the retina and cause it to fully detach (see schematic in Fig. 6.8(a)). There are three main causes of retina detachment: exudative, tractional, and regmatogenous (regma from the Greek 'rupture'). Retina detachment can occur when the gelatinous substance that fills the posterior cavity of the eye and supports the retina against the eye wall, becomes liquefied with aging, promoting a shrinking of the vitreous that induces tractional forces that pull the retina into the posterior cavity, allowing the liquid to penetrate the subretinal space dissecting the retina layer until it becomes completely detached.

According to the Medline Plus organization, a retina can tear on its own without any external cause or injury. In addition, according to the National Eye Institute, trauma to the head or eye, complications of cataract surgery, 'a family history of retina detachment', and other eye disorders can cause retina detachment. Diabetes and severe myopia, or nearsightedness, may also cause a retina to become detached. Retina detachment typically happens in only one eye; however, retinal detachment from one eye may indicate the likelihood of subsequent retina detachment in the other eye.

Symptoms of a detached retina include bright flashing lights in the peripheral vision, blurred vision, partial blindness, and 'floaters' in the visual field. The vitreous gel of the eye pulling on or bumping the retina causes the flashing lights associated with a detached retina. 'Floaters,' which may appear as dark spots floating in the visual field are caused by condensed vitreous gel. Another symptom of a detached retina resembles a shadow over part of the visual field. All the symptoms mentioned above are cause for an immediate examination by an eye doctor, and surgery soon after symptoms appear. A detached retina can occur in people of all ages, but is most common among Caucasian males over the age of 40. Retina detachment can lead to blindness if not properly treated.

6.4.3 Conventional current treatment of retina detachment

The two major current surgical treatments for retina detachment are: 1) scleral buckling, for which a sponge of silicone is placed on the outside of the eye and sewn in place (the scleral buckle is very small and not visible after surgery), to

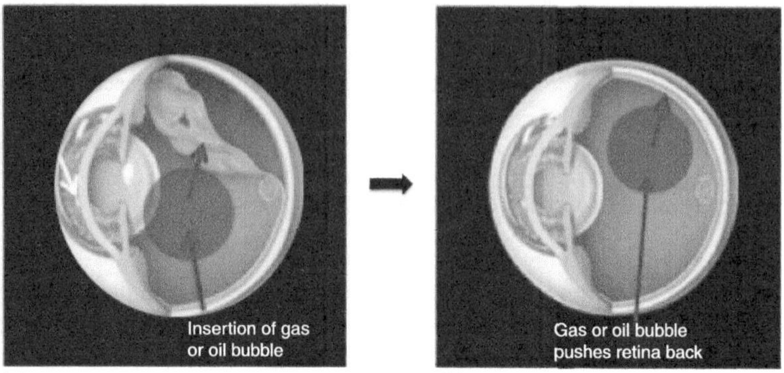

(a) (b)

6.8 (a) Schematic of retina detachment and insertion of gas or oil bubble to push retina back onto the inner eye wall. (b) Gas or oil bubble pushes retina back onto the inner eye wall for laser treatment for final re-attachment.

push the sclera toward the tear in the retina; however, drawbacks of this approach are an increased rate of subretinal hemorrhage, diplopia due to damage of the extra-ocular muscles refractive changes and rupture of the sclera buckling; 2) pneumatic retinopexy, a less severe treatment, for which the surgeon injects a gas or oil bubble inside the vitreous cavity (Fig. 6.8(a)). The bubble pushes the retina against the inner wall of the eye (Fig. 6.8(b)), allowing the tear to seal against the eye wall for subsequent laser treatment to complete the retina re-attachment.

Pneumatic retinopexy works well when the retina tear is on the upper part of the eye. However, when the retina detachment happens on the bottom part of the eye, the patient has to keep their head upside-down for several days, for the bubble to push on the retina, because the bubbles always move upwards. This condition results in problems for the treatment because patients do not follow guidelines properly. In addition, the patient cannot travel in planes for some time because the gas bubble would be subjected to dangerous pressure variations that can have damaging effects in the eye.

6.4.4 Novel nanotechnology-based treatment of retina detachment

Nanotechnology represents the technological revolution of the 21st century. Nanotechnology deals with manipulation and control of matter at the scale between 1 and 100 nm, pursuing the development of new products by taking advantage of new physical properties that arise as the scale goes down from the molecular to the atomic scale. In this sense, nanoparticles are among the first truly nanotechnology products already in the market, and specifically metal-oxide nanoparticles of about 10–50 nm in diameter, based on Fe_3O_4 nanocrystals, where iron appears in its Fe^{+3} and Fe^{+2} valence state, forming a crystal network with O atoms, commonly known as magnetite, have drawn a lot of attention both from industry and academia because of their many applications. Among these applications, biotechnology and medicine are two fields in which magnetic nanoparticles have found a wide variety of uses, including bioseparation, as contrast agents for MRI, therapeutic agents in hyperthermia and drug delivery, and recently as nanosensors and nanoactuators for lab on a chip devices.[12] Magnetic nanoparticles can be used as nanoactuators, as they are nanoscale magnets that can be manipulated by magnetic fields. The nanomagnets are represented by the nanoparticles with a large net magnetic moment. Each magnetic nanoparticle contains only one magnetic domain. In the absence of magnetic fields, the nanoparticles are oriented randomly due to thermal fluctuations that are significant at the nanoscale (superparamagnetic regime). When an external magnetic field is applied in the vicinity of magnetic nanoparticles a strong torque is produced, which can overcome random thermal fluctuations orienting the magnetic nanoparticles in the direction of the magnetic field. In the case where the applied magnetic field has a gradient (magnetic field strength varies with position), this will exert a force on the magnetic nanoparticles so that they tend to move toward the area of highest magnetic field gradient. The intensity of the force depends on the magnetic moment of the nanoparticles (the nanoparticle size) and the gradient of the magnetic field, which is determined by the configuration of the magnets in place. This concept of 'magnetic pulling' based on magnetization of magnetic nanoparticles under an external magnetic field can be harnessed to produce a device for the treatment of several human disorders. Among such disorders, retina detachment is one that can be treated very efficiently with magnetic nanoparticles.

Research work by a University of Buenos Aires-Hospital Austral-Centro Atómico Bariloche (all three in Argentina)-Argonne National Laboratory (USA) collaboration demonstrated a novel approach for treatment of retina detachment, using superparamagnetic nanoparticles (particles that become magnetized in the presence of a magnetic field, but lose the total net magnetization of the whole upon magnetic field removal).[13] This new retina detachment treatment involves attaching a rare earth magnet array on the outside wall of the eye at the location where the retina detachment occurs (Fig. 6.9), and then injecting superparamagnetic nanoparticles (~15 nm in diameter) inside the eye (Fig. 6.9(a)). The external magnet produces a magnetic field gradient that induces a magnetic force in the superparamagnetic nanoparticles, which are then agglomerated and pulled towards the detached retina section to push the retina back against the inner wall of the eye (Fig. 6.9(b)) for subsequent laser treatment for final re-attachment.

Once the detached retina has been pushed back onto the inner eye wall, a laser is applied that seals the gap existing between the retina layer and the rest of the eye wall. The new retina detachment treatment described in this section, based on the integrated magnet/superparamagnetic action provides a novel approach for retina detachment treatment, which has several advantages over prior treatments described

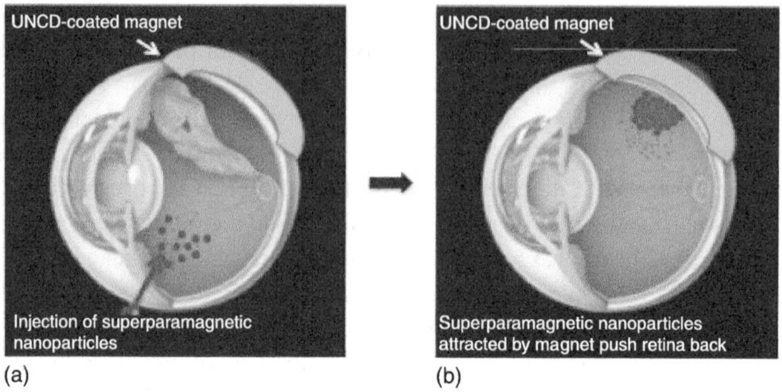

6.9 (a) Schematic showing retina detachment, attachment of a flexible magnet (this magnet can be coated with UNCD to make it more biocompatible, although it may not be absolutely necessary because of the short-term attachment that may be needed to re-attach the retina) and injection of superparamagnetic Fe_3O_4 nanoparticles with patented functionalization, produced in the Centro Atómico Bariloche-Argentina, by R. Zysler's group. (b) The magnetic field generated by the external magnet pulls the nanoparticles agglomerating them to exert enough force to push the retina back on the inner wall of the eye.

in Section 6.4.3: 1) the new treatment can be applied to the more difficult case of lower eye retina detachment without putting the patient upside-down; 2) the magnetic nanoparticles are biocompatible and biodegradable and once they come into contact with phagocytic cells they can be absorbed and degraded intra-cellularly and recycled to the iron intracellular storage compartment (ferritin)[14,15] by the eye once the magnet is taken off and the particle dispersed again; 3) the magnet can be coated with a UNCD film to make it highly bioinert and biocompatible, while implanted. It is important to note that the superparamagnetic nanoparticles only agglomerate under the influence of an external magnetic field and disaggregate after removing it. This property ensures that no magnetic embolus will be generated by agglomeration of the particles once the external magnetic field is switched off.

The animal pre-clinical trials performed in the collaboration described in this section demonstrated that the new retina detachment treatment using the integrated magnet/superparamagnetic nanoparticles provides an order of magnitude better approach than those based on conventional treatments described in Section 6.4.3. However, further work currently under way is necessary to optimize the new retina detachment treatment.

6.5 Conclusions

The new paradigm in biomaterials and medical treatments described in this chapter is enabling a new generation of implantable biomedical devices to treat a broad range of human disorders affecting the eye. The integration of physiology, new biomaterials and micro/nanofabrication technologies are enabling the development of new devices and nanoparticles implantable in the human eye for diagnosis, monitoring, and/or therapeutic treatment of vision degraded or lost either through genetically induced degenerative conditions, or traumatic events. The novel UNCD coating technology developed and patented at Argonne provides a unique bioinert/biocompatible material for a new generation of long life implantable devices in the eye. In addition, the new superparamagnetic nanoparticles developed and patented by the group in the Centro Atómico Bariloche–Argentina, and the clinical procedures developed in the Argentina–USA Institutional collaboration are opening the way for a new generation of micro and nanodevices based on magnetic nanoparticles. It is foreseen that both UNCD and magnetic nanoparticle technologies will have a major impact in healthcare in future.

6.6 Acknowledgments

This work was supported by U.S. Department of Energy, Office of Science, Office of Basic Energy Sciences-Materials Science, under contract DE-AC02-06CH11357 and DARPA under contracts MIPR 06-W238. Use of the Center for Nanoscale Materials was supported by the U. S. Department of Energy, Office of Science, Office of Basic Energy Sciences, under Contract No. DE-AC02-06CH11357. The TEM work was performed at the Electron Microscopy Center of Argonne National Laboratory.

The authors acknowledge the great contributions of the many scientists, students and postdoctorals who contributed to the science and technology of UNCD films during the past 20 years, namely: J.A. Carlisle (Initially Argonne National Laboratory and currently CTO of Advanced Diamond Technologies, Inc, special thanks for his leadership in bringing the UNCD technology to commercialization), A. R. Krauss, D. M. Gruen, A. V. Sumant, Y. C. Chen, B. Kabius, J. M. Hiller, B. Shi, X. Xiao.

The submitted manuscript has been created by UChicago Argonne, LLC, Operator of Argonne National Laboratory ('Argonne'). Argonne, a U.S. Department of Energy Office of Science laboratory, is operated under Contract No. DE-AC02-06CH11357. The U.S. Government retains for itself, and others acting on its behalf, a paid-up non-exclusive, irrevocable worldwide license in said article to reproduce, prepare derivative works, distribute copies to the public, and perform publicly and display publicly, by or on behalf of the Government.

6.7 References

1. M. S. Humanyun, 'Intraocular Retinal Prosthesis', *Tr. Am. Ophth. Soc.* 99 (2001) 271.
2. D. D. Zhou and E. Greenbaum (Eds). *Implantable Neural Prostheses vols. 1 and 2 Techniques and Engineering Approaches*, Springer (2010).

3. F. Stuart, D. Edell, A. Guzelian, Y. *et al.* 'Plasma-enhanced Chemical Vapour Deposited Silicon Carbide as an Implantable Dielectric Coating', *J. Biomedical Mater. Res. A* 67 (2003) 856.
4. J. Seo, S. Kim, H. Chung, *et al.* 'Biocompatibility of Polyimide Microelectrode Array for Retinal Stimulation', *Mater. Sci. Engin. C* 24 (2004) 185.
5. H. Hammerle, K. Kobuch, K. Kohler, W. *et al.* 'Biostability of Micro-photodiode Arrays for Subretinal Implantation', *Biomaterials* 23 (2002) 797.
6. O. Auciello and A. V. Sumant, 'Status Review of the Science and Technology of Ultrananocrystalline Diamond' (UNCD™) Films and Application to Multifunctional Devices, *Diamond and Related Materials* 19 (2010) 699.
7. X. Xiao, J. Wang, J. A. Carlisle, *et al.* '*In Vitro* and *In Vivo* Evaluation of Ultrananocrystalline Diamond for Coating of Implantable Retinal Microchips', *J. Biomedical Materials* 77B (2) (2006) 273.
8. K. S. Lim, B. D. Allan, A. W. Lloyd, *et al.* 'Glaucoma Drainage Devices; Past, Present and Future', *Br. J. Opthalmol.* 82 (1998)1083.
9. Y. C. Chen, X. Y. Zhong, A. R. Konicek, *et al.* 'Synthesis and Characterization of Smooth Ultrananocrystalline Diamond Films via Low Pressure Bias-Enhanced Nucleation and Growth', *Appl. Phys. Lett.* 92 (2008) 133113.
10. X. Y. Zhong, Y. C. Chen, N. H. Tai, *et al.* 'Effect of Pretreatment Bias on the Nucleation and Growth Mechanisms of Ultra-nanocrystalline Diamond Films via Bias-Enhanced Nucleation and Growth: An Approach to Interfacial Chemistry Analysis via Chemical Bonding Mapping', *J. Appl. Phys.* 105 (2009) 034311.
11. MedicineNet.com.
12. M. Tang, P. J. Rusell, and A. Khatri, 'Magnetic Nanoparticles: Prospects in Imaging and Therapy', *Discovery Medicine* 7 (38) (2007).
13. J. M. Vargas and R. D. Zysler, 'Tailoring the Size in Colloidal Iron Oxide Nanoparticles', *Nanotechnology* 16 (2005) 1474.
14. J. Wang, Y. Chen, B. Chen, *et al.* 'Pharmacokinetic Parameters and Tissue Distribution of Magnetic Fe_30_4 Particles in Mice', *Int. J. Nanomedicine* 5 (2010) 860.
15. J. D. Lopez-Castro, A. V. Maraloiu, J. J. Delgado, *et al.* 'From Synthetic to Natural Nanoparticles: Monitoring the Biodegradation of SPIO(P904) into Ferritin by Electron Microscopy', *Small* 3 (11) (2011) 4597.

7 Ultrananocrystalline diamond (UNCD) for neural applications

Y-C. CHEN, National Hsinchu University of Education, Taiwan and Harvard Medical School, USA, D-C. LEE, Institute of Cellular and System Medicine, Taiwan, N-H. TAI, National Tsing-Hua University, Taiwan, I-M. CHIU, Institute of Cellular and System Medicine, Taiwan, National Chung Hsing University, Taiwan and The Ohio State University, USA

DOI: 10.1533/9780857093516.2.171

Abstract: Diamond films have been considered as ideal candidates for protective coatings on bioimplants, as bioimplants themselves or as a guide for neural differentiation, because of their excellent mechanical properties, functional amenability, biocompatibility, and unique nanostructures. We separate nanocrystalline diamond films into two categories based on growth chemistries, nanostructure, and properties: nanocrystalline diamond (NCD) and ultrananocrystalline diamond (UNCD). UNCD is suitable for application as a hermetic coating for protection of implantable artificial retina medical devices, and also contributes to improvement of neural stem cell (NSC)-based cell transplantation, tissue engineering for neural tissue repair and regeneration and study of neural cell differentiation.

Key words: ultrananocrystalline diamond (UNCD), neuron cell, diamond films, neural and retinal prostheses.

7.1 Introduction

Diamond has long been considered as 'the biomaterial of the 21st century', and diamond films have been considered as ideal candidates for protective coatings on bioimplants, as bioimplants themselves or as a guide for neural differentiation, because of their excellent mechanical properties, functional amenability, biocompatibility and unique nanostructures.[1,2] The term 'diamond' has a specific meaning in physics, referring to the cubic crystalline form of carbon, space group *Fd3m2*. In this chapter, we separate nanocrystalline diamond films into two categories based on the growth chemistries, nanostructure (crystalline size), and properties: Nanocrystalline diamond (NCD) films, which are generally grown in hydrogen-rich chemical vapor deposition (CVD) growth environments, and ultrananocrystalline diamond (UNCD) films, which are generally grown in argon-rich and hydrogen-poor CVD environments.[3] NCD and UNCD have very different crystalline microstructures. NCD has grain sizes beginning with the size and density of the nucleating diamond particles and ranging up to 100–300 nm with very low to moderate amounts of sp^2-bonded carbon trapped at defects or grain boundaries. Some forms of NCD grown with very high methane concentration may contain as much as 50% non-diamond carbon phase.[4] The distinction between NCD and micro- or polycrystalline diamond is somewhat arbitrary and relates to the grain size and thickness of the films. On the other hand, UNCD thin films are synthesized using microwave plasma enhanced chemical vapor deposition (MPECVD) with argon-rich Ar/CH_4 plasma chemistries. UNCD consists of diamond grains ~5 nm in diameter and grain boundaries of 0.4–0.6 nm (Fig. 7.1(a)). This unique nanostructure results in a very smooth as-deposited surface (typical root-mean-squared (RMS) roughness of about 10–20 nm) that has excellent mechanical properties and is chemically inert.[5] NCD films are now being explored for not only a wide range of biomedical applications, such as artificial joints, retinal implants and nerve conduit for peripheral injury, but also further can be used to conduct different differentiation directions of neural stem cells (NSCs) (Fig. 7.1(b–d)).

For artificial retinal implants that use silicon microchips based on the complementary metal oxide semiconductor technology, the deposition/processing temperature of hermetic coatings on microchips should be lower than 400°C in order to avoid the failure of connections and materials inside microchip.[6] Thus, a very important distinction between the UNCD and the conventional diamond (NCD/MCD) deposition process is that UNCD can be grown at 400°C with growth rates similar to those observed for high temperature growth.[6,7] Furthermore, the capability to covalently functionalize the surface of UNCD makes it amenable to a specific physiological environment, which substantially improves its biocompatibility and also induces different differential directions of NSCs.[8,9] The combination of all these properties makes UNCD suitable as a hermetic coating for the protection of implantable artificial retina medical devices, and also contributes to improvement of NSC-based cell transplantation, tissue engineering for neural tissue repair and regeneration and study of neural cell differentiation.

7.2 Mechanism aspects of ultrananocrystalline diamond (UNCD)/neural cell interactions

Nanostructured materials provide a new insight into interaction with biological systems that takes place on a sub-cellular level with a high degree of specificity. The use of these materials for culturing cells has advantages over using a defined polystyrene dish in biocompatibility and low cytotoxicity. They allow cell growth and development adapted to a specific application without using potentially harmful chemicals in the human body. The mechanistic basis of the nano-topographical effects on cells could be discussed in indirect (biochemical signal-mediated) and direct (force-mediated) mechano-transduction. The interaction of nano-sized particles with living cells transgresses the framework laid down by previous known macroscopic interactions. The excellent biocompatibility,

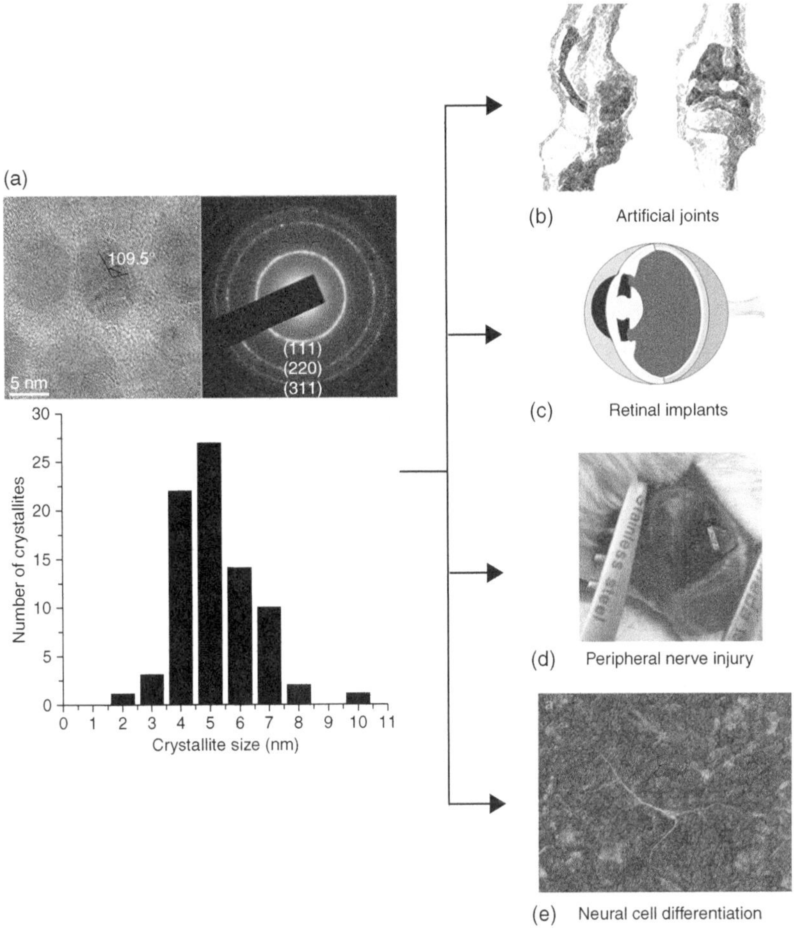

7.1 Possible medical applications of nanocrystalline diamond (NCD) films. (a) High resolution transmission electron microscope (TEM) image of NCD films reveals individual crystallites having the lattice spacing of diamond of 0.206 nm. The corresponding selected area electron diffraction (SEAD) pattern shows diffraction rings corresponding to {111}, {220} and {311} planes of diamond. The NCD films could be used in developing artificial joints (b), retinal implants (c), repair of peripheral nerve injury or neural diseases (d), and studies of neural cell differentiation (e).

extreme mechanical, adjustable electrical properties and chemical inertness make diamond a prime candidate for developing medical applications.[4,10,11] Many studies have been performed by plating cells on NCD or UNCD surfaces to investigate the suitability of these biomaterials as growth supporters to determine which surface characteristic properties are suitable for cell growth and proliferation.

Thalhammer and co-workers investigated the suitability of nanodiamond (ND) monolayers as a platform for neuronal growth.[12] Neurons cultured on various ND-coated substrates perform remarkably well, and similar to those grown on standard protein-coated materials with respect to their initial cell attachment, sustained neurite outgrowth, cell-autonomous neuronal excitability and functionality of the resulting electrical networks.[12] ND layering provides an excellent growth substrate on various materials for functional neuronal networks and bypasses the necessity of protein coating, which promises great potential for chronic medical implants. Surfaces of different materials, no matter if glass, NCD or Si, coated with monolayers of monodispersed detonation-derived nanodiamonds displayed promising similarity to the protein-coated materials regarding neuronal cell attachment, neurite outgrowth and functional network formation. Importantly, the neurons were able to grow in direct contact with the ND-coated material and could be easily maintained in culture for an extended period, equal to those on protein-coated substrates. Given the biocompatibility of NDs, and their potential for surface functionalization, ND layering might prove a valuable material technique for implants on a wide range of substrates. In this study, neuronal cells cultured on ND films exhibited cell morphology similar to those cultured on regular chemicals. However, the physiological function study would need to be carried on and followed up.

In 2005, Ariano *et al.* cultured rat hippocampal neurons and chick ciliary ganglia for several days on oxygen- and hydrogen- terminated NCD (O-NCD and H-NCD) surfaces preserving their morphology and electrical properties. The mixtures of adhesion molecules (poly-d-lysine, poly-dl-ornithine, laminin) are used as organic substrates to anchor the cells to the diamond surface.[13,14] In the presence of adherent chemical molecules, rat hippocampal neurons plated on O-NCD surface survive and preserve their synaptic activity and somatic Ca^{2+} current densities. Chick ciliary ganglion neurons adhere, survive and are functional on H-NCD surface as well. The tested biocompatibility of central and peripheral neurons with NCD diamond surfaces indicates that NCD electrodes are suitable for interfacing with different types of neuronal networks and can be used for wide-spectrum pharmacological screenings. These results highlight the potential of functionalized diamond surfaces as substrates for constructing microelectrode arrays for multiparametric recording of electrical activity and optical signals in neuronal networks.

Furthermore, Ariano *et al.* presented a study on the adhesion, growth, and viability of GT1-7 neuronal cells on diamond surfaces with different topography and surface terminations.[15,16] Cells were maintained in the presence of 10% fetal bovine serum (FBS), and the proteins present in this medium may have been adsorbed on the surface and influence cell adhesion and survival. However, GT1-7 cells, like most neuronal models, cannot attach, survive and maintain their functional properties for several days in a simple serum-free medium; some addition, such as B27 supplement is generally necessary. This procedure, in turn, adds to the extracellular environment proteins and other molecules of unknown nature.[15] Cells plated on NCD samples adhere, proliferate and preserve their somatic Ca^{2+} activity, whatever the chemistry of the diamond surface (H- or O-terminated), whereas the adhesion and growth of cells on homo-epitaxial diamonds significantly depend on the surface termination (the more hydrophilic, the more biocompatible is the surface).[15] With respect to homo-epitaxial samples, the roughness at the sub-micrometer scale allows a larger surface contact area, allowing an efficient interface with electrically excitable cells. From the AFM analysis, it was found that neuronal cell adhesion is promoted on NCD, the surface roughness of which is within 90 nm RMS. Cell adhesion is much lower on flat homo-epitaxial diamonds surfaces with RMS smaller than 1 nm. These results indicate that nano-topography of diamond surfaces should have better protein-repellent properties than those of pure and flat diamond, and was also observed in other cell lines such as osteoblasts (SAOS-2).[17] Thus, optimized primary substrate roughness with specific morphology, combined with extraordinary NCD properties such as mechanical stability and chemical resistance, will promote better interaction with cells.

UNCD with grains of ~5 nm and a very smooth surface of 10–20 nm possesses the desirable properties of diamond and can be deposited as a smooth and conformal coating using chemical vapor deposition at low temperature as used in biomedical applications. Bajaj *et al.* compared cell adhesion, proliferation, and growth of rat pheochromocytoma cells (PC12) on UNCD films, silicon, and platinum films substrates.[18] Fluorescence images showed that PC12 cells were growing characteristic neuronal processes and these processes were interacting with each other on both platinum and UNCD surfaces, yet, on the silicon surface they were forming closely packed islands without processes. This effect can be interpreted as indicative of the affinity of the PC12 cells on platinum and UNCD surfaces under study, exhibiting a distinctive outgrowth of axons and dendrites on the surfaces. The maximum PC12 cell numbers and spreading were again observed on the UNCD surface, followed by the platinum and the silicon surfaces.[18] Their results showed that UNCD films exhibited superior characteristics including cell number, total cell area, and cell spreading. The results could be attributed to the nanostructured nature or a combination of nanostructure/surface chemistry of UNCD, which provides a high surface energy, hence promoting adhesion between the receptors on the cell surface and the UNCD films. According to published data,[6,15,18] neuronal cells grown on NCD or UNCD films exhibited proliferation activity, neurite outgrowth, and electrophysiology activity.

Recently, Chen *et al.* showed that UNCD could be used in guiding neural stem cell differentiation and also demonstrated a novel role for H-UNCD films in promoting differentiation of NSCs through activation of Fak-Erk1/2 through integrins.[8,9] H-UNCD films were compared with standard grade polystyrene in terms of their impact on the differentiation of NSCs. When

NSCs were cultured on these substrates in medium supplemented with low concentration of serum and without any differentiating factors, H-UNCD films spontaneously induced neuronal differentiation on NSCs. By direct suppression of a mitogen-activated protein kinase/extracellular signaling-regulated kinase 1/2 (MAPK/ERK1/2) signaling pathway in NSCs using U0126, known to inhibit the activation of Erk1/2, we demonstrated that the enhancement of the ERK1/2 pathway is one of the effects of H-UNCD-induced NSC differentiation. Moreover, a functional-blocking antibody directed against integrin β1 subunit inhibited neuronal differentiation on H-UNCD films. This result demonstrated the involvement of integrin β1 in H-UNCD-mediated neuronal differentiation. Mechanistic studies revealed the cell adhesion to H-UNCD films associated with focal adhesion kinase (Fak) and initiated MAPK/ERK1/2 signaling. Chen *et al.* demonstrated that H-UNCD film-mediated NSCs differentiation involves fibronectin-integrin β1 and pFak/MAPK/ERK1/2 signaling pathways in the absence of differentiation factors.[9] The confocal immunofluorescence image showed the spatial relationship of cellular signaling molecules, FAK and ERK1/2 (Fig. 7.2). These observations raise the potential for the use of UNCD as a biomaterial for central nervous system transplantation and tissue engineering.

NSCs are found in the brain and can differentiate into three types of cells: neurons, astrocytes, and oligodendrocytes.[19] The two major aims of biomaterials used in stem cell biology are to provide cues for directed differentiation and retaining proliferation capacity before differentiation. The ability to control stem cell differentiation or proliferation using topography alone has focused on the focal adhesions, which were the sites of cell attachment to underlying substrates.[20–23] Focal adhesions play a pivotal role in all subsequent cell actions in response to nanotopography. The focal adhesion kinase (FAK) localizes at focal adhesions or focal contacts and can regulate cellular transcription, leading to sequential posttranslational modification.[24] The integrin dependent signaling pathway is mediated by non-receptor tyrosine kinase, most notably Fak, which is constitutively associated with β-integrin subunit.[24–26]

Rezek and colleagues investigated adsorption of FBS, a crucial component for cell growth, on intrinsic CVD mono-crystalline diamond with H- or O-terminations.[27,28] They concluded that the proteins contained in FBS are present on both H/O-diamond surfaces. The adhered proteins do not form covalent bonds to the diamond surface with either H- or O-termination. FBS is adsorbed in about the same monolayer thickness (2–4 nm) on both H/O-diamond surfaces. As the cell morphologies are slightly different,[29] it is likely that the protein compositions that adhere to H-diamond and O-diamond surfaces are different. Integrins and other cell adhesion molecules act as interconnectors between cells and the extracellular matrix or the surface of cell growth support such as a polystyrene Petri dish. Using NCD or UNCD films as cell growth surfaces, the proteins present

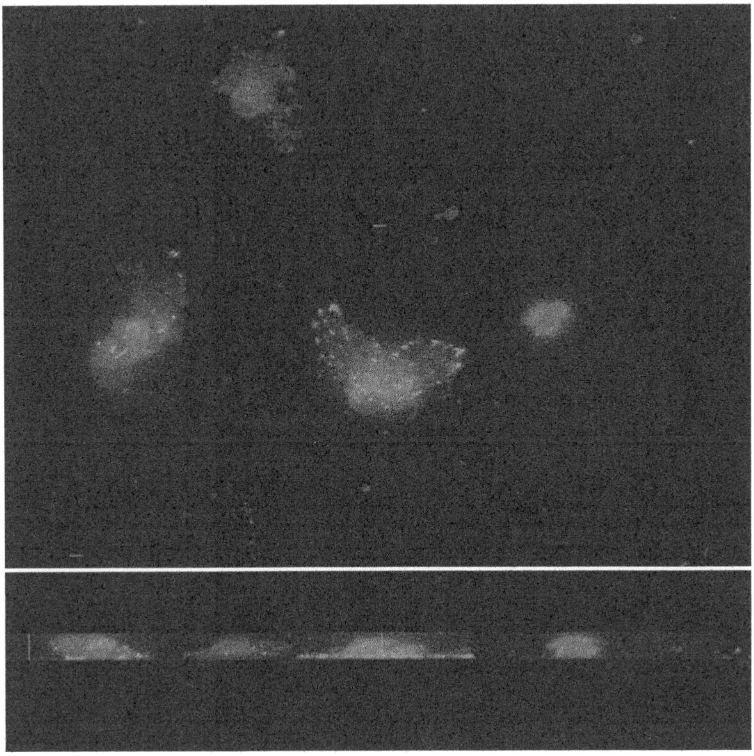

7.2 Confocal immunofluorescence image showing the spatial relationship of cellular signaling molecules FAK and ERK. The neural stem cells grown on the H-UNCD film in the regular medium without any differentiating reagents were stained with anti phospho-FAK antibody labeled with Alexafluor 594 (red) and anti phospho-ERK labeled with DyLight 488 (green).The dual colors of phospho-FAK and phospho-ERK were detected in the cells simultaneously and localized to their proper subcellular positions. In the quadrant of stacking images, phospho-FAK was observed in basal cell membrane adherent to HUNCD films, whereas phospho-ERK was shown assembled in the cytoplasm.

in medium may be adsorbed on the surface and influence cell behaviors. The integrin–ligand complex formation could trigger intracellular signaling cascades and thereby regulate cellular phenotype, motility, proliferation, and differentiation. We also studied the interactions of proteins adhered to UNCD films in mediating NSC differentiation. Via LC-MS/MS study, fibronectin, transferrin, and apolipoprotein were identified preferentially absorbed onto UNCD films, but not on the Petri dish polystyrene surface (Fig. 7.3).

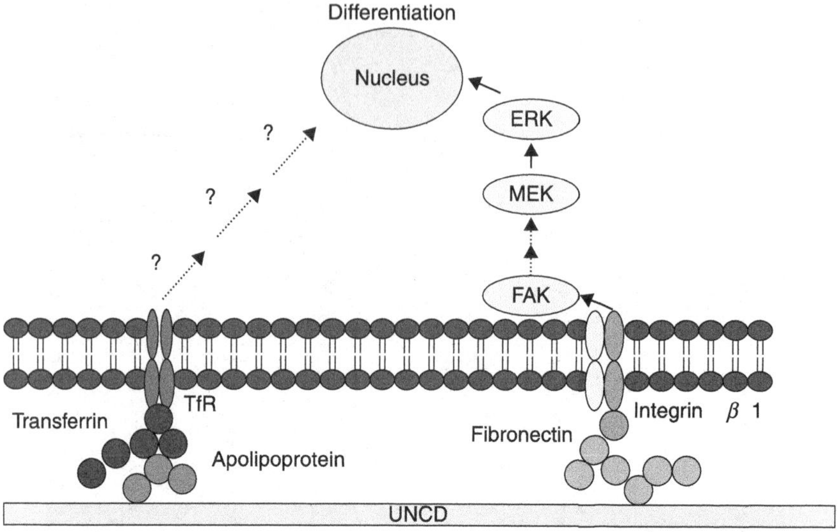

7.3 Possible interactions of proteins adhered to UNCD films in mediating NSC differentiation. UNCD films could absorb fibronectin, transferrin, and apolipoprotein from medium that contains low concentration of serum and is free of differentiating reagents. The absorbed fibronectin on UNCD films activates cellular transmembrane receptor integrin β1, FAK and ERK 1/2 pathway, ultimately leading to neural differentiation from NSCs. Other than fibronectin, transferrin and apolipoprotein were detected in the UNCD absorbed protein profile. The possible mechanism of transferrin-induced signaling pathway has yet to be established.

7.3 Methods of guiding neurons

Characterization of the interaction between cells and contact surfaces is essential for cell-based biosensors, tissue engineering, and optimization of implant materials. Extensive efforts are made to construct a junction between neurons and electronic chips, i.e. a brain–machine interface. Cells recognize their environment and consequently start to modify it. The potential impact of such devices is enormous as they can be used to compensate for both sensory and motor deficits in the nervous systems, e.g. they could be used to restore vision, hearing and motor impairments as well as impaired autonomic functions.[6] This feat is, however, not trivial as the number of nerve cell processes and neurons are counted in the millions and efficient neuro-electronic junctions must be small. Thus they must have a high-spatial resolution; here nanotechnology may offer a solution. Besides guiding growth direction of neuronal cells, clinical applications require precise control of differentiation of NSCs *in vivo*, because most injuries to the central nervous system are caused by the loss or damage of a specific sub-population of the neural circuits. Thus, focusing on how to obtain neuronal and oligodendrocyte phenotype differentiation from NSCs is essential because of the central role of neurons and the supporting role of oligodendrocytes in the neurological system.[30,31]

Primary cultures of rodent neurons require a specially treated surface for initial attachment and survival, and this is routinely provided by the deposition of extracellular matrix (ECM) proteins. Specht *et al.* showed the ordered growth of mammalian neurons by micro-contact printing of specifically patterned proteins, laminin, on single crystalline diamond surfaces, exemplifying the necessity of protein coating for neuronal growth.[32] The fabricated pattern consisted of a grid of 5 μm lines at a 50 μm pitch. Neuron adhesion and outgrowth was specific for those areas of the diamond that had been stamped with laminin, resulting in ordered growth of high resolution. Neurons survived in culture for the duration of the experiment, and laminin patterns were stable for at least one week in culture.[32] Although protein coating is sufficient for *in vitro* experiments, *in vivo* implants, such as in neural prosthetics, will require biocompatible coatings that preferably will not introduce foreign proteins into the body.

Chen *et al.* investigated the interaction of UNCD with NSCs and found that controlling the surface properties of UNCD can manipulate the differentiation of NSCs.[8] When NSCs were cultured on these substrates in low serum and without any differentiating factors, H-UNCD films spontaneously induced cell proliferation and neuronal differentiation (Fig. 7.4(c)). Using high-resolution scanning electron microscope (SEM) images reveals that the cell-H-UNCD films contacts were filopodia/nano-diamond interactions all along cells (Fig. 7.4(a) and (b)). O-UNCD films were also shown to further improve neural differentiation, with a preference to differentiate into oligodendrocytes[8,9] (Fig. 7.4(d)). Hence, controlling the surface properties of UNCD could manipulate the differentiation of NSCs for different biomedical applications. These observations raise the potential for the use of UNCD as a biomaterial for central nervous system transplantation and tissue engineering.

These findings are exciting as they show the possibility of the application of diamond as a new biomaterial. Diamond is extremely inert and should therefore not lead to cytotoxicity caused by degradation products. This property makes diamond an attractive, widely biocompatible material. Therefore, diamond is a good candidate for neuronal implants and would be expected to perform well if not better than other materials *in vivo*. Hydrophobicity has been used by others to preferentially attach laminin and further to guide neuron growth. This technique could be exploited on diamond by varying the surface termination (and hence hydrophobicity) with extremely high resolution, without the involvement of further chemical modifications.

7.4 Neural and retinal prostheses

One of the key components in neural prosthetic systems is the microelectrode/microprobe, which interfaces with neurons for electrical and chemical signal

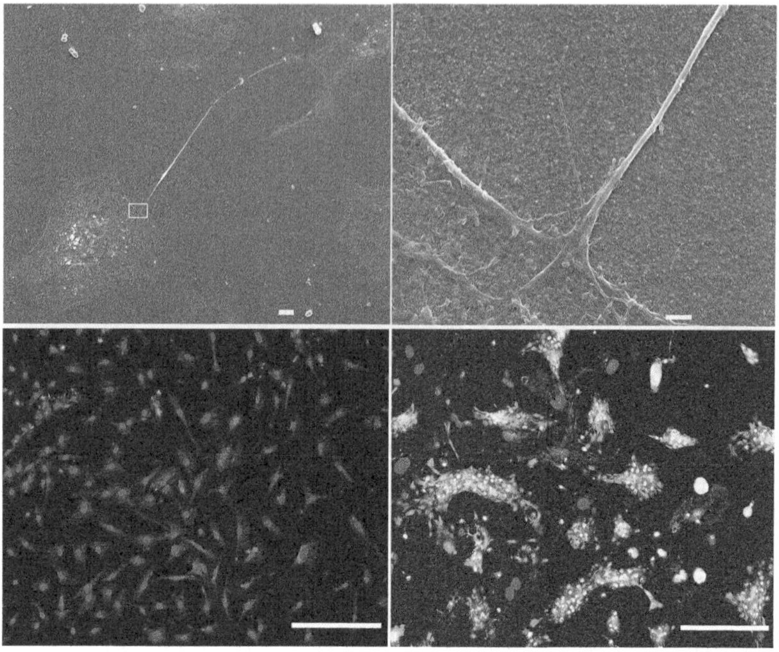

7.4 Neural differentiation of NSCs on UNCD films. NSCs were cultured on H-UNCD films without any differentiating reagents for seven days. Scanning electron microscope (SEM) images showed the interaction between cell and H-UNCD and cell and cell (a). Higher magnification of the box in (a) was performed to enlarge the contacting region of cells to UNCD films (b). TuJI immuno-reactive differentiated neurons could be observed on H-UNCD film (c) and Gale immuno-reactive differentiated oligodendrocytes could be observed on O-UNCD film (d). Scale bar: (a) 10 μm; (b) 1 μm; (c) 100 μm and (d) 100 μm.

recording and for stimulation. With the development of microelectromechanical systems technologies, sophisticated microprobes with electrode arrays have been developed and are widely used in neural activity studies, drug delivery, and cochlear implants.[4] They play an important role in several medical palliative treatments where electrical stimulation is required, such as for the Parkinson's disease.[33] More prospective projects are now aiming to alleviate disabilities with the possibility of providing disabled people with computer-driven motility or providing vision to the blind.[4,6] There are five criteria for diamond when exploring electrode materials for biosensors, and developing hermetic coatings for encapsulation of implantable medical devices, specifically for the microchip retinal implant: 1) bioinertness and biocompatibility; 2) mechanical robustness; 3) chemical and electrochemical inertness and electrical insulation; 4) tunable conductivity after doping; and 5) easy functionalization.[6]

Microprobe arrays have been fabricated, microassembled and integrated with a hybrid application-specific integrated circuit chip to build a three-dimensional (3D) microelectrode array.[34] Nevertheless, most are made of silicon as silicon-based microfabrication technology is well developed. Because of flexibility issues associated with Si probes, researchers have recently been studying the use of other materials in probe fabrication. The most important component on the microprobes is the metal site, which is used for signal recording and electrical stimulation. Commonly used site materials include platinum, gold, titanium nitride, and iridium oxide. For electrical stimulation, the electrode should have a large charge storage capacity and large charge delivery capacity in order to deliver a sufficient amount of charge in a small geometric area. Sites for electrical recording, on the other hand, should be fabricated from a highly conductive material (such as gold) and small double-layer capacitance in order to reduce thermal noise and minimize background noise (non-Faradaic current), respectively.[35] Therefore, in order to have a good signal to noise ratio (>3), the electrode should have low capacitance as well as a wide water potential window (i.e. a potential range in which there is no current caused by oxygen or hydrogen evolution).[35] Ariano *et al.* developed a device for recording the extracellular electrical activity for culturing neuronal networks based on H-terminated conductive diamond.[16] They further provided the first report of electrical activity from living neurons recorded by a H-terminated diamond electrode. The device is able to detect the spontaneous extracellular electrical activity of a neuronal cell line (GT1-7 cells), and can be used to monitor the effects of either changes in the extracellular medium such as ion substitution or addition of pharmacological agents, e.g. channel blockers. The time courses of these signals were in good agreement with those recorded by means of conventional microelectrode array (MEAs) and with the negative derivative of the intracellular action potentials recorded with the patch clamp technique from single cells.[15,16]

Yoshimi's group has mainly studied reward-induced burst firing of dopaminergic neurons in the primate midbrain.[36] Voltammetry allows high-speed detection of dopamine release in the projection area. Although voltammetry has revealed presynaptic modulation of dopamine release in the striatum, to date, reward-induced release in awakened brains has been recorded only in rodents. To make such recordings, it is possible to use conventional carbon fibers in monkey brains but the use of these fibers is limited by their physical fragility.[36,37] Constant-potential amperometry was applied to novel diamond microelectrodes for high-speed detection of dopamine. In primate brains during Pavlovian cue-reward trials, a sharp response to a reward cue was detected in the caudate of Japanese monkeys. Overall, this method allows measurements of monoamine release in specific target areas of large brains, the findings will expand the knowledge of reward responses obtained by unit recordings.

Chan *et al.* first demonstrated that the diamond probe received the stimulated neural signal at a signal to noise ratio of ~2.[35] There are several possible reasons for such low signal to noise ratio. One of the possible reasons is that the probe position may not be close enough to the body of the firing neurons. The strength of the neuron signal attenuates with increasing distance between the recording site and the target neurons. Moreover, since the resistivity of the boron-doped diamond interconnects (10^{-3} Ω-cm) is relatively high compared to metal interconnects, the total resistance of the diamond site along with the diamond interconnect becomes high, leading to more thermal noise.[35] It is also worth noting that due to the surface roughness of polycrystalline diamond films, the surface area of the electrodes is much higher than the metal films. The surface area of polycrystalline diamond can be approximately five times greater than that of smooth metals, which can result in greater background noise, compared to a metal electrode of the same size. Increasing the signal to noise ratio will be a priority in future works. For the first time, the design, fabrication, and testing of a novel polycrystalline diamond-based microprobe was reported for possible applications in neural prosthesis. The polycrystalline diamond probe has also been successfully implanted in the auditory cortex area of guinea pig brains for *in vivo* neural studies. The recorded signal amplitude was 30–40 μV and had a duration of 1 ms.[35]

Better understanding of the architecture of neural networks is developing, which will help the design of future *in vivo* prostheses. Novel microelectrode array prototypes combining a silicon array of high density and shape ratio (up to 1024 tips of 80 μm in height, separated by 50 μm spacing) with complete software interface and embedding signal treatment are now industrially developed. The development provides the ability to record neural activity, for example from spinal cords deposited on the high aspect ratio electrodes. However, when used for the stimulation of neurons, the voltage bursts often have destructive effects on the quality of the electrodes, especially after intensive use. Bonnauron's group proposed to use the same structure with a conductive boron-doped NCD layer on top of the high aspect ratio electrodes. They optimized a process enabling coating of 3D structures of micrometer tips with boron-doped NCD layer thin layers.

The other example is a retinal microchip used to restore vision lost because of retinal degeneration. The basic function of this implant is to translate visual information, captured by an externally worn camera, into a pattern of electrical stimulation pulses that is then applied to the retina. One prototype of this implant is a low-resolution device that contacts the retina with 16 electrodes. In clinical trials of this prototype, completely blind individuals were able to interpret the electrical stimulus from it as a visual sensation. An improvement in this field would involve developing an implantable microelectronic device that can stimulate the retina at hundreds of individual locations, in much the same way as a computer display uses a large number of pixels to create an image. Packaging this microchip is a significant technical challenge, as the package must simultaneously protect the microchip from the corrosive eye fluids, protect the eye from the chip materials, and allow the circuit to interface with the retina through microelectrodes.[6,3] Therefore, this microchip must be both biocompatible and bioinert. Specifically, it should not induce any adverse reaction by retina tissue that may influence its physiological function, and it should not have any electrochemical reaction with the physiological environment that might produce gas (e.g. oxygen or hydrogen) and lead to chemical attack of the microchip surface, thereby impairing its functionality. In most of the current generation of implantable retinal microelectronic devices, Si is used as the structural and functional material in the microchip.[3] However, Si is soluble in human fluids over a long period of time. Therefore, hermetic coatings with good biocompatibility and bioinertness are critically needed for encapsulation of bioimplantable devices composed of Si. Coating materials currently being evaluated for encapsulating artificial retinal prototype implants include SiO_2, SiN_x, SiC, and polyimide, but the dissolution and decay of SiO_2 passivation layer, structure defects, degenerations and leakage currents from devices have been found when implanted in animals up to several months. Xiao *et al.* demonstrated that UNCD is bioinert and biostable for at least 6 months *in vivo*. These tests involved implantation of the UNCD-coated Si chips in the eyes of rabbits.[6] These results demonstrated the potential of UNCD as a hermetic coating on implantable retinal microchips. Further work is ongoing to overcome the remaining technical barriers to fully integrate UNCD coatings into future generations of these biomedical devices.

7.5 References

1. Muller, R., Adamschik, M., Steidl, D., *et al.* (2004) Application of CVD-diamond for catheter ablation in the heart, *Diam. Relat. Mat.*, 13, 1080–1083, 10.1016/j.diamond.2003.12.012.
2. Butler, J. E., and Sumant, A. V. (2008) The CVD of nanodiamond materials, *Chem. Vapor Depos.*, 14, 145–160, 10.1002/cvde.200700037.
3. Auciello, O., Gruen, D. M., Krauss, A. R., *et al.* (2000) Science and technology of ultrananocrystalline diamond (UNCD) thin films for multifunctional devices. In *Smart Electronics and Mems Ii* (Abbott, D., Varadan, V. V., and Boehringer, K. F. eds.), Spie-Int Soc Optical Engineering, Bellingham. pp. XXI–XXXI.
4. Williams, O. A. (2011) Nanocrystalline diamond, *Diam. Relat. Mat.*, 20, 621–640, 10.1016/j.diamond.2011.02.015.
5. Naguib, N. N., Elam, J. W., Birrell, J., *et al.* (2006) Enhanced nucleation, smoothness and conformality of ultrananocrystalline diamond (UNCD) ultrathin films via tungsten interlayers, *Chem. Phys. Lett.*, 430, 345–350, 10.1016/j.cplett.2006.08.137.
6. Chen, Y. C., Zhong, X. Y., Konicek, A. R., *et al.* (2008) Synthesis and characterization of smooth ultrananocrystalline diamond films via low pressure bias-enhanced nucleation and growth, *Appl. Phys. Lett.*, 92, 133113, 10.1063/1.2838303.
7. Xiao, X. C., Wang, J., Liu, C., *et al.* (2006) In vitro and in vivo evaluation of ultrananocrystalline diamond for coating of implantable retinal microchips, *J. Biomed. Mater. Res. Part B*, 77B, 273–281, 10.1002/jbm.b.30448.
8. Xiao, X., Birrell, J., Gerbi, J. E., *et al.* (2004) Low temperature growth of ultrananocrystalline diamond, *J. Appl. Phys.*, 96, 2232–2239, 10.1063/1.1769609.
9. Chen, Y.-C., Lee, D.-C., Hsiao, C.-Y., *et al.* (2009) The effect of ultra-nanocrystalline diamond films on the proliferation and differentiation of neural stem cells, *Biomaterials*, 30, 3428–3435, 10.1016/j.biomaterials.2009.03.058.

10. Chen, Y.-C., Lee, D.-C., Tsai, T.-Y., *et al.* (2010) Induction and regulation of differentiation in neural stem cells on ultra-nanocrystalline diamond films, *Biomaterials*, 31, 5575–5587, 10.1016/j.biomaterials.2010.03.061.
11. Auciello, O., and Sumant, A. V. (2010) Status review of the science and technology of ultrananocrystalline diamond (UNCD (TM)) films and application to multifunctional devices, *Diam. Relat. Mat.*, 19, 699–718, 10.1016/j.diamond.2010.03.015.
12. Li, W., Kabius, B. and Auciello, O. (2010) Science and Technology of Biocompatible Thin Films for Implantable Biomedical Devices. In *2010 Annual International Conference of the IEEE Engineering in Medicine and Biology Society*. pp. 6237–6242.
13. Thalhammer, A., Edgington, R. J., Cingolani, L. A., *et al.* (2010) The use of nanodiamond monolayer coatings to promote the formation of functional neuronal networks, *Biomaterials*, 31, 2097–2104, 10.1016/j.biomaterials.2009.11.109.
14. Ariano, P., Baldelli, P., Carbone, E., *et al.* (2005) Cellular adhesion and neuronal excitability on functionalised diamond surfaces, *Diam. Relat. Mat.*, 14, 669–674, 10.1016/j.diamond.2004.11.021.
15. Erriquez, J., Gilardino, A., Ariano, P., *et al.* (2005) Calcium signals activated by arachidonic acid in embryonic chick ciliary ganglion neurons, *Neurosignals*, 14, 244–254, 10.1159/000088640.
16. Ariano, P., Budnyk, O., Dalmazzo, S., *et al.* (2009) On diamond surface properties and interactions with neurons, *European Physical Journal E*, 30, 149–156, 10.1140/epje/i2009-10520-9.
17. Ariano, P., Lo Giudice, A., Marcantoni, A., *et al.* (2009) A diamond-based biosensor for the recording of neuronal activity, *Biosensors & Bioelectronics*, 24, 2046–2050, 10.1016/j.bios.2008.10.017.
18. Broz, A., Baresova, V., Kromka, A., *et al.* (2009) Strong influence of hierarchically structured diamond nanotopography on adhesion of human osteoblasts and mesenchymal cells, *Physica Status Solidi a-Applications and Materials Science*, 206, 2038–2041, 10.1002/pssa.200982203.
19. Bajaj, P., Akin, D., Gupta, A., *et al.* (2007) Ultrananocrystalline diamond film as an optimal cell interface for biomedical applications, *Biomed Microdevices*, 9, 787–794, 10.1007/s10544-007-9090-2.
20. Lee, D. C., Hsu, Y. C., Chung, Y. F., *et al.* (2009) Isolation of neural stem/progenitor cells by using EGF/FGF1 and FGF1B promoter-driven green fluorescence from embryonic and adult mouse brains, *Mol Cell Neurosci*, 41, 348–363, 10.1016/j.mcn.2009.04.010.
21. Guilak, F., Cohen, D. M., Estes, B. T., *et al.* (2009) Control of Stem Cell Fate by Physical Interactions with the Extracellular Matrix, *Cell Stem Cell*, 5, 17–26, 10.1016/j.stem.2009.06.016.
22. Anselme, K., and Bigerelle, M. (2011) Role of materials surface topography on mammalian cell response, *International Materials Reviews*, 56, 243–266, 10.1179/1743280411y.0000000001.
23. Fisher, O. Z., Khademhosseini, A., Langer, R., and Peppas, N. A. (2010) Bioinspired Materials for Controlling Stem Cell Fate, *Accounts of Chemical Research*, 43, 419–428, 10.1021/ar900226q.
24. Li, D., Zhou, J., Chowdhury, F., *et al.* (2011) Role of mechanical factors in fate decisions of stem cells, *Regenerative Medicine*, 6, 229–240, 10.2217/rme.11.2.
25. Biggs, M. J. P., Richards, R. G., and Dalby, M. J. (2010) Nanotopographical modification: a regulator of cellular function through focal adhesions, *Nanomedicine-Nanotechnology Biology and Medicine*, 6, 619–633, 10.1016/j.nano.2010.01.009.

26. Bikle, D. D. (2008) Integrins, insulin like growth factors, and the skeletal response to load, *Osteoporosis International*, 19, 1237–1246, 10.1007/s00198-008-0597-z.
27. Docheva, D., Popov, C., Mutschler, W., and Schieker, M. (2007) Human mesenchymal stem cells in contact with their environment: surface characteristics and the integrin system, *Journal of Cellular and Molecular Medicine*, 11, 21–38, 10.1111/j.1582-4934.2007.00001.x.
28. Rezek, B., Ukraintsev, E., Michalikova, L., *et al.* (2009) Adsorption of fetal bovine serum on H/O-terminated diamond studied by atomic force microscopy, *Diam. Relat. Mat.*, 18, 918–922, 10.1016/j.diamond.2009.02.009.
29. Ukraintsev, E., Rezek, B., Kromka, A., *et al.* (2009) Long-term adsorption of fetal bovine serum on H/O-terminated diamond studied in situ by atomic force microscopy, *Physica Status Solidi B-Basic Solid State Physics*, 246, 2832–2835, 10.1002/pssb.200982257.
30. Armstrong, R. J., and Svendsen, C. N. (2000) Neural stem cells: from cell biology to cell replacement, *Cell Transplant*, 9, 139–152.
31. Bithell, A., and Williams, B. P. (2005) Neural stem cells and cell replacement therapy: making the right cells, *Clin Sci (Lond)*, 108, 13–22, 10.1042/CS20040276.
32. Specht, C. G., Williams, O. A., Jackman, R. B., and Schoepfer, R. (2004) Ordered growth of neurons on diamond, *Biomaterials*, 25, 4073–4078, 10.1016/j.biomaterials.2003.11.006.
33. Baron, M. S., Vitek, J. L., Bakay, R. A. E., *et al.* (1996) Treatment of advanced Parkinson's disease by posterior GPi pallidotomy: 1-year results of a pilot study, *Annals of Neurology*, 40, 355–366, 10.1002/ana.410400305.
34. Le Van Quyen, M., and Bragin, A. (2007) Analysis of dynamic brain oscillations: methodological advances, *Trends Neurosci*, 30, 365–373, 10.1016/j.tins.2007.05.006.
35. Chan, H.-Y., Aslam, D. M., Wiler, J. A., and Casey, B. (2009) A Novel Diamond Microprobe for Neuro-Chemical and -Electrical Recording in Neural Prosthesis, *Journal of Microelectromechanical Systems*, 18, 511–521, 10.1109/jmems.2009.2015493.
36. Yoshimi, K., Naya, Y., Mitani, N., *et al.* (2011) Phasic reward responses in the monkey striatum as detected by voltammetry with diamond microelectrodes, *Neuroscience Research*, 71, 49–62, 10.1016/j.neures.2011.05.013.
37. Phillips, P. E., Stuber, G. D., Heien, M. L., *et al.* (2003) Subsecond dopamine release promotes cocaine seeking, *Nature*, 422, 614–618, 10.1038/nature01476.

8

Nanodiamonds for drug delivery systems

A. E. MENGESHA, Drake University, USA and B-B. C. YOUAN, University of Missouri-Kansas City, USA

DOI: 10.1533/9780857093516.2.186

Abstract: Nanodiamonds offer a potential novel template for drug delivery and targeting, because of their small primary particle size, purity, excellent properties, facile surface functionalization, high biocompatibility, and inexpensive large-scale synthesis. However, nanodiamond properties such as aggregation state, surface chemistry, and presence of impurities, as well as the localization and accumulation behavior at the organism level, must be controlled to maintain safety and retain efficacy of conjugated therapeutic agents. A clinically applicable approach requires investigation of biocompatibility, biodistribution, and biological fate of the nanodiamond as well as its conjugates.

Key words: nanodiamonds, small molecules, peptides, proteins, gene delivery, targeting.

8.1 Introduction

This chapter presents a brief overview of the potential of nanodiamonds as novel template for drug delivery and targeting. Drug delivery has typically focused on optimizing drug therapy by simplifying administration of drugs, improving effectiveness, and clinical safety. Systems with controlled rate delivery offer substantial advantages over conventional dosage forms such as minimized *in vivo* fluctuations of drug concentrations, with potential for reduced side effects and reduced dosing frequency, and improved patient compliance. For a drug to exert its desired effect, it needs to interact with its physiological target, such as a receptor, but many drugs do not have inherently high specificity for reaching and interacting with their targets. Site-selective drug delivery systems face a new challenge to deliver the drug to the right place at the right time. To achieve this, drug delivery systems must satisfy a number of essential requirements, such as not to be removed too rapidly from circulation, to retain their drug content until they reach the target site, and to supply native drug at the required rate and amount for a desired period to effectively and safely treat the pathological condition (Petrak, 2005).

With the rapid development of nanoscience and nanotechnology, a wide variety of carbon nanomaterials have been synthesized and utilized in drug delivery (Thostenson *et al.*, 2001). Because of their excellent properties, facile surface functionalization (which enables bioconjugation), high biocompatibility, and inexpensive large-scale synthesis, diamond-based materials have recently gained global attention as a novel template for drug and vaccine delivery into target cells or specific tissues. Fusion of material science and drug delivery technologies led to the emergence of nanotechnology as a novel alternative for efficient transporting and translocating of therapeutic molecules.

Nanodiamonds represent an emerging class of materials with important clinical applications in medicine. Their consistent dimensions, unique surface properties, facile processing parameters and scalability, and innate biocompatibility and applicability as imaging/diagnostic and therapeutic platforms, make them an ideal foundation for therapeutic and diagnostic approaches.

In this chapter, we summarize the recent development of nanodiamonds as a novel template for drug delivery and targeting. Some of the physicochemical properties of nanodiamonds that significantly influence safety and their application as novel drug delivery systems are reviewed. The focus will be on nanodiamonds and their surface modified analogs used as drug delivery for proteins, nucleic acids, and water-insoluble low molecular weight therapeutic agents. The development, route of administration, safety, and efficacy of these nanodiamond-based drug delivery systems will be discussed. Finally, the future directions and challenges of nanodiamond-based research in engineering, medicine, and biotechnology are overviewed.

8.1.1 Nanodiamonds: definition and physicochemical properties

Nanodiamonds are members of the family of nanocarbons, which include nano-sized amorphous carbon, fullerenes, diamondoids, tubes, onions, horns, rods, cones, peapods, bells, whiskers, platelets, and foam (Shenderova *et al.*, 2002).

Definition of nanodiamonds

Nanodiamonds are carbon nanoparticles with truncated octahedral architecture (Fig. 8.1) that are about 2–8 nm in diameter and can deliver a wide range of therapeutics, including small molecules, proteins, and nucleic acids (Zhang *et al.*, 2009b, Chen *et al.*, 2009). Nanodiamond particles with the smallest monocrystalline size (about 4 nm), also called detonated nanodiamonds are produced by detonation of carbon-containing explosives followed by purification as shown in Fig. 8.1 (Osawa, 2008).

The unique optical, chemical, and biological properties of diamond nanoparticles have generated incredible clinical interest in several applications including drug and gene delivery. The attractive features of diamond nanoparticles include their surface properties and their non-toxic nature that can be exploited to provide an effective and selective platform to obtain a targeted intracellular release of some

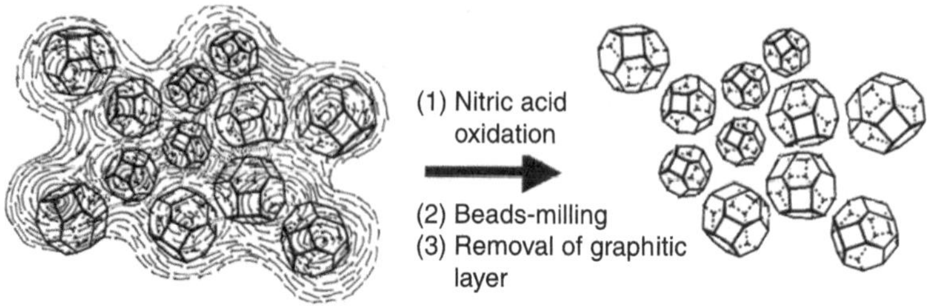

8.1 Illustrations of the purification process of nanodiamonds produced by detonation. Taken with some modifications from Osawa, E. (2008) 'Mono disperse single nanodiamond particulates,' *Pure and Applied Chemistry* 80(7), 1365–1380, with permission.

substance. The use of diamond nanoparticles can also increase the stability of the payload.

Physicochemical properties of nanodiamonds

In addition to retaining the properties inherent to diamond, nanodiamonds exhibit a number of specific features, both in structure and in physicochemical characteristics. Critical features such as particle size, size distribution, particle morphology, particle composition, surface area, surface chemistry, and particle reactivity in solution are important factors that must be defined to accurately understand nanodiamonds and predict their biological properties (Boverhof and David, 2010). In addition, it is important to determine the degree of chemical purification of diamond from the graphite phase (i.e. sp^2/sp^3 ratio of hybridized carbon atoms) as well as the presence and type of impurities in the bulk and on the surface of the nanodiamond aggregates.

The aggregation of the primary nanodiamonds and the formation of stable aqueous colloidal solutions are derived properties that mainly depend on the physical and chemical properties of the nanodiamonds and, in turn, significantly influence the application of these materials. Primary nanodiamond particles are rarely found in isolated forms in dispersion. Apparently, aggregation among nanodiamonds is a critical feature that governs their physicochemical properties as well as associated health hazards. The presence of a persistent form of aggregation in nanodiamonds and associated health hazards have been described and reviewed (Shenderova *et al.*, 2002). Krüger and his colleagues named this special form of aggregation of the primary particles of nanodiamonds, which consist of core particles 60–200 nm in size, as agglutination (Krüger *et al.*, 2005). Conglomerates of core agglutinates that may grow to microns in diameter can be readily dispersed in water upon vigorous stirring. Pulverization methods such as wet beads mill can produce primary nanodiamond particles from their agglutinates (Krüger *et al.*, 2005). Successful disintegration of tight aggregates by stirred-media milling with microbeads provided a stable colloidal solution of nanodiamond (4 nm), but the colloid is colored deep black because of a graphitic partial surface induced by strong collision with beads during the milling process (Eidelman *et al.*, 2005).

Fractal dimension is generally useful in the characterization of aggregate morphology based on Eq. 8.1:

$$N_p = A\left(\frac{R_g}{R_o}\right)^{D_f} \qquad [8.1]$$

where D_f is the fractal dimension, N_p is the number of primary particles in the aggregate, A is a dimensionless prefactor, R_o is the primary particle radius, and R_g is the characteristic radius of the aggregate, which we take to be the radius of gyration. Eq. 8.1 is a result of the power law dependence of the density–density correlation function for the primary particles in an aggregate on distance from a selected reference point. The value of D_f is divided into three groups: 1) fractal-like aggregates with $1.35 < D_f < 1.89$; 2) possibly non-fractal particles with $D_f > 2$; and 3) particles of mixed morphology.

Values of D_f were determined experimentally from an analysis of aggregate photomicrographs (Xiong and Friedlander, 2001). Taking the logarithm of both sides of Eq. 8.1 gives Eq. 8.2:

$$logN_p = logA + D_f logR_g - D_f logR_o \qquad [8.2]$$

where R_g is the radius of gyration = $[(1/M)\Sigma(m_i\, r_i)]^{1/2}$, m_i is the mass of the *i*th primary particle, M is the total aggregate mass Σm_i, and r_i is the distance of the *i*th primary particle from the center of mass. The corresponding log–log plot of N_p versus the normalized radius of gyration allows D_f to be obtained as the slope of the log–log plot, and the log of A as the Y intercept (Xiong and Friedlander, 2001). Aggregates with chain-like structures are formed by collisions of smaller chains described by certain collision algorithms that lead to values of D_f between 1.5 and 2.0. Like D_f, the prefactor A is important in computations of the dynamics of aggregation processes. In the absence of measured values, A is usually assumed to be unity. However, experimental values of A may vary significantly around unity (Xiong and Friedlander, 2001). Overall, the fractal dimension is useful in estimating agglomerate transport rates, light scattering, and chemical reactivity.

Diffusion characteristics and the importance of high stability of aqueous colloidal solution of nanodiamonds have been reported (Blagoveshchenski *et al.*, 2011). Interfacial interactions which could be charge–dipole as in the case of hydration (Huang *et al.*, 2008a) or charge–charge type are critical factors for the colloidal stability of nanodiamond dispersions. The interfacial interaction between nanodiamonds and cationic drugs, such as the ammonium salt of doxorubicin, is strong, and because of this interaction the nanodiamonds could serve as a potential drug carrier (Huang *et al.*, 2007).

Advanced instrumental techniques such as X-ray diffractometry, small-angle X-ray, Raman and IR spectroscopy, high resolution transmission electron microscopy and scanning electron microscopy, electron spin resonance and nuclear magnetic resonance have been utilized to characterize and study nanodiamonds. Application of these methods to define nanodiamond particles, their structures, defects, and impurities are reviewed elsewhere (Shenderova *et al.*, 2002, Shames *et al.*, 2002, Panich *et al.*, 2006, Komatsu *et al.*, 2007, Alexenskii *et al.*, 2001, Hong *et al.*, 2009, Korobov *et al.*, 2010).

8.1.2 Emerging nanodiamond applications in drug delivery and targeting

The possibility of incorporating carbon-based nanomaterials into living systems has opened the way for investigation of their potential applications in the emerging field of nanomedicine. A wide variety of different nanomaterials based on allotropic forms of carbon, such as nanotubes, nanohorns, and nanodiamonds are currently being explored in different biomedical applications (Bianco *et al.*, 2008). The most important and well-known application of nanodiamonds is as a novel drug carrier to improve efficacy and reduce toxicity of therapeutic agents (Huang *et al.*, 2007, Lam *et al.*, 2008, Chen *et al.*, 2009). Table 8.1 summarizes selected applications of nanodiamonds in drug delivery and targeting.

One of the main characteristic advantages of nanodiamonds is a multipole facet that one nanocrystal can carry several drug molecules (Barnard and Sternberg, 2007). Moreover, the nanodiamond–drug complex forms a tight gel that forms a network of aggregated nanodiamond particles. Nanopores having diameters of 8–10 nm are formed within aggregates, and drug molecules are trapped within the nanopore providing a stronger nanodiamond–drug interaction.

Nanodiamonds are very attractive carriers for smart dosage forms that are responsive to stimuli and release their payload on demand. Guan and co-workers described the application of nanodiamonds as a pH-responsive drug delivery system (Guan *et al.*, 2010). An anticancer drug cisplatin (cis-dichlorodiammineplatinum (II) CDDP) was loaded onto nanodiamond by adsorption and complexation. CDDP was released from the composite in phosphate-buffered saline (PBS) of pH 6.0 at a rate higher than in PBS of pH 7.4. As a result, it is predicted that the nanodiamond vehicle would deliver low concentrations of CDDP in the blood, but release much more drug after integration into the acidic cytoplasm, thereby reducing toxic side effects. The complexation between CDDP and the carboxyl groups on the nanodiamond surface is responsible for the pH-responsive release property (Guan *et al.*, 2010).

Nanodiamond materials can serve as highly versatile platforms for controlled functionalization and delivery of a wide spectrum of therapeutic elements. Huang *et al.* (2007) showed the conjugation of doxorubicin on nanodiamonds (2–8 nm) and preserved efficacy of the drug.

Table 8.1 Applications of nanodiamond in drug delivery and targeting

Therapeutic agents	Physicochemical nature of nanodiamonds (ND)	Applications/ *in vitro* or *in vivo* results	References
Cisplatin (cis-dichloro-diammineplatinum (II), CDDP)	ND–CDDP composite	pH-responsive release of CDDP and active *in vitro* against human cervical cancer cells	Guan *et al.*, 2010
Dexamethasone	ND (2–8 nm)-multilayer nanofilm with positively charged poly-L-lysine	Monitor the inflammation of RAW 264.7 murine macrophage using genetic analysis (RT-PCR)	Huang *et al.*, 2008b
Dexamethasone and 4-hydroxytamoxifen	ND–drug complex	Enhance water dispersion of water-insoluble drugs	Chen *et al.*, 2009
Doxorubicin HCl (Dox)	Red fluorescent ND, ~140 nm	Dox delivery HeLa cells via clathrin-dependent endocytosis pathway	Li *et al.*, 2011
Doxorubicin HCl (Dox)	Nanodiamonds (2–8 nm)	Improve anticancer efficacy by reducing drug-efflux-based chemoresistance	Merkel and DeSimone, 2011, Ma *et al.*, 2011, Chow *et al.*, 2011, Huang *et al.*, 2007
Doxorubicin HCl (Dox)	Microfilm architecture consists of Dox–ND (2–8 nm) conjugates	Localized, stable, and continuous slow release of Dox for at least 1 month	Lam *et al.*, 2008
Folic acid (FA)	Fluorescent ND–FA conjugate	Receptor-mediated targeting of cancer cells	Zhang *et al.*, 2009a
Paclitaxel	ND (3–5 nm)–paclitaxel conjugate	*In vitro* mitotic arrest and apoptosis in A549 human lung carcinoma cells	Liu *et al.*, 2010

Enhancing chemotherapeutic efficiency through improved drug delivery would facilitate treatment of chemoresistant cancers. Drug efflux by adenosine triphosphate-binding cassette (ABC) transporter proteins, such as MDR1 and ABCG2, is the most common mechanism of chemoresistance. One way to improve drug delivery through inhibition or retarding drug efflux is through the use of nanodiamond-based therapies, which are both scalable and biocompatible. Chow *et al.* (2011) examined the efficacy of nanodiamond-conjugated chemotherapeutic agents in mouse models of liver and mammary cancer. A complex of nanodiamonds and doxorubicin overcame drug efflux and significantly increased apoptosis and tumor growth inhibition compared with free drug. Unmodified doxorubicin treatment represents the clinical standard for most cancer treatment regimens and the complex could significantly decrease toxicity *in vivo*. Thus, nanodiamond-conjugated chemotherapy represents a promising, biocompatible strategy for overcoming chemoresistance and enhancing chemotherapy efficacy and safety (Chow *et al.*, 2011, Merkel and DeSimone, 2011).

Aqueous dispersible detonation nanodiamonds were assembled into a closely packed nanodiamond multilayer nanofilm with positively charged poly-L-lysine via the layer-by-layer deposition technique (Huang *et al.*, 2008b). The biofunctionality and preserved drug efficacy of the nanodiamond film as an anti-inflammation drug matrix have been demonstrated by dexamethasone anti-inflammatory transfer to the interfaced murine macrophages.

In general, because of their superior chemical and physical properties as well as biocompatibility, diamond-based nanostructures have emerged as promising alternative materials for biomedical applications. The attractive properties of nanodiamonds could be exploited for development of therapeutic agents for diagnostic probes, delivery vehicles for gene therapy, tissue scaffolds, and development of novel medical devices.

8.1.3 General requirements for use of diamond-based materials

To achieve maximum pharmacological effects with minimum side effects, drugs should be delivered to target sites without significant distribution to non-target areas. Pharmaceutical nanocarrier systems including nanodiamonds provide useful drug delivery platforms for improving target specificity, therapeutic activity, and reducing toxicity. Safety and retaining efficacy of the drug are the basic requirements for any nanocarrier system (Youan, 2008).

Safety of nanodiamonds

As the applications and industrial production of nanodiamonds increase, there is an increase in the potential risk to humans and the environment from exposure and additional concerns about short- and long-term toxicological effects. To explore the application of nanodiamonds as drug delivery vehicles, the issues of biocompatibility, cytotoxicity, and genotoxicity have been highlighted in several papers (Boverhof and David, 2010, Chao *et al.*, 2007a, Li *et al.*, 2010, Xing *et al.*, 2011, Zhang *et al.*, 2010, Chao *et al.*, 2006, Chao *et al.*, 2007b, Yuan *et al.*, 2010, Schrand *et al.*, 2007).

While attempting to evaluate the safety of nanodiamonds, cytotoxicity studies could be affected by various factors that need to be carefully controlled. The need to characterize nanodiamonds in solution before assessing *in vitro* toxicity is a high priority. Particle size, size distribution, particle morphology, particle composition, surface area, surface chemistry, and particle reactivity in solution are important factors which need to be defined to accurately assess the toxicity of nanodiamonds (Murdock *et al.*, 2008, Vippola *et al.*, 2009).

The results of toxicological studies of nanodiamonds may also be varied based on agglomeration changes in the presence or absence of serum in cell culture media. Toxicity data revealed that the addition of serum to cell culture media can, in some cases, have a significant effect on particle toxicity possibly as a result of changes in agglomeration or surface chemistry. The significance of serum proteins in cell culture medium has been discussed by Li and co-workers (Li *et al.*, 2010). When cells were exposed to nanodiamonds dispersed in complete cell culture medium, no cytotoxicity was detected. However, severe cell death was found after exposure to nanodiamonds dispersed in serum-free medium. It was also necessary to characterize the impact of sonication, which is implemented to aid in particle dispersion and solution mixture. It has been observed that dispersion of nanomaterials in solution rarely leads to distribution at the primary particle size. This agglomeration raises concerns when considering size-dependent toxicity, specific surface area toxicity, and dose-dependent toxicity for *in vitro* experiments (Murdock *et al.*, 2008, Krüger *et al.*, 2005, Jingkun *et al.*, 2009).

Retention efficacy of drug-loaded nanodiamond-based delivery templates

For any drug delivery system, maintaining the efficacy of the loaded drug is a basic requirement. Diamond-based material should not affect the activity or functionality of the conjugated therapeutic agents. As exemplified by the work of Perevedentseva and co-workers, investigation of the activities as well as structural stability of the therapeutic agents after conjugation on nanodiamond particles have dramatic influence on the success of drug delivery (Perevedentseva *et al.*, 2011). They found that the activity of lysozyme as a model protein upon adsorption depends on the nanodiamond's size and surface properties. Lysozyme adsorbed onto nanodiamonds of 100 nm and larger maintains comparable activity within experimental error to lysozyme in solution; whereas activity decreases significantly when adsorbed onto 5–50 nm. This phenomenon clearly indicates the need to select appropriate size and surface properties of nanodiamonds that do not alter the functional properties of therapeutic agents.

8.2 Surface modification of diamond nanoparticles for drug delivery and targeting

Nanodiamonds with a modified surface offer the most significant potential for biological and medical applications (Krueger, 2008). Fabrication of biologically amenable functionalized nanomaterials provides a platform for safe delivery of biomimetic and therapeutically active substrates (Huang *et al.*, 2009).

The design of nanoparticles that are suitably functionalized for applications in biology or medicine is an ongoing challenge for both chemists and biologists. Carbon-based nanomaterials offer, in addition to their remarkable physical properties, the possibility of being functionalized by biomolecules; this makes them suitable for sensing, detection, diagnostic, and/or therapeutic applications.

In addition to biomedical applications, surface modification of nanodiamond could provide an opportunity for ease of handling and processing. Surface modification of nanodiamonds with hydrogen gas has been reported to prevent formation of aggregates and clusters (Williams *et al.*, 2010). By annealing aggregated nanodiamond powder in hydrogen gas, large (>100 nm) aggregates are broken down into their core particles (4 nm). Dispersion of these particles into water via high power ultrasound and high speed centrifugation, results in a monodisperse nanodiamond colloid, with exceptional long time stability in a wide range of pH. The large change in zeta potential resulting from this gas treatment demonstrates that nanodiamond particle surfaces are able to react with molecular hydrogen at relatively low temperatures, a phenomenon not witnessed with larger (20 nm) diamond particles or bulk diamond surfaces (Williams *et al.*, 2010).

8.2.1 Surface modification and functionality

Surface modification and functionalization of nanodiamonds for their application as drug carriers that can form covalent or electrostatic binding to the active biomolecules have been reviewed (Zhang *et al.*, 2009b, Shimkunas *et al.*, 2009, Martin *et al.*, 2009, Liu *et al.*, 2008, Vial *et al.*, 2008, Chen *et al.*, 2009). Inherent properties of nanodiamonds could be improved to increase biocompatibility, cellular uptake and loading capacity. Fenton treatment of nanodiamonds reduces the amount of amorphous soot matter and the process maintains crystallinity, reduces the particle size to about 4 nm, increases the surface hydroxyl population, and increases water solubility. All these changes are beneficial for subsequent covalent functionalization (Martín *et al.*, 2010).

A triethylammonium-functionalized nanodiamond acts as a gene delivery system permitting a plasmid to cross a cell membrane, something that does not occur for the plasmid alone without the assistance of polycationic nanodiamonds (Martín *et al.*, 2010). Functionalization of nanodiamond with N,O-carboxymethyl chitosan for protein drug delivery has been reported (Wang *et al.*, 2010).

Imparting multiple functions to nanoparticles through organic functionalization has attracted significant interest, particularly in terms of biomedical applications. Diamond nanoparticles have been recognized as one of the best platforms, due to their ability to create covalent bonding with introduced functionalities. Takimoto *et al.* (2010) showed multistep organic transformations on the nanodiamond surface that accumulated the requisite functions layer by layer through covalent bonds. They incorporated hydrophilic and fluorescent properties onto the nanodiamond surface by adding polyethylene glycol (PEG) and fluorescein segments that can be used in cellular imaging.

Surface-modified nanodiamonds also provide conformational stabilization, as well as a high degree of surface exposure to protein antigens (Kossovsky *et al.*, 1995). By enhancing the availability and activity of the antigen *in vivo*, a strong, specific immune response can be elicited. Surface-modified diamond nanoparticles as antigen delivery vehicles improved the immune response against Mussel adhesive protein (Kossovsky *et al.*, 1995). Vial *et al.* (2008) described the preparation and stabilization of peptide-grafted nanodiamonds that provide aqueous colloidal suspension for drug delivery.

8.3 Development of nanodiamond-based drug delivery for proteins

Protein pharmaceuticals have become powerful and indispensable in combating human diseases because they have high specificity and activity even at relatively low concentrations. Specific uses of nanodiamonds in both non-conjugated and conjugated forms as drug carriers for proteins have been considered. Amino acids and small peptides coupled to the diamond surface are potentially useful for the synthesis of surface-bound peptides and proteins, and for the attachment of biologically active compounds (Kruger *et al.*, 2006).

Examples of nanodiamond-based drug delivery for proteins and related biomedical applications are mentioned in Table 8.2. Fluorescent nanodiamonds covalently linked with transferrin have been reported as an attractive vehicle for receptor-mediated specific cellular uptake and targeting of cancer cells (Li and Zhou, 2010). The conjugate enters the cells through receptor-mediated endocytosis, which is dependent on the ATP of the environment.

In addition to drug delivery, nanodiamond surface–protein interactions via silane linkage and electrostatics have been explored for applications such as extraction in proteomics. The functionalization of nanodiamond with aminophenylboronic acid allows selective capture of glycoproteins from unfractionated protein mixtures, providing a method for isolation and detection (Yeap *et al.*, 2008).

Table 8.2 Examples of nanodiamond-based products for protein and peptide delivery

Therapeutic agents	Physicochemical nature of nanodiamonds (ND)	Applications/*in vitro* or *in vivo* results	References
Growth factor α (TGF-α) antibody (Ab)	ND–Ab complex	pH-triggered *in vitro* release of the active Ab	Smith *et al.*, 2011
Protein (egg white lysozyme)	ND–lysozyme complex	Fluorescence-based assay of enzymatic activity	Perevedentseva *et al.*, 2011, Chao *et al.*, 2007a
Enzyme glucose oxidase (GOX)	GOX-functionalized ND films	Sensitive glucose sensor	Pedro *et al.*, 2011
Dipeptide (Phe-Lys) conjugated doxorubicin HCl	Carboxylated ND	Device for controlled drug release	Huang *et al.*, 2011
Transferrin	Transferrin-coupled fluorescence NDs	Cellular uptake and targeted drug delivery	Li and Zhou, 2010, Mao-Feng *et al.*, 2009
Immunoglobulin (IgGI), bovine serum albumin (BSA) and rabbit antimouse (RAM) antibody	ND–IgGI125 and RAM–ND–BSAI125 complexes	Delivery of biologically active substances	Purtov *et al.*, 2010
Bovine insulin	ND–insulin complex	pH-dependent protein delivery	Shimkunas *et al.*, 2009
Glycoproteins	Aminophenylboronic acid (APBA) functionalized NDs	Selective capture of glycoproteins from unfractionated protein mixtures during MALDI assay	Yeap *et al.*, 2008
Fluorescent thiolated peptide	ND (35 nm) coated by silanization	Improve aqueous colloidal suspension stability, provide *in vitro* and *in vivo* targeting	Vial *et al.*, 2008

alpha-Bungarotoxin (α-BTX)	Carboxylated ND–α-BTX conjugate	cND–α-BTX blocks the function of α7-nicotinic acetylcholine receptor	Liu *et al.*, 2008
Yeast cytochrome c	ND (4–6 nm)–poly-L-lysine conjugate	Adsorption and immobilization of the protein onto ND surfaces	Huang and Chang, 2004
Mussel adhesive protein (MAP)	ND (5–300 nm)–MAP conjugate	The conjugate provides conformational stabilization, as well as a high degree of surface exposure to the protein antigen	Kossovsky *et al.*, 1995
Chlorotoxin-like peptide from the venom of *Buthus martensii* Karsch (BmK CT)	Fluorescent ND–BmK CT conjugate	Inhibit migration of rat C6 glioma cells	Yuejun *et al.*, 2011

The latest development of protein engineering allows production of proteins with desired properties and large potential markets, but clinical advances of therapeutic proteins are still limited by their fragility. Numerous investigations have shown that nanocarriers can improve the stability of therapeutic agents against enzymatic degradation and achieve desired therapeutic levels in target tissues for the required duration (Di Marco *et al.*, 2010).

Recognition of antigens by immunocompetent cells involves interactions that are specific to the chemical sequence and conformation of the epitope (antigenic determinant). Adjuvants enhancing immunity to antigens tend to either alter the antigen conformation through surface adsorption or shield potentially critical determinants, for example functional groups. Surface-modified diamond nanoparticles provide conformational stabilization, as well as a high degree of surface exposure to protein antigens (Kossovsky *et al.*, 1995). By enhancing the availability and activity of the antigen, a strong, specific immune response can be elicited.

8.4 Development of nanodiamond-based drug delivery for genes

The design and synthesis of safe efficient non-viral vectors for gene delivery has attracted significant attention in recent years primarily because of the severe side effect profile reported with the use of their viral counterparts. Previous experiments have revealed that strong interaction between the carriers and nucleic acids may well hinder the release of the gene from the complex.

Gene therapy holds great promise for treating diseases ranging from inherited disorders to acquired conditions and cancers. However, effective and safe gene delivery remains a challenge. Nanodiamonds are rapidly emerging as promising carriers for gene delivery. Zhang and co-workers demonstrated the effectiveness of nanodiamonds as vectors for *in vitro* gene delivery via surface-immobilization with 800 Da polyethyleneimine (PEI800) and covalent conjugation with amine groups. Nanodiamond–PEI800 composite possesses low cytotoxicity and exhibits high transfection efficiency. The authors demonstrated that DNA-functionalized nanodiamonds represent an efficient opportunity toward gene delivery and serve as a rapid, scalable, and broadly applicable gene therapy strategy (Zhang *et al.*, 2009b). Polycationic-functionalized nanodiamonds that contains surface triethylammonium groups react electrostatically with a plasmid and act as a gene delivery system permitting the plasmid to cross cell membranes (Martín *et al.*, 2010).

The application of nanodiamond to deliver nucleic acids such as plasmid DNA, antisense oligonucleotides, and siRNA is described in Table 8.3.

Controlled gene delivery systems, acting as localized depots of genes, provide an extended sustained release of genes, giving prolonged maintenance of the therapeutic level of encoded proteins. They also limit the DNA degradation in the

Table 8.3 Examples of the application of nanodiamonds in gene delivery and targeting

Therapeutic agents	Physicochemical nature of nanodiamonds (ND)	Applications/*in vitro* or *in vivo* results	References
Small interfering RNA (siRNA)	NDs coated with cationic polymer	Delivery of siRNA into Ewing sarcoma cells	Alhaddad *et al.*, 2011
Plasmid having the green fluorescent protein gene	Thionine functionalized fenton-treated ND (4 nm)	Gene delivery, HeLa cell	Martín *et al.*, 2010
Plasmid DNA	ND–PEI800 (800 Da polyethyleneimine)	Gene delivery *via* DNA-functionalized ND to HeLa cells	Zhang *et al.*, 2009b
DNA oligonucleotides	Carboxylated NDs–poly(L-lysines)–DNA oligonucleotide conjugate	Facilitates the isolation, concentration, purification, digestion, and analysis of DNA oligonucleotides	Kong *et al.*, 2005

nuclease-rich extracellular environment. Although attempts have been made to adapt existing controlled drug delivery technologies, more novel approaches are being investigated for controlled gene delivery. Surface-modified nanodiamonds such as poly-L-lysine-coated diamonds have been explored for DNA oligonucleotide binding (Kong *et al.*, 2005).

Strong interaction between the carriers such as nanodiamonds and nucleic acid may also hinder the release of the gene from the complex in the cytosol, adversely affecting transfection efficiency. However, surface modification and incorporation of reducible disulfide bonds within the delivery systems themselves, which are then cleaved in the glutathione-rich intracellular environment, may help in solving this puzzle (Defang *et al.*, 2009).

8.5 Development of nanodiamond-based drug delivery for low molecular weight therapeutic agents

The conjugation of a wide range of small molecule therapeutic agents with diamond nanoparticles has been a major theme of many studies (Guan *et al.*, 2010, Huang *et al.*, 2008b, Ma *et al.*, 2011, Merkel and DeSimone, 2011, Li *et al.*,

2011, Chow *et al.*, 2011, Liu *et al.*, 2010, Chen *et al.*, 2009, Lam *et al.*, 2008). This interest has been stimulated by the capability of the diamond nanoparticles to bind a wide range of organic molecules, their low level of toxicity, and their strong and tunable optical absorption. The facets present on the nanodiamond surface have been shown to possess charge properties that enable potent water binding for dispersability and sustained therapeutic release (Korobov *et al.*, 2007, Ōsawa *et al.*, 2009). Smart dosage forms that deliver drug to selected target at selected time improve the drug efficacy and safety. In this respect, Guan and co-workers reported nanodiamonds to be a pH-responsive vehicle for the anticancer drug, cisplatin (Guan *et al.*, 2010).

Nanoparticle-conjugated anticancer drug provides a novel strategy for cancer therapy. Liu *et al.* (2010) covalently linked paclitaxel to the surface of 3–5 nm sized nanodiamonds. Nanodiamond–paclitaxel conjugation induced both mitotic arrest and apoptosis, and markedly blocked the tumor growth and formation of lung cancer in experimental animals. The conjugate was taken into lung cancer cells in a concentration-dependent manner and localized in the microtubules and cytoplasm (Liu *et al.*, 2010).

Similarly, doxorubicin was reversibly bound to nanodiamonds with sodium hydroxide chemical treatment, which provides a sustained release profile both *in vitro* and *in vivo*. The resulting nanodiamond drug delivery system improved both drug retention in tumor cells and treatment safety and efficacy in murine cancer models, suggesting that nanodiamonds are a promising drug delivery platform for chemoresistant tumors (Chow *et al.*, 2011).

A broad array of water-insoluble compounds has displayed therapeutically relevant properties toward a spectrum of medical and physiological disorders, including cancer and inflammation. However, the continued search for scalable, facile, and biocompatible routes toward mediating the dispersal of these compounds in water has limited their widespread application in medicine. Water-dispersible, nanodiamond cluster-mediated interactions have been utilized to enhance dispersion of poorly water soluble therapeutic agents and improve the stability of the suspension while preserving the agents' functionality (Chen *et al.*, 2009). The dispersal of poorly water-soluble drugs using carbon-based strategies, such as PEGylated nanographene oxides, has been explored for the delivery of otherwise problematic drugs (Zhuang *et al.*, 2008).

8.6 Biocompatibility, biodistribution and biological fate of nanodiamonds

The biocompatibility of detonated nanodiamonds from the standpoint of cell viability and proliferative behavior has been assessed. Zhang and colleagues investigated the biodistribution of nanodiamonds using radiotracer techniques and evaluated acute toxicity in mice after intratracheal instillation (Zhang *et al.*, 2010). The biodistribution showed that, besides having the highest retention in the lung, nanodiamonds distribute mainly in the spleen, liver, bone, and heart. An analysis of histological morphology and biochemical parameters indicated that nanodiamonds could induce dose-dependent toxicity.

Mode of absorption and biodistribution of nanodiamonds is highly linked with surface property and conjugation. Receptor-mediated active transport has been elucidated for nanodiamonds that are covalently linked with transferrin. Receptor-mediated endocytosis of the conjugate was found to be ATP-dependent and can be competitively inhibited (Li and Zhou, 2010). Nanodiamonds are not trapped by the endosomes, which is a promising result for future potential as drug delivery systems (Faklaris *et al.*, 2008).

8.7 Conclusions

Effective drug delivery systems for biopharmaceuticals, such as small molecules, peptide-based drugs, proteins, vaccines, and nucleic acids still present major challenges in providing safe and effective targeting of intracellular locations. Smart dosage forms that deliver drug to selected target at selected time improve the drug's efficacy and safety. Nanodiamonds appear to be a promising candidate for biomedical use because of their small primary particle size (2–8 nm), purity, excellent properties, facile surface functionalization (which enables bioconjugation), high biocompatibility, and inexpensive large-scale synthesis. The fabrication of biologically amenable functionalized nanodiamonds provides a platform for safe and effective delivery of therapeutic agents. However, attributes of nanodiamonds such as aggregation state, surface chemistry, presence of impurities, as well as the localization and accumulation behavior within the body have to be controlled to maintain safety and retain efficacy of conjugated therapeutic agents. A clinically applicable approach requires investigation of biocompatibility, biodistribution, and biological fate of the nanodiamond as well as its conjugates.

This chapter described the application of nanodiamonds in both non-conjugated and conjugated forms as drug carriers. Small molecule therapeutic agents such as doxorubicin hydrochloride, dexamethasone, cisplatin, 4-hydroxytamoxifen, paclitaxel and folic acid (Table 8.1) were successfully conjugated/coated on nanodiamond platforms and introduced into living cells. The safety and efficacy of these nanodiamond conjugates were elucidated. The application of nanodiamonds as drug delivery for a wide variety of proteins such as growth factors, enzymes, peptides, antibodies, insulin, glycoproteins, and toxins (Table 8.2) has been discussed. The development of gene delivery including plasmid, siRNA, and DNA oligonucleotides (Table 8.3) using functionalized nanodiamonds also has been reported. In summary, nanodiamonds could play a key role in drug delivery by providing sustained drug release, and improved stability and compatibility, as well as targeting a specific receptor for biomedical applications.

8.8 References

Alexenskii, A. E., Baidakova, M. V., Dideikin, A. T., *et al.* 2001. Effect of chemical treatment on the structure of ultradisperse diamond and onion-like carbon. *AIP Conference Proceedings*, 590, 425.

Alhaddad, A., Adam, M.-P., Botsoa, J., *et al.* 2011. Nanodiamond as a Vector for siRNA Delivery to Ewing Sarcoma Cells. *Small (Weinheim An Der Bergstrasse, Germany)*, 7, 3087–3095.

Barnard, A. and Sternberg, M. 2007. Crystallinity and surface electrostatics of diamond nanocrystals. *Journal of Materials Chemistry*, 17, 4811–4819.

Bianco, A., Kostarelos, K. and Prato, M. 2008. Opportunities and challenges of carbon-based nanomaterials for cancer therapy. *Expert Opinion on Drug Delivery*, 5, 331–342.

Blagoveshchenski, N. M., Novikov, A. G., Rozhkova, N. N. and Osawa, E. 2011. Diffusion Characteristics of Water in the Vicinity of Single-Nano Buckydiamond as Revealed by Quasi-Elastic Neutron Scattering. *Fullerenes, Nanotubes and Carbon Nanostructures*, 19, 52–57.

Boverhof, D. R. and David, R. M. 2010. Nanomaterial characterization: considerations and needs for hazard assessment and safety evaluation. *Analytical and Bioanalytical Chemistry*, 396, 953–961.

Chao, J.-I., Perevedentseva, E., Chung, P.-H., *et al.* 2007a. Nanometer-sized diamond particle as a probe for biolabeling. *Biophysical Journal*, 93, 2199–2208.

Chao, J. I., Chang, C. C. and Cheng, C. L. 2006. Interaction and toxicity of nanodiamonds in human cells. *Faseb Journal*, 20, A75.

Chao, J. I., Liu, K. K., Cheng, C. L. and Chang, C. C. 2007b. Toxicity and detection of carboxylated nanodiamonds on human lung epithelial cells. *Faseb Journal*, 21, A267.

Chen, M., Pierstorff, E. D., Lam, R., *et al.* 2009. Nanodiamond-Mediated Delivery of Water-Insoluble Therapeutics. *Acs Nano*, 3, 2016–2022.

Chow, E. K., Zhang, X. Q., Chen, M., *et al.* 2011. Nanodiamond therapeutic delivery agents mediate enhanced chemoresistant tumor treatment. *Sci Transl Med*, 3, 73ra21.

Defang, O., Shah, N., Hong, Z., *et al.* 2009. Reducible Disulfide-Based Non-Viral Gene Delivery Systems. *Mini Reviews in Medicinal Chemistry*, 9, 1242–1250.

Di Marco, M., Shamsuddin, S., Razak, K. A., *et al.* 2010. Overview of the main methods used to combine proteins with nanosystems: absorption, bioconjugation, and encapsulation. *International Journal of Nanomedicine*, 5, 37–49.

Eidelman, E. D., Siklitsky, V. I., Sharonova, L. V., *et al.* 2005. A stable suspension of single ultrananocrystalline diamond particles. *Diamond and Related Materials*, 14, 1765–1769.

Faklaris, O., Garrot, D., Joshi, V., *et al.* 2008. Detection of Single Photoluminescent Diamond Nanoparticles in Cells and Study of the Internalization Pathway. *Small*, 4, 2236–2239.

Guan, B., Zou, F. and Zhi, J. F. 2010. Nanodiamond as the pH-Responsive Vehicle for an Anticancer Drug. *Small*, 6, 1514–1519.

Hong, Z. C., Perevedentseva, E., Treschev, S., *et al.* 2009. Surface enhanced Raman scattering of nano diamond using visible-light-activated TiO. *Journal of Raman Spectroscopy*, 40, 1016.

Huang, H., Dai, L., Wang, D., *et al.* 2008a. Large-scale self-assembly of dispersed nanodiamonds. *Journal of Materials Chemistry*, 18, 1347–1352.

Huang, H., Pierstorff, E., Osawa, E. and Ho, D. 2007. Active nanodiamond hydrogels for chemotherapeutic delivery. *Nano Letters*, 7, 3305–3314.

Huang, H., Pierstorff, E., Osawa, E. and Ho, D. 2008b. Protein-mediated assembly of nanodiamond hydrogels into a biocompatible and biofunctional multilayer nanofilm. *Acs Nano*, 2, 203–212.

Huang, H. J., Chen, M., Bruno, P., *et al.* 2009. Ultrananocrystalline Diamond Thin Films Functionalized with Therapeutically Active Collagen Networks. *Journal of Physical Chemistry B*, 113, 2966–2971.

Huang, L. C. and Chang, H. C. 2004. Adsorption and immobilization of cytochrome c on nanodiamonds. *Langmuir*, 20, 5879–5884.

Huang, S., Shao, J., Gao, L., *et al.* 2011. Adsorption of Cathepsin B-sensitive peptide conjugated DOX on nanodiamonds. *Applied Surface Science*, 257, 8617–8622.

Jingkun, J., Günter, O. and Pratim, B. 2009. Characterization of size, surface charge, and agglomeration state of nanoparticle dispersions for toxicological studies. *Journal of Nanoparticle Research*, 11, 77.

Komatsu, N., Kadota, N., Kimura, T. and Osawa, E. 2007. Solution-phase 13C NMR Spectroscopy of Detonation Nanodiamond. *Chemistry Letters*, 36, 398–399.

Kong, X., Huang, L. C. L., Liau, S. C. V., *et al.* 2005. Polylysine-coated diamond nanocrystals for MALDI-TOF mass analysis of DNA oligonucleotides. *Analytical Chemistry*, 77, 4273–4277.

Korobov, M. V., Avramenko, N. V., Bogachev, A. G., *et al.* 2007. Nanophase of Water in Nano-Diamond Gel. *Journal Of Physical Chemistry C*, 111, 7330–7334.

Korobov, M. V., Batuk, M. M., Avramenko, N. V., *et al.* 2010. Aggregate structure of 'single-nano buckydiamond' in gel and dried powder by differential scanning calorimetry and nitrogen adsorption. *Diamond and Related Materials*, 19, 665–671.

Kossovsky, N., Gelman, A., Hnatyszyn, H. J., *et al.* 1995. Surface-modified diamond nanoparticles as antigen delivery vehicles. *Bioconjug Chem*, 6, 507–511.

Krueger, A. 2008. New carbon materials: Biological applications of functionalized nanodiamond materials. *Chemistry-a European Journal*, 14, 1382–1390.

Krüger, A., Kataoka, F., Ozawa, M., *et al.* 2005. Unusually tight aggregation in detonation nanodiamond: Identification and disintegration. *Carbon*, 43, 1722–1730.

Kruger, A., Liang, Y. J., Jarre, G. and Stegk, J. 2006. Surface functionalisation of detonation diamond suitable for biological applications. *Journal of Materials Chemistry*, 16, 2322–2328.

Lam, R., Chen, M., Pierstorff, E., *et al.* 2008. Nanodiamond-Embedded Microfilm Devices for Localized Chemotherapeutic Elution. *Acs Nano*, 2, 2095–2102.

Li, J., Zhu, Y., Li, W., *et al.* 2010. Nanodiamonds as intracellular transporters of chemotherapeutic drug. *Biomaterials*, 31, 8410–8418.

Li, Y., Zhou, X., Wang, D., *et al.* 2011. Nanodiamond mediated delivery of chemotherapeutic drugs. *Journal of Materials Chemistry*, 21, 16406–16412.

Li, Y. Q. and Zhou, X. P. 2010. Transferrin-coupled fluorescence nanodiamonds as targeting intracellular transporters: An investigation of the uptake mechanism. *Diamond and Related Materials*, 19, 1163–1167.

Liu, K.-K., Chen, M.-F., Chen, P.-Y., *et al.* 2008. Alpha-bungarotoxin binding to target cell in a developing visual system by carboxylated nanodiamond. *Nanotechnology*, 19, 205102 (pp. 10).

Liu, K. K., Zheng, W. W., Wang, C. C., *et al.* 2010. Covalent linkage of nanodiamond-paclitaxel for drug delivery and cancer therapy. *Nanotechnology*, 21, 31510619 (pp. 14).

Ma, X.-W., Zhao, Y.-L. and Liang, X.-J. 2011. Nanodiamond delivery circumvents tumor resistance to doxorubicin. *Acta Pharmacologica Sinica*, 32, 543–544.

Mao-Feng, W., Su-Yu, C., Niann-Shiah, W. and Huan, N. 2009. Fluorescent nanodiamonds for specifically targeted bioimaging: Application to the interaction of transferrin with transferrin receptor. *Diamond and Related Materials*, 18, 587–591.

Martín, R., Alvaro, M., Herance, J. R. and García, H. 2010. Fenton-treated functionalized diamond nanoparticles as gene delivery system. *Acs Nano*, 4, 65–74.

Martin, R., Heydorn, P. C., Alvaro, M. and Garcia, H. 2009. General Strategy for High-Density Covalent Functionalization of Diamond Nanoparticles Using Fenton Chemistry. *Chemistry of Materials*, 21, 4505–4514.

Merkel, T. J. and DeSimone, J. M. 2011. Dodging drug-resistant cancer with diamonds. *Sci Transl Med*, 3, 73ps8.

Murdock, R. C., Braydich-Stolle, L., Schrand, A. M., *et al.* 2008. Characterization of nanomaterial dispersion in solution prior to In vitro exposure using dynamic light scattering technique. *Toxicological Sciences*, 101, 239–253.

Ōsawa, E. 2008. Monodisperse single nanodiamond particulates. *Pure And Applied Chemistry*, 80, 1365–1380.

Ōsawa, E., Ho, D., Huang, H., *et al.* 2009. Consequences of strong and diverse electrostatic potential fields on the surface of detonation nanodiamond particles. *Diamond and Related Materials*, 18, 904–909.

Panich, A. M., Shames, A. I., Vieth, H. M., *et al.* 2006. Nuclear magnetic resonance study of ultrananocrystalline diamonds. *European Physical Journal B — Condensed Matter*, 52, 397–402.

Pedro, V., Manoj, K. R., Humberto, G., *et al.* 2011. GOX-functionalized nanodiamond films for electrochemical biosensor. *Materials Science and Engineering C*, 31, 1115–1120.

Perevedentseva, E., Cai, P. J., Chiu, Y. C. and Cheng, C. L. 2011. Characterizing protein activities on the lysozyme and nanodiamond complex prepared for bio applications. *Langmuir*, 27, 1085–1091.

Petrak, K. 2005. Essential properties of drug-targeting delivery systems. *Drug Discovery Today (England)*, 10, 1667–1673.

Purtov, K. V., Petunin, A. I., Burov, A. E., *et al.* 2010. Nanodiamonds as Carriers for Address Delivery of Biologically Active Substances. *Nanoscale Research Letters*, 5, 631.

Schrand, A. M., Huang, H. J., Carlson, C., *et al.* 2007. Are diamond nanoparticles cytotoxic? *Journal of Physical Chemistry B*, 111, 2–7.

Shames, A. I., Panich, A. M., Kempiński, W., *et al.* 2002. Defects and impurities in nanodiamonds: EPR, NMR and TEM study. *Journal of Physics and Chemistry of Solids*, 63, 1993–2001.

Shenderova, O. A., Zhirnov, V. V. and Brenner, D. W. 2002. Carbon Nanostructures. *Critical Reviews in Solid State and Materials Science*, 27, 227.

Shimkunas, R. A., Robinson, E., Lam, R., *et al.* 2009. Nanodiamond-insulin complexes as pH-dependent protein delivery vehicles. *Biomaterials*, 30, 5720–5728.

Smith, A. H., Robinson, E. M., Zhang, X.-Q., *et al.* 2011. Triggered release of therapeutic antibodies from nanodiamond complexes. *Nanoscale*, 3, 2844–2848.

Takimoto, T., Chano, T., Shimizu, S., *et al.* 2010. Preparation of Fluorescent Diamond Nanoparticles Stably Dispersed under a Physiological Environment through Multistep Organic Transformations. *Chemistry of Materials*, 22, 3462–3471.

Thostenson, E. T., Ren, Z. and Chou, T. W. 2001. Advances in the science and technology of carbon nanotubes and their composites: a review. *Composites Science And Technology*, 61, 1899–1912.

Vial, S., Mansuy, C., Sagan, S., *et al.* 2008. Peptide-grafted nanodiamonds: Preparation, cytotoxicity and uptake in cells. *ChemBioChem*, 9, 2113–2119.

Vippola, M., Falck, G. C. M., Lindberg, H. K., *et al.* 2009. Preparation of nanoparticle dispersions for in-vitro toxicity testing. *Human and Experimental Toxicology*, 28, 377–385.

Wang, H. D., Yang, Q. Q. and Niu, C. H. 2010. Functionalization of nanodiamond particles with N,O-carboxymethyl chitosan. *Diamond and Related Materials*, 19, 441–444.

Williams, O. A., Hees, J., Dieker, C., *et al.* 2010. Size-Dependent Reactivity of Diamond Nanoparticles. *Acs Nano*, 4, 4824–4830.

Xing, Y., Xiong, W., Zhu, L., *et al.* 2011. DNA damage in embryonic stem cells caused by nanodiamonds. *Acs Nano*, 5, 2376–2384.

Xiong, C. and Friedlander, S. K. 2001. Morphological properties of atmospheric aerosol aggregates. *Proceedings of the National Academy of Sciences of the United States of America*, 98, 11851–11856.

Yeap, W. S., Tan, Y. Y. and Loh, K. P. 2008. Using detonation nanodiamond for the specific capture of glycoproteins. *Anal Chem*, 80, 4659–4665.

Youan, B.-B. C. 2008. Impact of nanoscience and nanotechnology on controlled drug delivery. *Nanomedicine (London, England)*, 3, 401–406.

Yuan, Y., Wang, X., Jia, G., *et al.* 2010. Pulmonary toxicity and translocation of nanodiamonds in mice. *Diamond and Related Materials*, 19, 291–299.

Yuejun, F., Na, A., Shuhua, Z., *et al.* 2011 BmK CT-conjugated fluorescence nanodiamond as potential glioma-targeted imaging and drug. *Diamond and Related Materials.* (October 2011), doi:10.1016/j.diamond.2011.10.010

Zhang, B., Li, Y., Fang, C. Y., *et al.* 2009a. Receptor-mediated cellular uptake of folate-conjugated fluorescent nanodiamonds: a combined ensemble and single-particle study. *Small*, 5, 2716–2721.

Zhang, X., Yin, J., Kang, C., *et al.* 2010. Biodistribution and toxicity of nanodiamonds in mice after intratracheal instillation. *Toxicol Lett*, 198, 237–243.

Zhang, X. Q., Chen, M., Lam, R., *et al.* 2009b. Polymer-functionalized nanodiamond platforms as vehicles for gene delivery. *Acs Nano*, 3, 2609–2616.

Zhuang, L., Robinson, J. T., Xiaoming, S. and Hongjie, D. 2008. PEGylated Nanographene Oxide for Delivery of Water-Insoluble Cancer Drugs. *Journal of the American Chemical Society*, 130, 10876–10877.

9
Diamond nucleation and seeding techniques for tissue regeneration

A. KROMKA, O. BABCHENKO, S. POTOCKY, B. REZEK, A. SVESHNIKOV and P. DEMO, Academy of Sciences of the Czech Republic, Czech Republic and T. IZAK and M. VARGA, Academy of Sciences of the Czech Republic, Czech Republic and Slovak University of Technology in Bratislava, Slovak Republic

DOI: 10.1533/9780857093516.2.206

Abstract: The growth of nanocrystalline diamond (NCD) thin films has become routine in labs and companies globally. This has been enabled by the fast progress of diamond nucleation and seeding in science and technology during the past decade, as a result of chemical vapour deposition (CVD) of NCD films requiring that a non-diamond substrate is treated by nucleation or seeding process prior to diamond growth. However, growth of ultrathin continuous NCD films (thickness <100 nm) with a sufficient quality of material by CVD on non-diamond substrates remains a proprietary know-how for each research group because of generally low nucleation efficiency.

Key words: diamond, nucleation, ultrasonic seeding, polymer composite, chemical vapour deposition, hot filament CVD, ion bombardment, microwave plasma, large area growth, linear antenna, SEM, AFM, XPS, nanotechnology, cell cultivation, tissue engineering.

This chapter compares the impact of three different pre-growth treatment processes on diamond growth by hot filament and microwave plasma chemical vapour deposition (CVD): 1) ion bombardment of substrate (bias enhanced nucleation in d.c. and a.c. mode); 2) ultrasonic treatment (seeding in suspension of diamond nanopowder and nanoparticles) on flat and geometrically shaped substrates; and 3) spin-coating of polymer composites on delicate substrates.

Combining these techniques with standard lithographic processes represents an effective way to directly grow microscopic diamond patterns on arbitrary substrates. Finally, novel trends and perspectives in diamond nucleation and growth are discussed.

9.1 Introduction

Carbon-based allotropes (e.g. graphene, fullerenes, carbon nanotubes – CNT, nanocrystalline diamond – NCD, etc.) are of especially high interest in the nanotechnology community because of their wide range of applications as smart multifunctional materials. In particular, nanocrystalline diamond (with carbon atoms bonded in sp^3 hybridization) is among those materials that display extremely high chemical inertness, the highest mechanical hardness and thermal conductivity, high electron and hole mobility, wide band gap, etc. These properties make NCD an extremely attractive candidate for advanced applications spanning from microelectronics through medicine to aerospace applications (Hsu *et al.*, 2010).

There are two principal technologies used to produce artificial diamonds. The high-pressure, high-temperature (HPHT) method applies high pressures (in orders of GPa) and high temperatures to obtain synthetic diamonds from carbonaceous materials, whereas low-pressure synthesis of diamond via plasma CVD uses a hydrocarbon gas mixture consisting of a carbon source and also hydrogen that selectively etches newly forming non-diamond structures.

CVD of diamond thin films is a complex process comprising several steps: 1) the activation of gases into radicals by appropriate source of energy; 2) gas phase chemical reactions between the activated species; 3) transport of the gas species to the substrate; and 4) reactions on the substrate (Yoshikawa *et al.*, 1990).

The type of energy source (thermal, plasma, flame, optical, etc.), the employed gas mixture (hydrogen or argon-rich mixture, oxygen containing species, etc.) and the temperature (gas and substrate temperature) are the most relevant parameters controlling the growth equilibrium. All these parameters have to be optimized to achieve the preferred formation of diamond. The diversity in carbon hybridizations makes the situation even more complex. From a thermodynamic point of view it means that successful diamond CVD growth has to prefer the formation of metastable diamond over more stable carbon forms (graphitic phases).

Nevertheless, any growth begins on an atomic and molecular level where a certain density of atoms results in the formation of a stable cluster. The formation of a stable cluster can start either from a gas phase or a solid state phase. The initialization or early stages of cluster formation are often known as the nucleation. The nucleation process is extremely important for diamond growth on foreign substrates (i.e. non-diamond substrates) because of the high surface energy of diamond. It influences not only the interlayer between diamond and substrate but also the size of formed grains and their crystallographic orientation, chemical purity (i.e. sp^3 to sp^2 ratio), adhesion to the substrate, etc. Thus, we can say that the nucleation process also controls film properties which directly determine their suitability for industrial uses. For example, smooth and continuous films are required for optical applications; high nucleation density is required for selective area deposition; large grains are crucial for heat spreading, etc. Generally, the nucleation yield depends on the specific nucleation enhancement method.

In the following sections the thermodynamic principles of nucleation and various experimental techniques used for diamond nucleation (and/or seeding) are reviewed. Experimental observations are correlated with theoretical predictions and advantages of each nucleation process are identified.

9.2 Diamond nucleation

As a result of random fluctuations, clusters of diamond-like structure are formed within an original, metastable phase (in this case, a supersaturated hydrocarbon gas) at a very early stage of evolution. Following Einstein's theory of fluctuations, the probability Prob(r) that a cluster of characteristic size r nucleates in the parent gaseous phase is proportional to:

$$\text{Prob}(r) \sim \exp\left(-\frac{\Delta G(r)}{kT}\right). \qquad [9.1]$$

where $\Delta G(r)$ represents Gibbs potential to form a diamond cluster of size r, k stands for the Boltzmann constant and T is thermodynamic temperature. Diamond clusters may randomly appear in the interior of metastable ionized hydrocarbon gas (homogeneous nucleation), or at preferential sites (in this case, the substrate) within the system (heterogeneous nucleation). According to Eq. 9.1, it is necessary to determine Gibbs energy required to form a diamond cluster of size r. (In fact, the specific form of $\Delta G(r)$ depends on the material under consideration, see e.g. Kožíšek and Demo, 1995; Demo *et al.*, 1999.)

Thermodynamically, $\Delta G(r)$ consists of two terms:

$$\Delta G(r) = \Delta G_v(r) + \Delta G_s(r), \qquad [9.2]$$

volumic (ΔG_v), which is related to the energy needed to rearrange freely moving carbon atoms into diamond structure, and surface (ΔG_s), connected with necessity to form a new interface between parent phase and diamond cluster. For the sake of simplicity, assume the spherical cluster of radius r (see Fig. 9.1).

In the case of *homogeneous nucleation* then

$$\Delta G_{\text{hom}} = -\frac{4}{3}\pi r^3 \frac{kT}{v} \ln S + 4\pi r^2 \sigma, \qquad [9.3]$$

where v is the volume of carbon atoms, σ stands for surface energy between the diamond cluster and the hydrocarbon gas, and S represents the degree of supersaturation of the gaseous phase by carbon atoms; usually,

$$S = \frac{P_{act}}{P_{eq}}, \qquad [9.4]$$

where P_{act} (respectively P_{eq}) is actual (respectively equilibrium) pressure within the system. The formation of a diamond is possible only for sufficiently high values of S ($S > 1$). Otherwise (i.e. for $S \leq 1$), the nucleation of diamond clusters is not thermodynamically favourable.

During *heterogeneous nucleation*, carbon atoms nucleate on a (usually non-diamond) substrate in the shape of a spherical cap with the contact

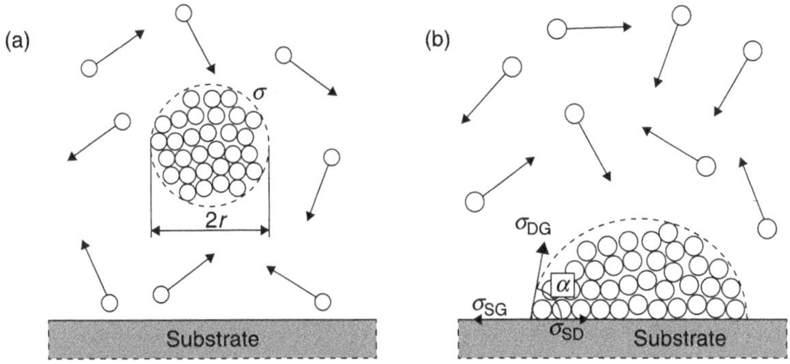

9.1 Schematic representation of homogeneous (a) and heterogeneous (b) nucleation. σ_{SG}, σ_{DG}, and σ_{SD} are surface energy between substrate and hydrocarbon gas, diamond cluster and hydrocarbon gas, and substrate and NCD cluster respectively.

angle α, expressing interplay between the three interfacial energies involved (see Fig. 9.1):

$$\cos\alpha = \frac{\sigma_{SG} - \sigma_{SD}}{\sigma_{DG}} \qquad [9.5]$$

As it may be readily proved (Vehkamäki, 2006), Gibbs energy, ΔG_{het}, required for heterogeneous nucleation is given by

$$\Delta G_{het}(\gamma) = \Delta G_{hom}(\gamma) f(\alpha), \qquad [9.6]$$

where

$$f(\alpha) = \frac{(2+\cos\alpha)(1-\cos\alpha)^2}{4}. \qquad [9.7]$$

As in most real cases, then $f(\alpha) \ll 1$ and – as follows from Eq. 9.1 – diamond nucleates mainly heterogeneously (see Fig. 9.2) (Demo *et al.*, 2000).

Newly formed diamond clusters are unstable below a certain critical size r_c, whose value may be determined from the extreme condition $\frac{\partial \Delta G}{\partial r} = 0$ to be

$$r_c = \frac{2v\sigma_{GD}}{kT \ln S}. \qquad [9.8]$$

Above the critical size r_c, the nanodiamond clusters become nuclei and tend to grow. Furthermore, at $r = r_c$, the so-called barrier of nucleation is given as

$$\Delta G_{het}(r_c) = \Delta G_{hom}(r_c) \cdot f(\alpha) = \frac{16\pi v^2 \sigma_{GD}^3}{3(kT \ln S)^2} \cdot f(\alpha). \qquad [9.9]$$

From Eqs 9.7 and 9.9, it is clear that the wettability of a substrate plays a very important role – via the contact angle α – in the diamond nucleation: the more

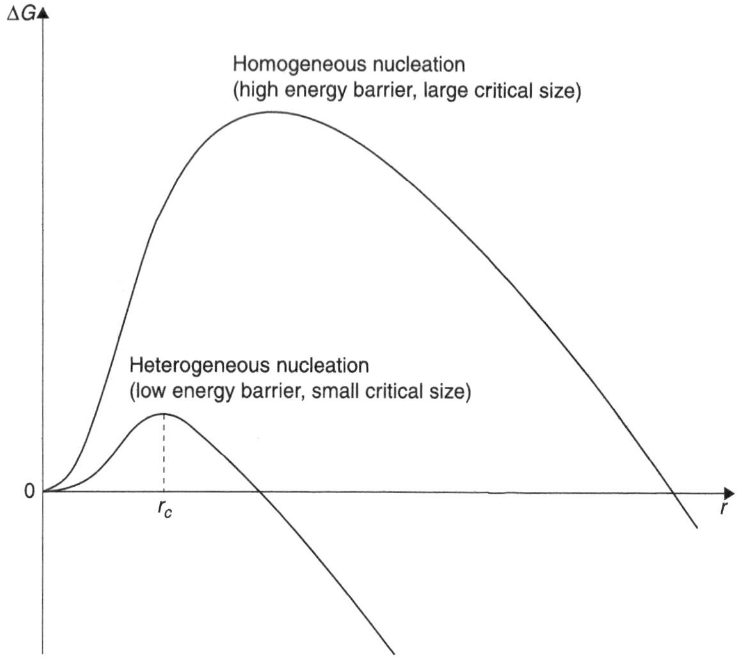

9.2 The nucleation barrier in heterogeneous versus homogeneous nucleation.

wettable the substrate (decreasing α), the lower the nucleation barrier for carbon atoms to nucleate the diamond. Consequently, at a constant temperature the formation rate of stable diamond clusters on a non-diamond substrate is strongly influenced by:

1. interactions between the diamond surface and its hydrocarbon environment (via surface energy σ_{GD});
2. the properties of the substrate (via contact angle α), which may be influenced by its pretreatment;
3. the degree of supersaturation (through S) of the gaseous phase by carbon atoms.

Three main growth modes can be distinguished, depending on the interaction strength of carbon adatoms with one another in comparison to the interaction strength of carbon adatoms with the substrate:

1. In the so-called Volmer-Weber mode of growth the interaction between carbon atoms is much stronger than their interaction with the substrate, which corresponds to $\sigma_{SD} \gg \sigma_{SG}$. From Eq. 9.5, it follows that the contact angle α is very high (bad wetting case). In this mode the nucleating diamond clusters

produce isolated three-dimensional (3D)-islands on the surface of the substrate. This mode represents the most accepted model for diamond growth.

2. The opposite situation of $\sigma_{SG} \gg \sigma_{SD}$ takes place when the interaction of carbon atoms with the substrate is relatively strong. In this, so-called Frank-van der Merwe mode of growth, the contact angle α is very small and the diamond nucleates one atomic layer at a time. This mode of growth is two-dimensional and is not known for diamond growth.
3. The intermediate situation, when both adatom–adatom and adatom–substrate interactions are comparable in strength ($\sigma_{SG} \sim \sigma_{SD}$), occurs in the Stranski-Krastanov mode of growth. The morphology of the surface in this case is a combination of the above two morphologies. Up to a certain critical thickness the layer grows predominantly in two-dimensional (2D)-mode, after which the formation of 3D islands becomes the main mechanism of nucleation. This situation was also observed during the early stages of diamond growth on seeded substrates.

9.3 Methods for diamond nucleation and seeding

It is well known that substrate features such as surface defects, surface energy, surface and bulk diffusion of atoms and chemical reactivity significantly contribute to the diamond nucleation process. Fig. 9.3 shows an example of diamond grains preferentially formed near the *energetically favourable sites* like substrate defects and/or scratching lines. In this case, no nucleation process was applied. Silicon substrates were loaded in the process chamber (the hot filament (HF) CVD

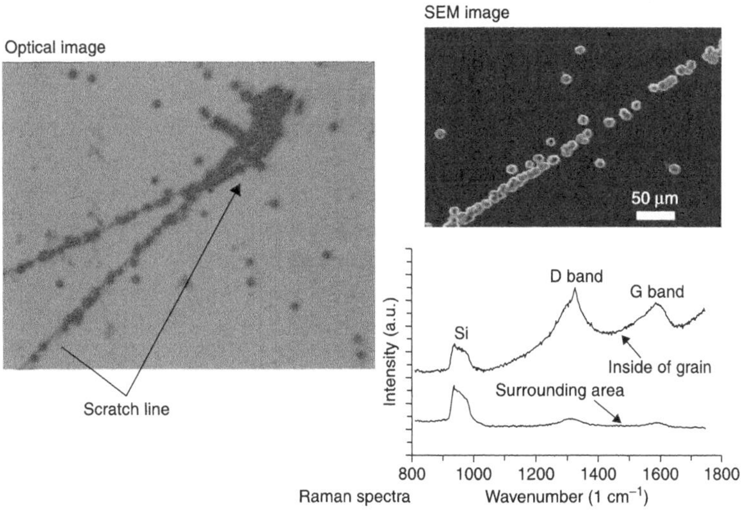

9.3 Optical image and surface morphology of Si substrate after the CVD diamond growth for 480 min. Raman spectra from grains (crystals) and surrounding area.

process) (Kromka, 2001). Generally, a few microscopic grains are observed across the substrate surface by optical microscopy. The density of these grains did not increase with the deposition time, only their size increased. The Raman spectrum inside the grains (dark points) shows two broad bands centred at 1310 and 1585 cm^{-1} with a left shoulder, which are assigned to presence of sp^2 bonded carbon labelled as D and G bands (Wang *et al.*, 1996; Bühlmann *et al.*, 1999). The diamond characteristic line is centred at 1331 cm^{-1}. Except for a few isolated crystals, the area surrounding these lines seems to be featureless. However, the Raman measurements revealed a spectrum consisting of two carbon bands (1300 and 1590 cm^{-1}) and a signal from the substrate material (silicon).

These results clearly confirm and demonstrate that nucleation of a diamond on a mirror-polished Si surface without applying any surface treatment (nucleation) would require a long incubation time (i.e. the time period required to initialize the diamond growth over the whole substrate). This restriction clearly limits any practical uses of diamond films. Therefore we need substrate pretreatment, which considers aspects such as 1) kinetic and thermodynamic principles of diamond nucleation; 2) the compatibility/suitability of the nucleation process with the chosen substrate; and 3) individual chemical and physical processes participating during the early stages of the diamond CVD growth (temperature, gas chemistry, etc.).

The efficiency of the nucleation process is standardly quantified by two parameters: surface nucleation density N_d (cm^{-2}) and surface nucleation rate N_r ($cm^{-2}*h^{-1}$). The surface nucleation density is the number of nuclei developed per unit of substrate surface. It is often obtained from Scanning Electron Microscope (SEM) or Atomic Force Microscope (AFM) morphological images. The nucleation density depends on several aspects, mainly on the nucleation procedure and the density of energetically favourable (activated) sites on the substrate surface.

As discussed in further detail later, the substrate (its bulk and surface), nucleation type and CVD growth conditions are the primary parameters influencing nucleation density. In the early stages of diamond growth, the size of the *primary* nuclei increases with the process time. In specific process conditions, new nuclei can also be continuously formed as a result of the presence of energetically favourable sites. At certain times, their density saturates and the nucleation ceases (the number of nucleation sites reduces to a negligible value). After this time period, the growth of diamond crystals starts to dominate the CVD process.

The diamond nucleation on non-diamond substrates can be summarized as follows (Spitsyn *et al.*, 1981):

- nucleation is mostly initialized on energetically favourable sites such as substrate defects and/or scratching lines, grain boundaries, dislocations, local strains, etc. (for instance nano-scratches are characterized by local high pressure values and a lower number of atoms is required to form a stable nuclei);
- the nucleation rate varies from 10^3 to 10^8 $cm^{-2}*h^{-1}$ and depends on the substrate material, pretreatment technique and CVD growth conditions;

- nucleation is lower on smooth single-crystalline substrates than on rough polycrystalline substrates;
- nucleation is higher on carbide-forming substrates (Si, Mo, Ti) than on chemically inert substrates (Cu, Au, Al_2O_3).

The pretreatment methods enhancing the diamond nucleation on various substrates can be classified as (Liu and Dandy, 1995; Das and Singh, 2007):

1. mechanical pretreatments
   - substrate scratching with abrasive material, often large diamond crystals are used;
   - ultrasonic seeding with diamond powders and composites;
2. bombardment and irradiation of surface
   - electron or ion bombardment (known as bias enhanced nucleation – BEN);
   - ion implantation of substrate;
   - pulsed laser irradiation;
   - ion etching of substrate;
3. modification of surface by thin layer or by chemical reactions
   - deposition of carbon layer (graphite, fullerenes, carbon fibres, DLC, hydrocarbon oil, polymer composites, etc.);
   - deposition of carbon forming metal film (Ti, W, Si);
   - thermally stimulated carbonization of substrate;
   - wet chemical etching of substrate;
   - modifications and combinations of the aforementioned methods.

Fig. 9.4 schematically summarizes the most commonly used pretreatment methods used to enhance the diamond nucleation on foreign substrates. Detailed information on the advantages and disadvantages of each individual treatment can be found in several reviews (Spitsyn *et al.*, 1981; Liu and Dandy, 1995; Das and Singh, 2007). Briefly, substrate scratching is the oldest and simplest technique.

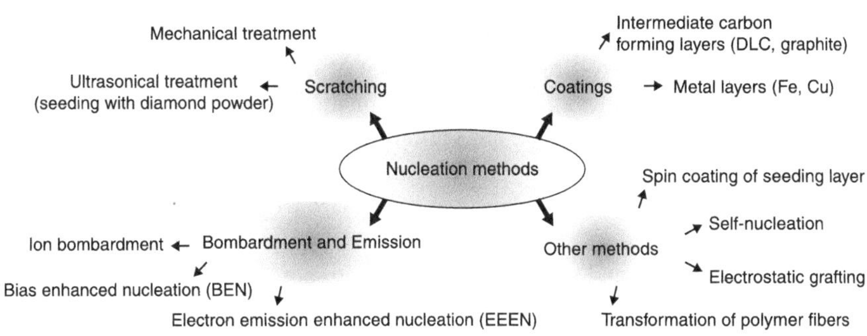

9.4 Commonly used pretreatment methods enhancing the diamond nucleation.

This process leads to mechanical damage and contamination of the substrate surface, which can also enhance the nucleation density. In recent years, ultrasonic treatment using ultradispersed detonation diamond represents the most perspective pretreatment method that is easily applied to substrates with a complex geometry and shape (Williams *et al.*, 2007; Kromka *et al.*, 2009a). From the broad range of bombardment and irradiation pretreatments, ion bombardment is the most promising alternative allowing the heteroepitaxial growth of diamond films on iridium substrates (Schreck *et al.*, 1997). Unfortunately, this technique is limited to use only on flat and electrically conductive substrates. Modification of the surface by a thin layer is also a potential alternative to mechanical scratching, especially as industrially acceptable thin films are used, which can be deposited over large areas (DLC, Ti, etc.) (Muller *et al.*, 1998; Daenen *et al.*, 2009; Lu *et al.*, 2012). Similarly, polymer–nanoparticle composites and polyelectrolyte–nanoparticle bi-layers have recently been developed (Kromka *et al.*, 2009b, 2009c; Scorsone *et al.*, 2009).

The inverse problem to the aforementioned enhancement of the nucleation is preventing the diamond film growth on certain areas of a substrate. This process is also known as selective area nucleation or selective area deposition and it is discussed in more detail later.

9.4 Bias enhanced nucleation in hot filament chemical vapour deposition

Bombardment of a substrate surface by electrons (Sawabe and Inuzuka, 1985) or ions (International Conference on the Applications of Diamond Films and Related Materials and Feldman, 1995) is a generally accepted method for enhancing the nucleation density. In addition to using a suitable substrate, the process parameters that influence the nucleation density and nucleation rate are: current density and applied voltage, gas composition (mainly methane concentration), total pressure and total time. The electron bombardment of the substrate, that is positive bias is applied to the substrate, was proposed to enhance decomposition of hydrocarbon species at the substrate surface (e.g. $CH_4 \rightarrow CH_3 \rightarrow CH_2 \rightarrow CH \rightarrow C$) (Sawabe and Inuzuka, 1985; Feldman, 1995; Liu and Dandy, 1995). A direct decomposition of hydrocarbons on the substrate surface was assumed to be more effective for the diamond nucleation as they are already on the substrate. The nucleation enhancement by gas species coming from the gas phase seems to be less important. Growth of heteroepitaxial diamond films on substrates pretreated by electron bombardment has not yet been achieved.

A more attractive and also more effective treatment for nucleation is ion bombardment, that is the substrate is negatively biased. The origin of nucleation enhancement is attributed to the increased flux of positively charged ions (mainly $C_xH_y^+$) to the surface, which is possibly followed by subsequent steps including 1) forming initial *carbon* clusters or a thin layer on the substrate; 2) increasing the surface mobility of adsorbed species as a result of a direct impact of ions; and 3) enhanced chemical reactions and concentration of dissociated hydrocarbons and atomic hydrogen near the substrate surface (Feldman, 1995; Liu and Dandy, 1995; Arnault, 2003; Chavanne *et al.*, 2011).

9.4.1 Filament carburization

The HF CVD process is an optimal choice for applications in which ultra-clean diamond films are not mandatory (i.e. optimal for overcoating of cutting inserts for tribology). The main limitation of the HF CVD method is the low chemical stability of the filaments and contamination of the growing diamond film by the filaments. The filament materials typically used are refractory metals such as W, Ta or Mo. At the beginning of the diamond growth, the dissociated methane and molecular hydrogen first react with the filaments. This leads to their carburization and embrittlement. It is therefore important to 'chemically stabilize' the filaments using a metal–carbide composite before the diamond growth (Kromka *et al.*, 2001a). The filament carburization can be simply monitored by measuring resistivity of filaments. Carburization of tungsten filaments is often started by heating them up to ~1500°C/3 min to outgas any impurities at the background pressure (see point A of the curve in Fig. 9.5). Then, a gas mixture of 1% methane diluted in hydrogen is introduced into the vacuum chamber and the filament temperature slowly increased

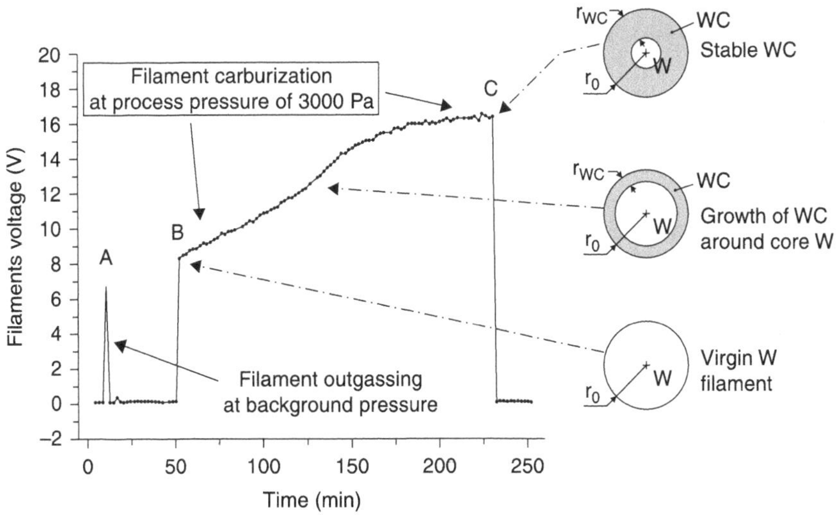

9.5 Time dependence of filament voltage (i.e. filament resistivity when the filament current is kept at a constant value) during the carburization process.

by increasing the d.c. current flow through filaments. We experimentally observed that finding the optimal *starting filament temperature* is very important. At a certain temperature (in our case voltage), the filament automatically starts to increase its resistivity due to forming tungsten carbide (WC) (point B). The formation of WC was confirmed by XRD, Raman and SEM measurements (Kromka *et al.*, 2001a). As the formed WC layer becomes thick enough, the carburization is a self-stopping process (point C). It should be mentioned that the carburization time can be shortened by using higher methane concentrations or higher starting temperatures. However, in our setup we observed that employing a fast carburization process (i.e. high filament temperature, methane concentration higher than 3% or d.c. plasma assisted environment) resulted in significant shortening of the filament lifetime or filament breaking during the diamond growth.

9.4.2 Single biasing

The bias controlled CVD process was shown as a promising way to overcome the problem of low nucleation density for applications where extremely smooth and clean surfaces are needed (Lee *et al.*, 1990). Several plasma-assisted HF CVD modifications have been developed and tested to improve diamond nucleation, for example a hollow cathode HF CVD system (Li *et al.*, 1997) or the direct pulsed BEN process (Hassan *et al.*, 1999). The direct bombardment of a substrate by ions is not a simple task because of 1) the requirements for large-area homogeneity; and 2) a controllable ion flux to substrate at relatively high pressures (3000 Pa). In the simplest setup, the BEN process is achieved by applying a d.c. power supply between the filaments and the substrate holder. However, this setup has several limitations, the first being that it behaves like the Schottky diode. Fig. 9.6 shows

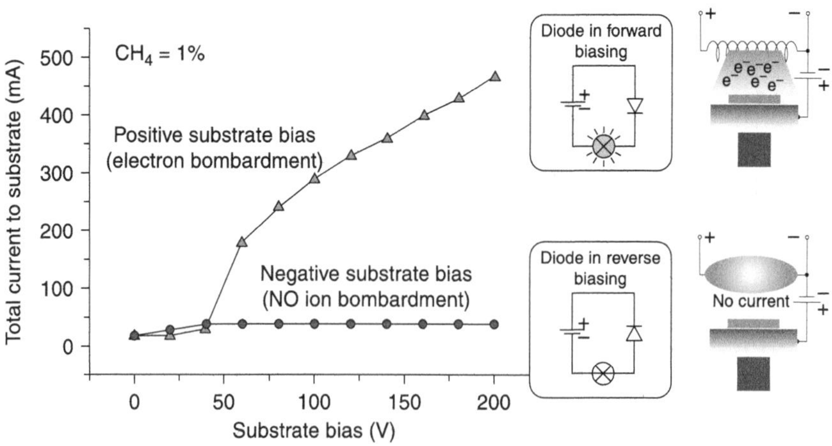

9.6 Dependence of substrate current on direct d.c. substrate bias and electronic scheme of the circuit.

the dependence of the substrate current on the substrate bias voltage (U_S). Current–voltage (I–V) measurements were accomplished using a molybdenum substrate. When the negative bias is applied to the substrate, no substrate current is measured for voltages up to 200V. In this case, thermally emitted electrons from hot filaments are *forced* back to their surface by the electrical field gradient and the situation is similar to the diode bias in 'reverse' mode. As the direction of the bias is changed, that is substrate is positively biased; a steep current increase is achieved at voltage as low as 50V. In this biasing mode, the system behaves as a diode in the 'forward' mode.

9.4.3 Double biasing

To overcome the previously mentioned limitations of applying the direct bias voltage to the substrate, we developed the hybrid HF CVD technique (Kromka, 2001). In this system, a graphite grid is located above the heated filaments. This setup enables the ignition of stable plasma at low voltages and essentially extends the ability of the standard HF CVD technique. The standard HF CVD system produces only radicals via thermal activation over the heated filaments and no ions are produced. In the present hybrid arrangement, positively charged ions are also formed. Thus, the gas mixture is activated via hot filaments and plasma. The second d.c. power supply is then connected between the filaments and the substrate holder to control bombardment of the substrate surface by either positively charged ions or electrons. This means that both types of plasma can be ignited simultaneously and, therefore, we labelled the system as the 'double bias HF CVD process'. The produced ions and/or ions bombarding the substrate can enhance gas activation, gas-phase dynamics, substrate-surface reactions, growth rate, etc.

The use of the double-plasma setup represents a unique method for controlling the nucleation process and/or formation of nanocrystalline diamond films. It should be noted that such a system has been independently developed and presented by Zhou *et al.* (Zhou *et al.*, 2000).

Double bias HF CVD is a reservoir of ions produced by igniting plasma between the filaments and the grid (U_G) in *forward* biasing. Ions are extracted from this plasma reservoir using a negative bias applied to the substrate. The current–voltage characteristics are shown in Fig. 9.7. As in the aforementioned experiment, I–V measurements were accomplished at full coverage of the substrate holder by the substrate material (Mo or Si) to suppress unwanted influences such as 1) holder memory effect (due to its overcoating by diamond and/or other carbon phases); and 2) non-homogenous distribution of the electric field over the substrate (Kromka, *et al.*, 2003a). When zero grid voltage was applied ($U_G = 0V$), the situation was similar to a previously discussed case when no current flow was achieved to the substrate (Fig. 9.6). Previously, we have shown that applying a grid voltage of 75V is required to measure the current flow

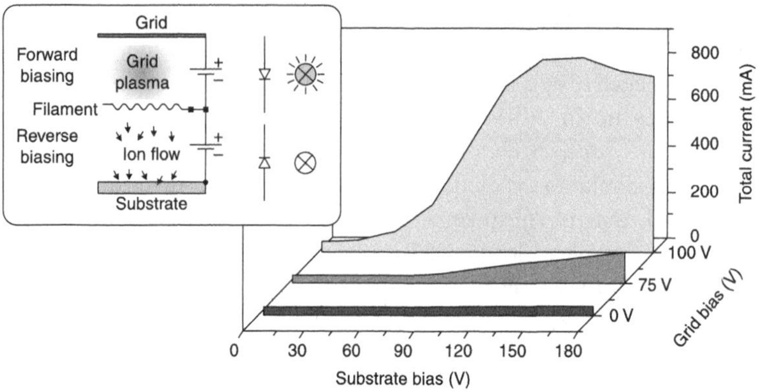

9.7 Current flow to the substrate as a function of substrate bias (0–180 V) for grid bias (0, 75 and 100 V) and schematic view of electronic circuit consisting of two diodes (left).

at a substrate bias of 100 V. When the grid voltage was 100 V, applying a substrate bias of as low as 40 V is high enough to measure the current flow (i.e. to achieve ion bombardment of the substrate). This result confirms that plasma produced above the filaments can be used as the reservoir of ions, which can more easily be 'extracted' from this plasma by applying a negative voltage to the substrate. Finally, they are accelerated to a certain energy level due to the potential gradient between filaments and the substrate. Ions bombarding the substrate participate in several ways in the diamond nucleation, as discussed in the following.

It is important to note that, during the nucleation step performed at a constant substrate bias, the total substrate current will vary with time. A representative time evolution of the substrate current is shown in Fig. 9.8. At the beginning of the BEN process the current to the substrate does not change for a certain time (incubation time). During this time period, the substrate is bombarded by energetic ions and there are still not enough stable diamond nuclei. Depending on the substrate material, a carbon interlayer can be formed such as graphite, DLC, amorphous carbon or even a carbide layer (i.e. SiC) (Zhou *et al.*, 2000; Kromka *et al.*, 2001b).

Under optimal BEN conditions, the number of sp^3 bonded carbon (nuclei or clusters) increases with the process time and reaches a certain level at which electron emission is substantially enhanced from these sp^3 features. Emitted electrons can additionally ionize atoms located near the substrate and thereby further increase the ion bombardment of the substrate. The substrate coverage with carbon layer (mixture of sp^2 and sp^3 carbon) increases too. When a nearly continuous *carbon layer* is deposited on the substrate, the current becomes stable or can even slightly decrease as a result of the re-nucleation processes. At this time, the BEN nucleation should be stopped. The CVD process can continue in the growth regime where diamond crystals get larger with the deposition time. This current variation in time is a common feature in BEN nucleation, that is the measured current–time curves are characteristic for the microwave plasma BEN process.

It should be noted that most researchers define the nucleation time (in our case 120 min) including the incubation period, some authors omit this time period. Uncertainty in the definition of the nucleation time makes experimental work less reproducible and disputable conclusions are presented.

When the ion bombardment is not stopped and the BEN nucleation still continues, the growing diamond layer can be damaged by the graphitization of diamond grains and re-nucleation can dominate the CVD growth. In such cases, the size of the diamond crystals is limited to nanoscale dimensions and does not increase with a prolonged deposition time (Zhou *et al.*, 2002; Vojs *et al.*, 2005).

The time constant from the substrate current curve can be extracted by applying the Avrami model, which expresses the time dependence of the transformed material fraction during crystallization (Avrami, 1939; Perng *et al.*, 2002). The formula is as follows:

$$\chi(t) = 1 - \exp[-(t-t_0)^n/C] \qquad [9.10]$$

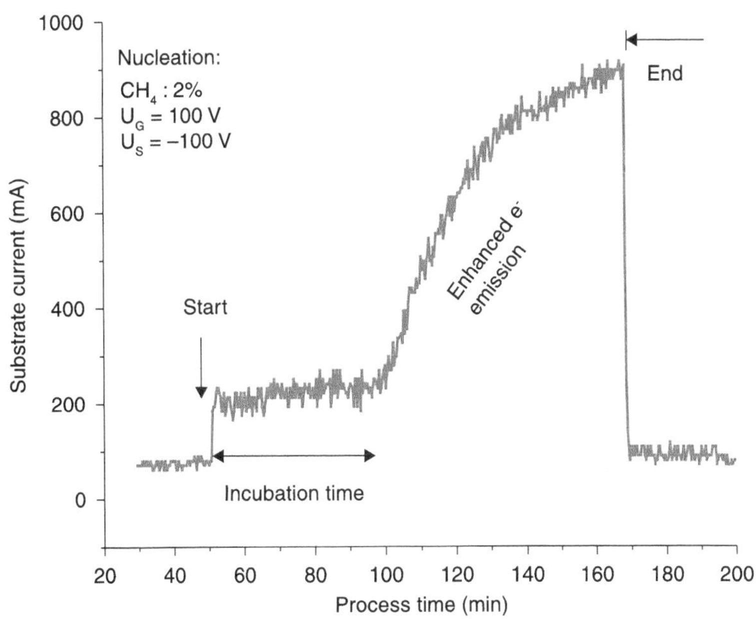

9.8 Time dependence of total current flow to the substrate during the BEN nucleation.

where t_0 is the incubation time for nucleation, *1/C* is the formation rate, and *n* expresses the nucleation type (*n=3* for continuous nucleation, *n=2* site saturation). For the curve shown in Fig. 9.8, the extrapolated incubation time was 50.6 min with $n = 0.68$.

It was shown that the current flow to the substrate depends on the grid and substrate bias. It is therefore expected that the incubation time will be significantly related to the applied substrate bias and process conditions. Our previous experiments performed at 0.5% CH_4 have confirmed this expectation (Kromka *et al.*, 2003a). For the negative substrate bias 100 V and lower, no current was measured. It means that after the CVD growth (20 h), only isolated diamond grains were formed. The nucleation took place at $Us = 120$ V and the extrapolated incubation time was 64 min. The diamond layer grown for 20 h exhibited rectangular-like crystals. The extrapolated incubation time monotonically decreases with an increasing substrate bias. For $Us = 180$ V, the incubation time was approximately 20 min. However, in this case the diamond layer consisted of randomly oriented crystals, and the growth rate was lower. The dependence of the incubation time on the substrate bias is summarized in Fig. 9.9.

The extrapolated value *n* monotonically decreases from 3.02 ($Us = 120$ V) to 0.68 ($Us = 180$ V) (Kromka *et al.*, 2003a). This variation of the *n* value can be assigned to the nucleation change from continuous to site saturation. At higher substrate bias the ion bombardment of the substrate and the energy of the impinging ions are also higher, and chemical reactions at (or near) the substrate

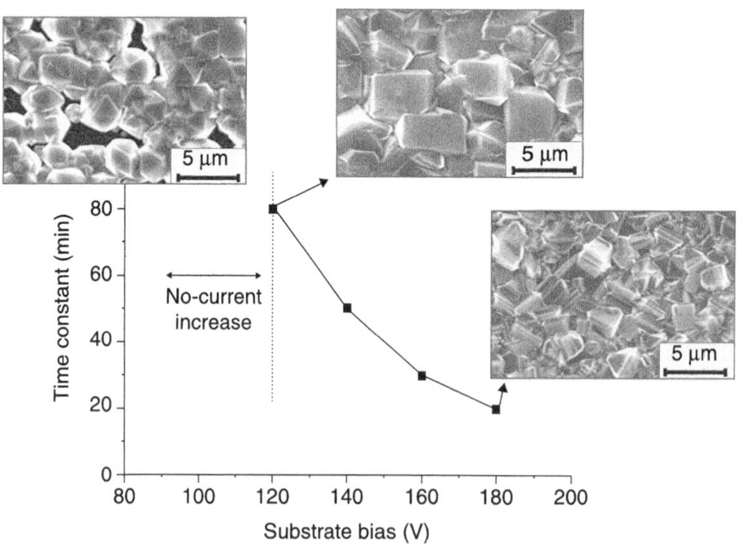

9.9 Time dependence of the total current flow to the substrate (0.5% CH_4, $U_G = 100$ V, p = 3000 Pa, nucleation time = 2 h).

surface should be faster. In such cases, inhomogeneous *regions* with a higher density of new nuclei, defects or impurities can be formed (Castro *et al.*, 1999). Therefore, we assume that the BEN nucleation at 180 V for 2 h is too long because the degradation of sp^3 nuclei and re-nucleation are competitive processes to the crystal growth. For our experimental setup, optimal BEN conditions (not discussed here) were following: *Us* = 120 V, 0.5% CH_4 in H_2, p = 3000 Pa.

The BEN process is not a trivial process and has attracted the attention of many researchers. Ion impinging of the substrate surface can increase the surface mobility of absorbed species (Stoner *et al.*, 1992), adatom diffusion (Jiang *et al.*, 1994) or initialize the formation of the transient interlayer (Robertson *et al.*, 1995). Generally, no significant change to the gas species was observed by Cui and Fang (Cui and Fang, 1996). Yugo *et al.* proposed that the hydrogen-enriched amorphous carbon layer could stabilize the diamond nuclei (Yugo *et al.*, 1991). The most complex model was presented by Lifshitz *et al.* (Lifshitz, 2002), who concluded that the BEN process is controlled by energetic species and that the nucleation process consists of four basic steps: 1) the formation of an ultrathin hydrogenated amorphous carbon layer (1–2 nm); 2) followed by spontaneous precipitation of sp^3 carbon clusters from this layer; 3) annealing and stabilization of the defective clusters; and 4) growth of the formed clusters by consuming the amorphous carbon layer that surrounds the diamond clusters.

The main advantage of the BEN process is that only this technique is able to initialize heteroepitaxial nucleation in the microwave plasma process followed by the heteroepitaxial diamond growth on iridium substrate (Schreck *et al.*, 1997). However, it was shown that the heteroepitaxial BEN process is very sensitive to optimal process conditions and even their slight change results in non-epitaxial diamond growth.

The main advantage of double bias HF CVD nucleation is controllable bombardment of the substrate by positively charged ions in reproducible and stable conditions, which is applicable for relatively high pressures (3000 Pa) and can be scaled up to large areas (limited only by the filament geometry). Next, the double bias HF CVD nucleation can make the *optimal process window* larger while the ion bombardment (dose and ion energy) is controlled, not only by the substrate bias, but also by 1) grid voltage; 2) by process conditions (gas composition – methane concentration, total gas pressure, etc.); and 3) by geometrical setup (distance of the filaments-to-grid, distance of the filaments-to-substrate). The variability of the process conditions is schematically illustrated in Fig. 9.10. At a low methane concentration (0.5%), a non-continuous layer was formed at d.c. substrate bias of 100 V. As the methane concentration increased from 0.5% to 2% or the total pressure decreased from 3000 to 1000 Pa, a continuous diamond layer is formed.

Finally, it has to be mentioned that double bias HF CVD nucleation is suitable for electrically non-conductive substrates (glass, ceramic) by applying an a.c. substrate bias (Kromka *et al.*, 2003b). Generally, higher substrate bias voltages

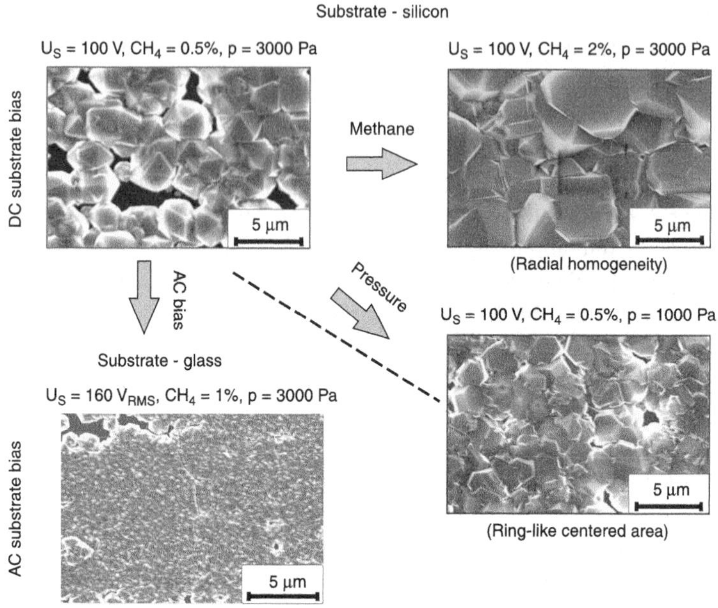

9.10 Schematic overview of the nucleation processes and process conditions and of their impact on resulting diamond thin film morphology (characterized by SEM).

(160 V_{RMS}) were required to achieve a nucleation efficiency comparable to the d.c. biasing at 120 V. The a.c. BEN pretreatment, which is still a largely unexplored field, potentially represents a promising solution for diamond growth on three-dimensionally shaped non-conductive materials.

9.5 Ultrasonic seeding

Another popular nucleation strategy is nucleation via ultrasound agitation in diamond powder suspension. This strategy descended from the use of embedding or the attachment of nano-sized fragments of diamond grit to the substrate to act as growth sites. Diamond nuclei are formed by adhering diamond particles from diamond powder solution to substrates by van der Waals interactions (Sumant *et al.*, 2007) or electrostatic forces based on zeta potential. The zeta potential of diamond particles can be changed to obtain a monodisperse nanodiamond colloid with an exceptionally long time stability in a wide range of pH and with a high positive zeta potential (>60 mV) (Williams *et al.*, 2010).

At first, substrate polishing (abrasion) using diamond paste was mainly used (Wang *et al.*, 1992; Higa *et al.*, 1996). Then, ultrasound nucleation in diamond powder suspension with micrometer or sub-micrometer large diamond grains became popular (Bienk and Eskildsen, 1993). Recently, the application of nano-sized crystals has become even more popular (Williams *et al.*, 2007; Kromka *et al.*, 2009a). The liquids used for suspensions are mostly alcohols (ethanol, methanol, isopropyl alcohol) or water. Ultrasonic seeding allows nucleation of non-conductive substrates with various 3D geometries and no specialized deposition apparatus is needed (Varga *et al.*, 2011).

Nowadays, ultrasonic seeding seems to be the most progressive and universal technique that allows very high nucleation densities up to 10^{12} cm^{-2} (Williams *et al.*, 2007; Kromka *et al.*, 2008a). Also, it can be easily used for selective area nucleation and deposition with a combination of lithography and polymer structures (Kromka *et al.*, 2009b). High nucleation densities were achieved for the first time in a so-called new nucleation process (NNP) introduced in 1999 by Rotter (Rotter, 1999), and further modified and studied by Butler's group (Sumant *et al.*, 2007). Recently there has been increased study into the ultrasonic seeding of diamond with various properties, using diamond particles in liquid solutions. For example, the size of used diamond particles can influence nucleation density and homogeneity (Kromka *et al.*, 2009a), as well as the mentioned zeta potential (Williams *et al.*, 2010).

For our study of diamond nuclei (seeds) distribution over the substrate surface, we used three types of diamond powders (DP) marked as S1, S2 and S3, all commercially available as fine-grained diamond powders with an average grain size of 5 nm. Type S1 is a dry nanocrystalline diamond powder, which was diluted in isopropyl alcohol. S2 and S3 are diamond powders delivered as liquid suspensions in deionized (DI) water. Although all diamond powders used were specified by suppliers as fine-grained, the *real* optical particle-size distributions, measured by dynamic light scattering (DLS) method, differ from the nominal because of the known tendency of clustering of the diamond nanoparticles (Ōsawa, 2008).

We used polished silicon (100) oriented wafers cut to a size of $15\times15\,cm^2$. To diminish any possible contamination and predefine initial surface properties, before nucleation treatment, the substrates were cleaned using the standard RCA cleaning process. Next, samples were pretreated by substrate immersion into the ultrasonic bath with S1, S2 or S3 suspension for 1 or 40 min. Nucleated substrates were thereby characterized using AFM surface analytical techniques. The influences of the powder type, pretreatment time and DP composition on the seeding density on silicon were examined.

9.5.1 Particle size distribution

Figure 9.11 shows the particle size distributions measured by DLS in liquid, related to the type of diamond powder used. Suspension S1 consists of particles (or agglomerates) with a broad size distribution centred at around 900 nm. In this case, DLS measurements do not exhibit any sign of primary nanoparticles (i.e. particles sized between 5 and 10 nm). The reason for this is probably that the

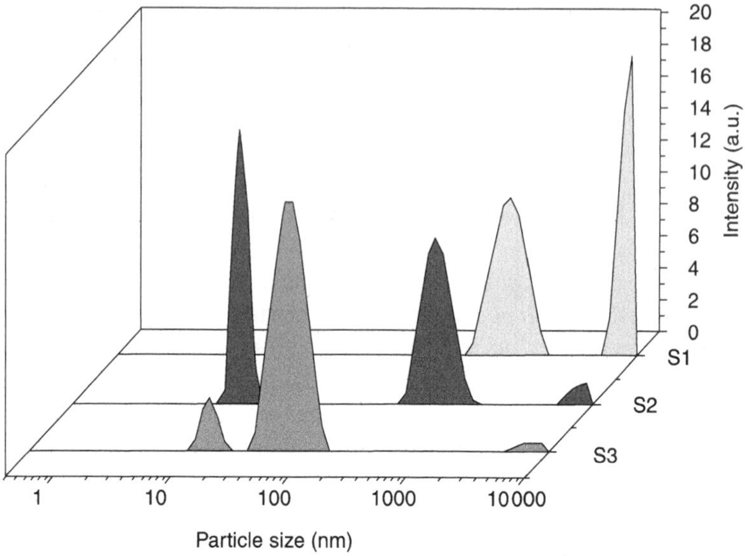

9.11 The dependence of a particle size distribution curve on the diamond powder suspension used (S1–S3), as measured by the DLS technique.

suspension was prepared from the dry powder, that is particles were strongly agglomerated. The particle size distribution curve was significantly different for suspensions S2 and S3. In these two cases particle size distributions were shifted to the nanoscale range. The DLS measurement of S2 suspension exhibited a sharp peak centred at around 10 nm and a broad peak centred at 460 nm. Figure 9.11 shows a particle distribution in S3 suspension, where the presence of nano-sized particles is also observed and light scattering on 13 nm particles is detectable. There was an additional band centred at 77 nm. What is remarkable is that the particle size distribution was not significantly sensitive either to ultrasonic or sonication processes. Only a slight shift in the particle size to lower values was observed for S2 and S3 suspensions.

A certain amount of each nucleation suspension was used for a sedimentation test. The suspension was captured immediately after mixing (Fig. 9.12(a)), and after five days of sedimentation (Fig. 9.12(b)). These results provide complementary information to DLS measurements about the stability of diamond powder colloid suspensions. As shown in Fig. 9.12, suspension S1 exhibited weak sedimentation and remains milky-yellow in colour. Suspension S2 exhibited the strongest sedimentation and the two separate phases are clearly distinguishable. The S3 suspension exhibited almost no sedimentation. The obvious, larger and heavier diamond particles are more likely to precipitate than smaller ones in the same liquid. On the other hand, the surface polarity strongly influences the colloid stability of suspension, however, even for large particles (Ōsawa, 2008). This

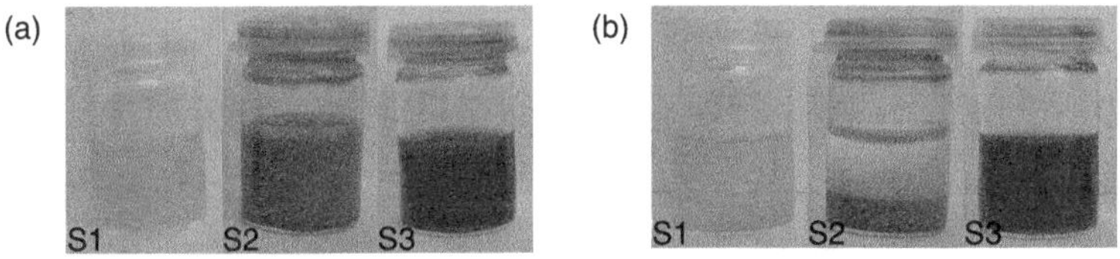

9.12 Sedimentation of diamond powder in suspension S1–S3 on (a) first day, (b) fifth day.

probably took place in the case of the S1 suspension (isopropyl alcohol). In the S1 suspension even quite large particles (900 nm) are not precipitate, whereas smaller particles in S2 (460 nm and even 10 nm) dropped to the sediment. The employed liquid (alcohol versus water) could also play a role. When comparing the second water-based suspension S3, it is clearly evident, that the larger particles of S1 suspension could remain in the colloid mainly because of the surface polarity. The nano-sized particles of the S3 suspension almost did not precipitate compared with the S1 and S2 suspensions. This proves that the best colloid stability and resistance to agglomeration is deduced from DLS.

After the nucleation of the substrates, the S1 type diamond powder showed higher light scattering as observed by the naked eye. These features were identified as large blocks of diamond powder coalesced in hillock-like structures. It is interesting to note that these surface non-homogeneities adhered well to the substrate and it was not possible to remove them by ultrasonic washing. On the other hand, Si substrates ultrasonically pretreated by S2 and S3 suspension revealed better homogeneity in the sense of optical reflectance from the mirror-polished silicon surface.

9.5.2 Morphology of seeded Si substrates

The surface morphologies and root mean square (RMS) roughness of the seeded silicon substrates measured by AFM are shown in Fig. 9.13. The flat areas were assigned to a clean Si surface and the protruded features were assumed to be diamond seeds. The AFM measurements on a sample pretreated for 1 min in the S1 suspension (Fig. 9.13(a)) revealed poor coverage of the substrate surface with diamond seeds, which is also the reason for the low RMS roughness (2.9 nm). Prolonging the treatment time up to 40 min (Fig. 9.13(d)) increases the surface coverage with diamond seeds. On the other hand, the RMS roughness also increases. Nevertheless, the seeding layer remains non-continuous.

For the water-based diamond suspensions (S2 and S3) the situation was completely different. In these cases, the 1 min process resulted in a nucleation density higher than even the 40 min treatment in the S1 suspension (compare Fig. 9.13(b) and (c) with (d)). The RMS roughness measured on these two samples was also higher than that for the sample pretreated for 1 min in the S1. The

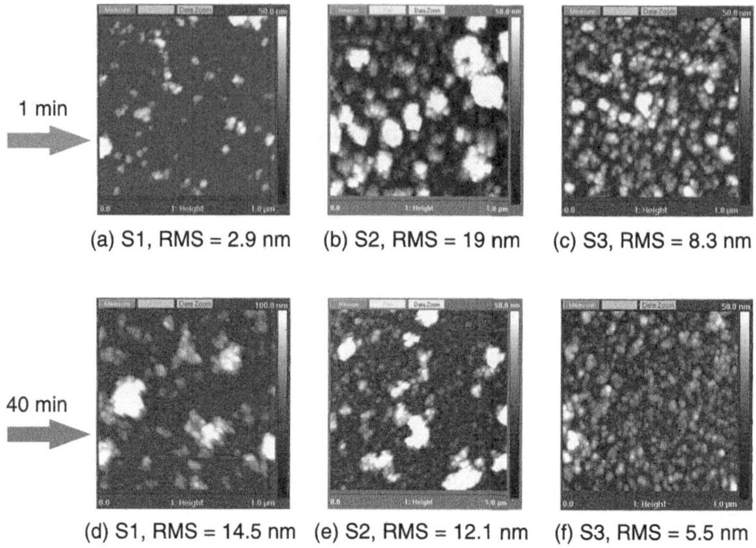

9.13 AFM surface morphologies (scan 1×1 μm^2) of silicon substrates pretreated in ultrasonic bath for 1 min (a, b, c) and for 40 min (d, e, f), where S1 is DP diluted in isopropyl alcohol, S2 and S3 diamond powder in DI water.

difference between the S2 and S3 pretreated samples can be seen from the AFM scan, and showed that the substrate nucleated by the S2 suspension (Fig. 9.13(b)) is covered by larger diamond seeds or aggregates than the substrate nucleated by S3 (Fig. 9.13(c)) and thus has an RMS roughness of at least two times higher. This issue could be explained by results from DLS measurements, which show that while the S2 suspension contains particles as large as 460 nm, the S3 suspension contains 13 nm and 77 nm large particles. Those large particles of the S2 suspension influence the RMS roughness.

As shown by AFM measurements (Fig. 9.13(e) and Fig. 9.13(f)), prolonging the treatment time in these suspensions results in a better homogeneity of surface coverage and, in addition, decreases the RMS roughness from 19 nm to 12 nm and from 8 nm to 6 nm for S2 and S3 suspensions, respectively. The reason for this decrease is explained by partially removing and decomposing larger aggregates during the long ultrasound treatment.

To calculate and validate the true seeding density from the observed AFM data, the following digression is essential. Fig. 9.14(a) shows a detailed morphology and phase profile across a diamond particle on a substrate. The height of the particle is about 5 nm, which corresponds to the size of the seeding particles, but the width of particle is about 20 nm. This is because the tip radius is comparable to the particle size and the observed morphology is a convolution of the tip and particle shapes. When the shapes of the tip and particle are approximated by

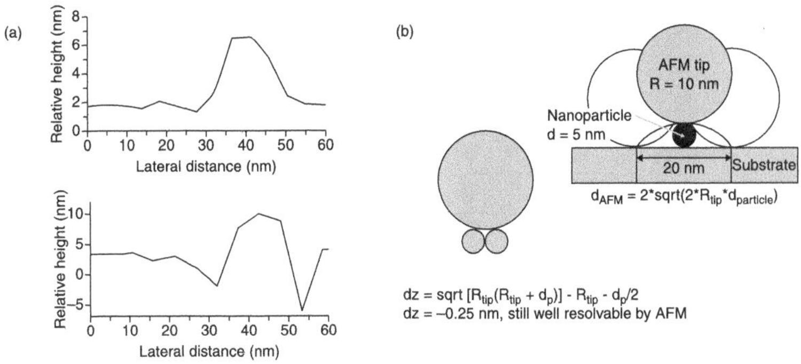

9.14 Proposed (a) detailed morphology and phase profile across a single particle on a substrate and (b) deconvolution of measurement.

spheres, the true width of particles can be calculated using geometry as $d_{particle} = d_{AFM}^2/8R_{tip}$ (Fig. 9.14(b)). For a 10 nm tip radius and 20 nm feature size detected by AFM the calculation yields a 5 nm particle size. The corresponding phase profile shows that the diamond particles typically have a 5 degrees larger phase lag than silicon substrate.

Figure 9.15(a,b) shows an AFM image and the height profile of the substrate pretreated for 40 min in the S3 suspension. The seeding particles are deposited in multilayers or aggregates of two to six particles' height. There are also some openings in the seeding layer, as indicated by the flat regions in the height profiles.

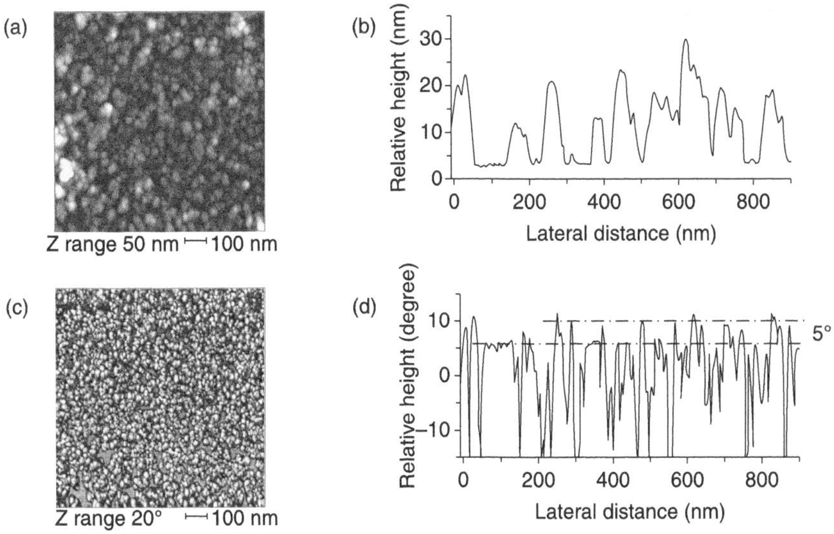

9.15 The AFM results of the height profile (a, b), and phase image (c, d) observed on a sample pretreated for 40 min in the S3 suspension.

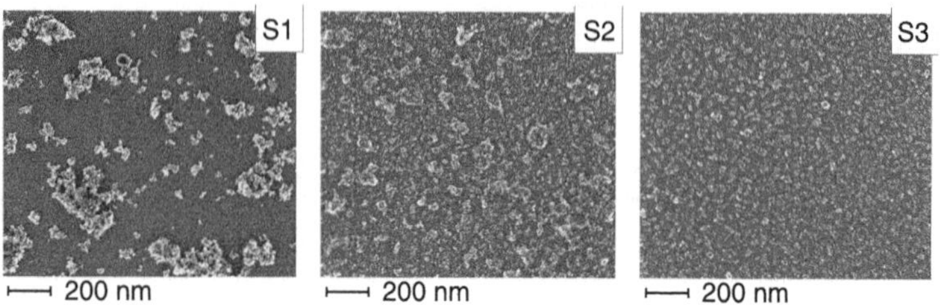

9.16 SEM images of silicon substrates pretreated in ultrasonic bath for 40 min: S1 is DP diluted in isopropyl alcohol, S2 and S3 diamond powder in DI water.

The phase image in Fig. 9.15(c,d) clearly resolves these irregular openings in the seeding layer with dimensions of <100 nm. Thus, as calculated from AFM measurements, when applied with pretreatment the S3 suspension results in a diamond nuclei surface coverage of 76%, that is a density in the order of 10^{12} cm^{-2} (as calculated for a particle diameter of 5 nm).

Figure 9.16 shows the SEM images of Si substrates after a 40 min nucleation in the S1–S3 suspensions. From these images it is evident that treatment in the S1 suspension (Fig. 9.16(a)) results in a poor seeding density with many areas completely free from diamond seeds. The other seeds are mainly aggregated into formations as large as 200 nm. Large formations could be observed on the surface of the sample pretreated with the S2 suspension as well (Fig. 9.16(b)). In contrast to the previous one, however, the space between these agglomerates is quite densely filled by the small diamond seeds (≤10 nm). Finally, as has already been shown by AFM the most efficient seeding was achieved on the sample pretreated with the S3 suspension (Fig. 9.16(c)). On this sample the homogeneous and dense diamond seeds cover the surface. In addition, the S3 suspension did not show the same aggregates as S1 and S2.

9.5.3 Chemical composition of seeded Si substrates

Table 9.1 summarizes the elemental composition obtained on the Si substrates after ultrasonic treatment by different DP suspensions for 1 or 40 min. The table includes four detected elements: O1s, C1s, Si2p and Zr3d. All these elements were measurable in a wide-range scan. As expected, in the near-surface region of the analyzed samples, carbon and silicon clearly dominate in the XPS spectrum. Surprisingly, a relatively high oxygen content is also present. Oxygen was detected in the carbon atoms as C-O bonds on diamond powder (Fig. 9.17), most probably as a result of the wet chemical cleaning procedure (Kruger *et al.*, 2005) and oxygen was also found to be chemically attached to the silicon surface (Si-O bond). In addition, traces of zirconium were found in detailed spectrum after a prolonged acquisition time over most of samples. The 'near–surface' contamination

Table 9.1 Surface composition of silicon substrate ultrasonically pretreated in suspensions of S1, S2 or S3 diamond powder for 1 or 40 min

DP suspension	Seeding time (min)	O	Si	Zr	Carbon		
		at. %	at. %	at. %	at. %	sp^2	sp^3
S1	1	33.8	41.8	0.3	24.1	75	25
	40	28.1	37.3	0	34.6	65	35
S2	1	25.8	24.8	0.5	48.9	58	42
	40	23.1	24.5	0.6	51.8	39	61
S3	1	29.6	29.2	0.7	40.5	54	46
	40	24.4	26.5	0.5	48.6	53	47

of the investigated surface by zirconium indicates that post-processing of diamond powder by a ball milling process was possibly used (Williams *et al.*, 2007; Ōsawa, 2008). The nitrogen content detected was a negligible amount and is therefore not included in Table 9.1.

The percentage of sp^3 hybridized carbon atoms in the analyzed volume of the ultrasonically seeded Si substrates was evaluated from the high resolution C 1s XPS spectrum (Fig. 9.17). The C 1s spectrum is asymmetric, indicating several C bonding states involved. The used fitting procedure of the C 1s characteristic peak is described elsewhere (Zemek *et al.*, 2006). In the presented C 1s XPS spectrum we can observe three maxima centred at 284.9 eV, 286.1 eV and 287.4 eV. The maxima centred at 284.9 and 287.4 eV are attributed to the sp^2 carbon bond and to C-O binding (Moulder *et al.*, 1995), respectively. The maximum centred at 286.1 eV is attributed to the sp^3 hybridized carbon bond. The chemical shift between sp^2 and sp^3 carbon bonds is ~1.2 eV, which is close to the previously calculated value of 1.1 eV (Titantah and Lamoen, 2005).

Based on the AFM and SEM results, the samples pretreated by the S3 suspension were further investigated for stability in hydrogen plasma. Samples were treated in microwave plasma in a focused ellipsoidal cavity resonator (Kromka *et al.*, 2008b). The process conditions were: microwave power 1100 W, pressure 30 mbar, H_2 gas flow 300 sccm and temperature 440°C. The times of treatment were 10 and 20 min. The results acquired by XPS are summarized in the form of the diagram in Fig. 9.18. Hydrogen plasma treatment leads to a clear decrease in Zr contamination. Surprisingly the Si signal also decreased from 27% to 9% (after 20 min treatment) in the whole spectrum. In contrast, the O signal in the XPS spectrum after 20 min plasma treatment increased from 24% to 33%. The increased amount of sp^2 (not shown here) could be explained by the graphitization of diamond seeds under the influence of plasma and temperature.

In summary, ultrasonic treatment is a very simple and low cost technique that is applicable to nearly all types of substrate materials without any restrictions for electrical properties. The sample pretreated in the S3 suspension (which includes the smallest diamond seeds) exhibits the most promising results in terms of low

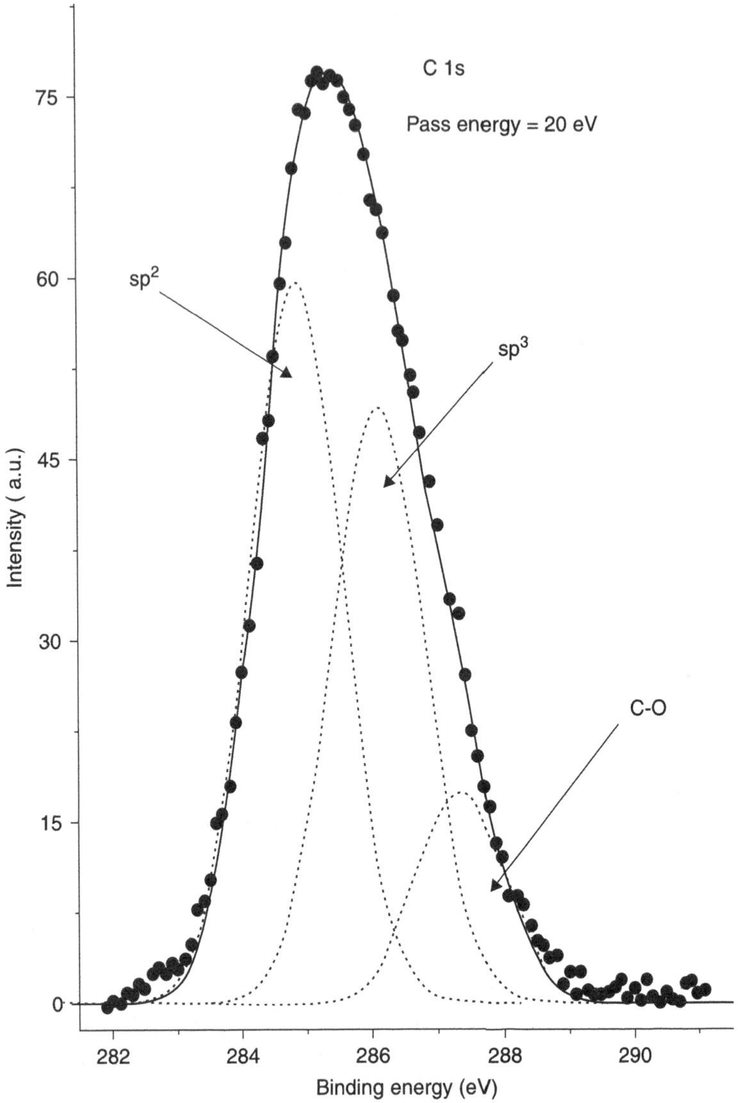

9.17 Detailed scan and C 1s peak fitting of XPS spectra acquired on substrate that was pretreated for 40 min in S3 suspension.

surface roughness and seeding density. The nucleation process using this suspension results in a seeding density of as high as 10^{12} cm^{-2} (Kromka *et al.*, 2008a). To our knowledge, this is the highest reported nucleation density achieved using ultrasonic treatment (Williams *et al.*, 2007; Lee *et al.*, 2011). This value is very close to the mathematically calculated value in the case of 10 nm nano-blocks. Achieving such a high nucleation density allows us to grow very thin (<100 nm), smooth and fully closed nanocrystalline diamond layers (Kromka *et al.*, 2008a;

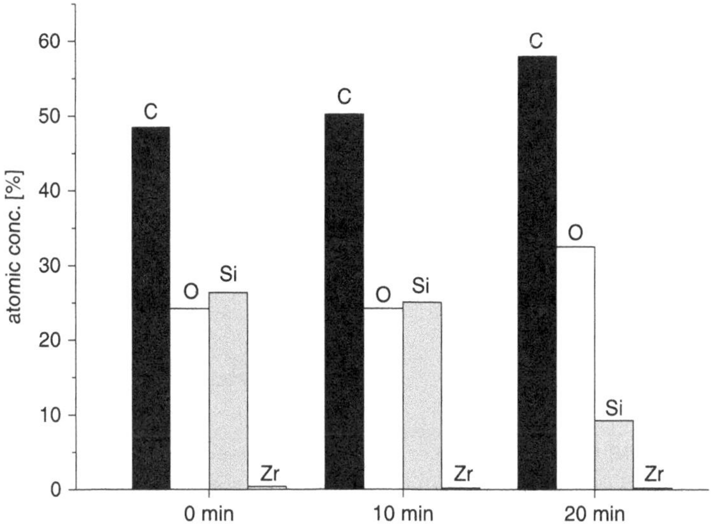

9.18 Comparative diagram from XPS measurements on substrates that were pretreated for 40 min in S3 suspension as a result of hydrogen plasma treatment.

et al., 2008a; Lee *et al.*, 2011) as well as to selectively grow submicron diamond structures (Babchenko *et al.*, 2012). Moreover, applying ultrasound nucleation is beneficial for three-dimensionally shaped geometries. In such cases, diamond films simply followed the topography of initially roughened Si substrate (Broz *et al.*, 2009; Kalbacova *et al.*, 2009; Kromka *et al.*, 2009a). The NCD films grown on such samples were found to be advantageous for living cell, proliferation, differentiation and adhesion to the surface. A further application of this nucleation technique is in the fabrication of coatings for three-dimensional optical elements used in the infrared reflection spectroscopy (Babchenko *et al.*, 2011).

9.5.4 Ultrasonic seeding with the assistance of non-diamond particles

In the previous section, ultrasonic seeding using diamond nanoparticles in solution was introduced as a universal and high efficiency tool to initiate diamond growth on diverse substrates and morphologies. Moreover, formation of nucleation centres can be improved by the addition of metal nano- or micro-particles into the solution with an ultra-dispersed diamond (UDD) powder (Fig. 9.19). The composition of the solution and properties of used particles are summarized in Table 9.2.

Buijnsters *et al.* (Buijnsters *et al.*, 2009) added metal particles such as Ti, Fe and W into solutions with nanodiamond powder. They concluded that the metal

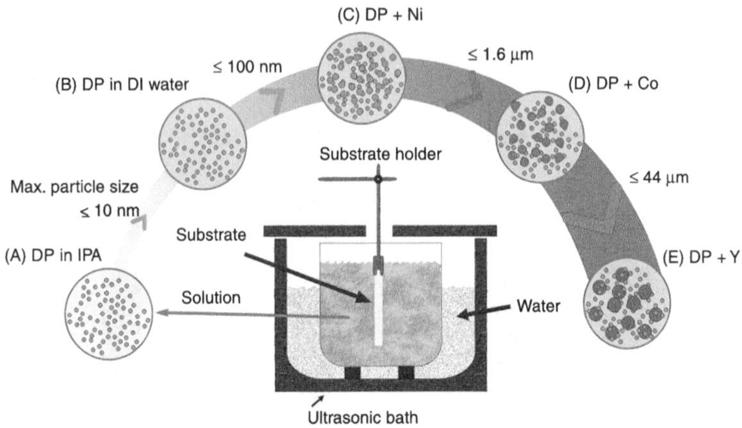

9.19 Schematic view of the ultrasonic seeding in different solutions. For definitions of samples A–E see Table 9.2.

particles have a strong influence on the nucleation density and homogeneity of the nucleation. The highest nucleation density was achieved for Ti nanoparticles combined with nanodiamond powder.

In our work (Varga *et al.*, 2011), we studied the effect of Ni, Co and Y metal powders with UDD powder on nucleation density. The result of such an investigation should be interesting as Ni and Co are commonly used as catalysts for diamond film growth in the HPHT technique (Liang *et al.*, 2005). The addition of Ni and Co catalysts allows HPHT pressures to run at lower temperatures than would otherwise be needed to produce a diamond. These catalysts dissolve carbon which facilitates diamond precipitation out of solution if other conditions for diamond formation are met. Yttrium has similar behaviour to Ti. Another application is described in the work of Zhang *et al.* (2008), in which synthesis of a single crystal diamond is presented using diamond seed particles electroplated with nickel film as a catalyst for the HPHT method. Moreover, Ni, Co and Y are commonly used as catalysts for the growth of carbon nanotubes (Kang *et al.*, 2008; Hsieh *et al.*, 2009).

We showed (Varga *et al.*, 2011) that use of Ni, Co and Y metal powders also results in an enhanced nucleation density, and these metal powders are the optimal solution for ultrasonic seeding. After 10 min growth, the nucleation is visible (Fig. 9.20). The best results were obtained using the nanodiamond powder solution with Ni particles. However, after 1 h of growth, more flat diamond layers were reached after nucleation in solutions containing Co and Y particles (Fig. 9.21). In this case, the homogeneous nucleation process and low growth rate resulted in a flatter diamond layer, but with low thicknesses.

Figure 9.22 shows Raman spectra of the deposited diamond layers after 10 min (Fig. 9.22(a)) and 1 h (Fig. 9.22(b)) of growth. After 10 min deposition there are two dominant bands, the wide G–band with sp^2 graphitic phases and the second order peak of Si, which is obvious as it is a thin, non-continuous layer. After a long

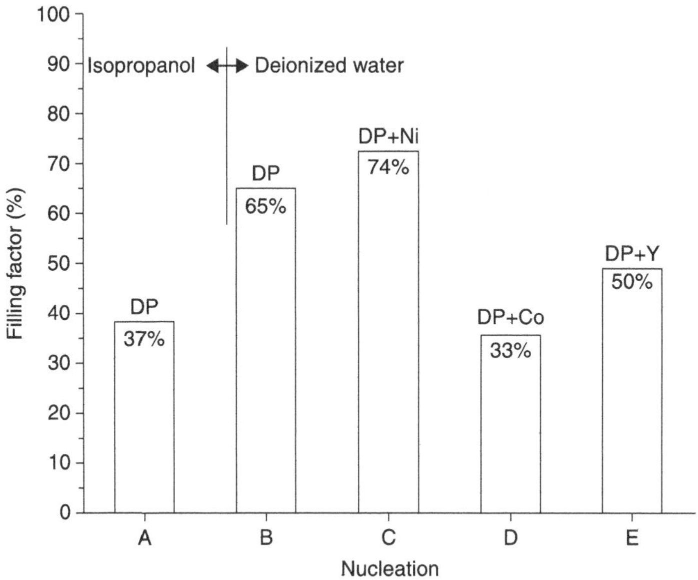

9.20 Histogram of percentual coverage of surface with diamond seeds after 10 min growth. Filling factor is defined as (covered area)/(covered area+not covered area). For definitions of samples A–E see Table 9.2.

period of deposition, the Raman spectra of each sample indicates high-quality diamond film (Fig. 9.22(b)). The ratio of diamond peak and G–band to the second order peak of Si substrate became higher because the diamond layers became thicker and continuous. When we compare the Raman spectra of samples prepared by different nucleation solutions, we can say that the highest quality of diamond was obtained with solution A and D, where the diamond peak is dominated on the G–band. However, in the case of the sample A, larger diamond grain size affects the Raman measurements, but this layer was not fully closed.

We can also conclude that ultrasonic abrasion with powder slurries increases the surface roughness due to the formation of nanoscale scratches (Varga *et al.*, 2011). The role of metal particles such as Ni, Co, Y is under discussion, yet it is

Table 9.2 Composition of the solutions used in the nucleation process

Solution	Powder	Particle size	Liquid
A	200 mg DP	≤10 nm	20 mL isopropyl alcohol + 5 mL DI water
B	200 mg DP	≤10 nm	25 mL DI water
C	200 mg DP + 200 mg Ni	Ni: ≤100 nm	25 mL DI water
D	200 mg DP + 200 mg Co	Co: <1.6 μm	50 mL DI water
E	200 mg DP +250 mg Y	Y: <44 μm	50 mL DI water

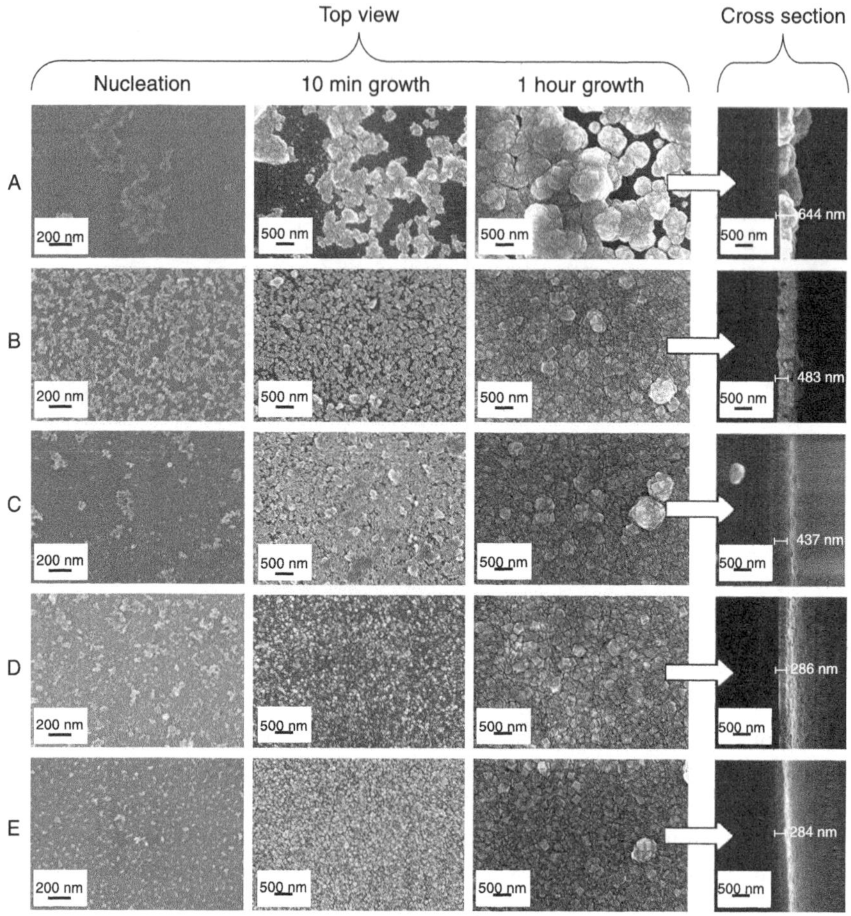

9.21 SEM images of prepared samples nucleated by ultrasonic seeding using different solutions, after 10 min and 1 h of diamond growth in a MW CVD reactor. For definitions of samples A–E see Table 9.2.

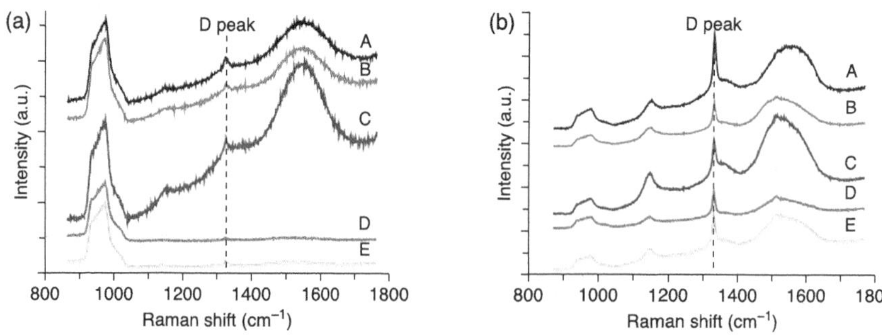

9.22 Raman spectra of diamond films deposited 10 min (a) and 1 h (b) after nucleation in various liquids. For definitions of samples A–E see Table 9.2.

obvious that they can influence the early stage of the diamond growth process as well. In summary, the combination of nano-sized diamond powder with micro-sized metal powders positively influences the nucleation and takes effect on diamond film growth.

9.6 Seeding using a polymer composite

An alternative route for diamond growth on non-diamond surfaces is the use of a polymer composite with UDD powder. This method is advantageous in cases where the treatment of mechanically soft and/or unstable substrates (polymers, ultra thin metals, etc.) is required. The dip technique (Ray *et al.*, 2003) has been tried as a soft seeding procedure for growing compact diamond films over large areas.

The earliest studies by Sun *et al.* (Sun *et al.*, 1997a, 1997b) showed that under heat treatment the polymer (phenylcarbyne) is converted into glassy carbon and under plasma treatment crystalline diamond can be grown. A two step mechanism was suggested with polymer decomposition followed by solid phase transition with atomic hydrogen playing an important role. Other studies have shown that using a polymer and/or spin-coated polymer on polished mirror or on scratched silicon substrates enhances the nucleation density (Wang *et al.*, 1997; Jingsheng *et al.*, 1999). The growth of isolated diamond crystals in sizes ranging from nanometres up to micrometres was presented. Applying other polymers as precursors did not, however, result in diamond growth at low substrate temperatures.

The polymer layer can be used as the functional surface for the electrostatic grafting of diamond nanoparticles onto 3D structures (Girard *et al.*, 2012). Diamond nanoparticles are spontaneously grafted onto the substrate surface via an ultrathin layer of polyelectrolyte (close to 3 nm). The principle of this method is based on electrostatic interactions between oxygen-terminated nanodiamond powder in colloidal solution with the coated substrate. It was proposed that the ultrathin polymer is immediately removed during the first seconds of the CVD diamond growth. A similar approach was reported for electrostatic grafting of hydrogen-annealed nanodiamonds onto silicon substrates (Hees *et al.*, 2011).

In our recent studies we focused on polymer composites, in which the neat polymer is mixed with UDD powders. Transfer of the composite polymer to the substrate can be achieved for instance by spin-coating of a thin film (Kromka *et al.*, 2009b, 2009c) or by electrospun nanofibrous textile (Potocký *et al.*, 2013). A slightly different method using separated components is the sequential deposition of polymer, UDD particles and polymer (Babchenko *et al.*, 2010). In all our experiments we have used the same type of UDD. Fig. 9.23 shows an overview of various pretreatment methods utilizing polymer composites. Each of these methods and results is presented and discussed in detail in the following sections.

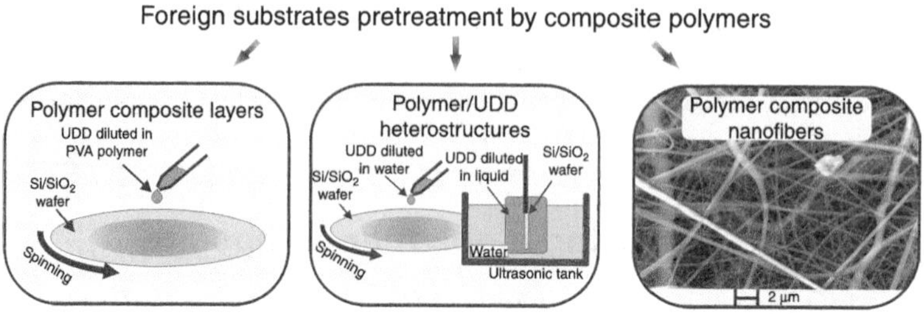

9.23 Various pretreatment methods utilizing polymer composites.

9.6.1 Polymer composite layers

Common silicon samples were used as substrates and cleaned using our standard methods (Kromka *et al.*, 2008b). They were then spin-coated with a polymer composite (4 wt% of polyvinyl alcohol (PVA) dissolved in 1 mL of deionized water and then 6.7 wt% of water solution containing UDD added to the PVA solution in 1:1 proportion), which was used as the seeding layer. The CVD deposition was performed in a microwave plasma-enhanced CVD reactor (Kromka *et al.*, 2008b) using standard process parameters: total gas pressure 30 mbar, 1% of methane diluted in hydrogen and two different substrate temperatures 430°C (growth time 20 h) and 830°C (growth time 2 h). The NCD film deposited at 430°C in the thickness of 370 nm was continuous without voids or openings. Randomly oriented and well-faceted diamond nanocrystals in sizes up to 200 nm were observed (see Fig. 9.24(a)). In addition, we observed that the diamond film surface coverage decreased when a thick polymer film was used as an interlayer (Kromka *et al.*, 2009c). In this case, small openings sized at approximately 200 nm were observed.

A different film quality was observed for the growth temperature of 830°C. In this case, a higher density of openings and crystal defects was observed (Fig. 9.24(b)). Moreover, the density and size of these openings increased significantly for films with the polymer interlayer.

The Raman spectra of the NCD films deposited at both temperatures exhibited one sharp diamond peak and two broad D- and G-bands (Kromka *et al.*, 2009b). The height of the films was around 200 nm for both temperatures.

It should be noted that using a Si substrate coated by a virgin flat PVA polymer without a seeding composite did not result in the growth of an NCD film. Thus, the diamond growth is clearly initialized due to the presence of fine-grained diamond powder in the PVA polymer composite as the morphology of the composite layer (thin film) does not enhance nucleation density.

In the previous paragraphs we described the process in which a thin NCD film was grown on a flat surface using a polymer composite nucleation layer. For further processing of the diamond film (e.g. structuring, fabrication of electronic devices) the use of a top-down lithography processes is typically necessary.

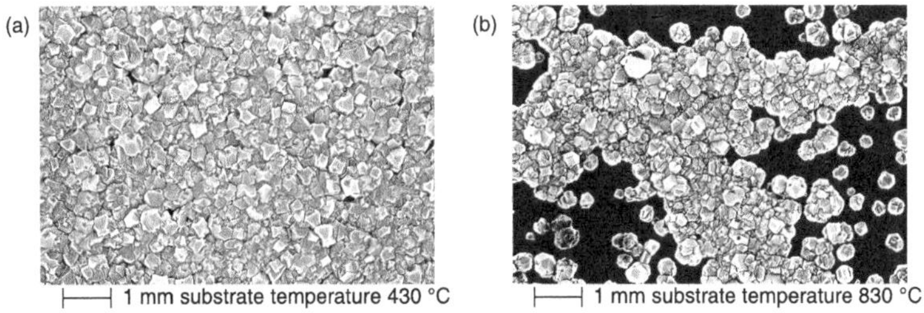

9.24 Surface morphology of NCD films grown at (a) low and (b) high substrate temperature with 600 nm thick PVA interlayer.

One can also manipulate the seeding process to directly grow three-dimensional NCD structures (layers, porous-like structures or self-assembled air bridges) using polymer composites. For these experiments, the same silicon samples protected by a SiO_2 layer were used as substrates and cleaned by our standard methods (Kromka *et al.*, 2009b). Then, they were spin-coated with an OFPR photoresist (Dynachem Ltd.), which was dried and photolithographically treated to realize linear stripes 30 μm in width, 1.5 μm in height and at a distance of 30 μm stripe-to-stripe. This polymer was labelled as the 'primary polymer'. The Si/SiO_2 substrates covered with the primary polymer stripes were seeded in four different ways. The sample labelled as 'low UDD' was spin-coated with the polymer suspension consisting of mixed PVA (4 wt.%) with UDD (6.7 wt.%) in ratio 1:1. Sample labelled as 'high UDD' was spin-coated with composite PVA (2.5 wt.%) and UDD (6.7 wt.%). Afterwards, standard CVD growth occurred in a microwave plasma CVD chamber.

Low temperature growth (410°C) – the CVD growth at low temperature, the sample seeded with low UDD concentration shows two different regions (Fig. 9.25). The first region exhibits a formation of fully closed diamond film (the region on the primary polymer stripe) and the second one which shows openings in the film (the region between the primary polymer stripes). In both regions, crystals in size of approximately 200 nm are observed. The height of the formed stripes was 130 nm as measured by AFM.

Increased UDD concentration in the seeding polymer resulted in a fully closed and hierarchically structured NCD film (Fig. 9.26). The region on a primary polymer stripe reveals a three-dimensional structure. Moreover, the final film structure is more complex. It consists of a fine-grained fully closed layer as the background, which is decorated by isolated grains growing on top. The size of isolated grains is up to 200 nm. The fine-grained layer replicates the morphology of the starting substrate character. The height of stripes is 300 nm.

High temperature growth (850°C) – the CVD growth at high substrate temperature differs from the growth at low temperature (Kromka *et al.*, 2009b). First, broadening of the primary polymer stripes and loss of the 3D geometry was observed for high temperature growth. Second, the grown layer was almost

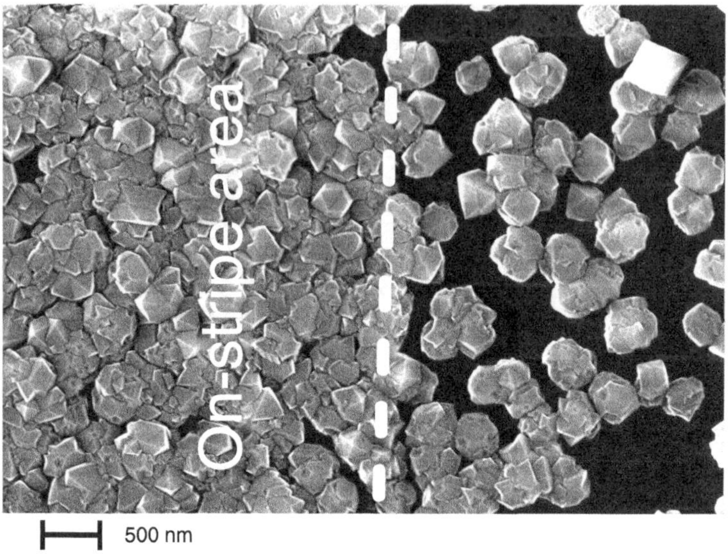

9.25 SEM morphology of 'low UDD' seeded sample after growth.

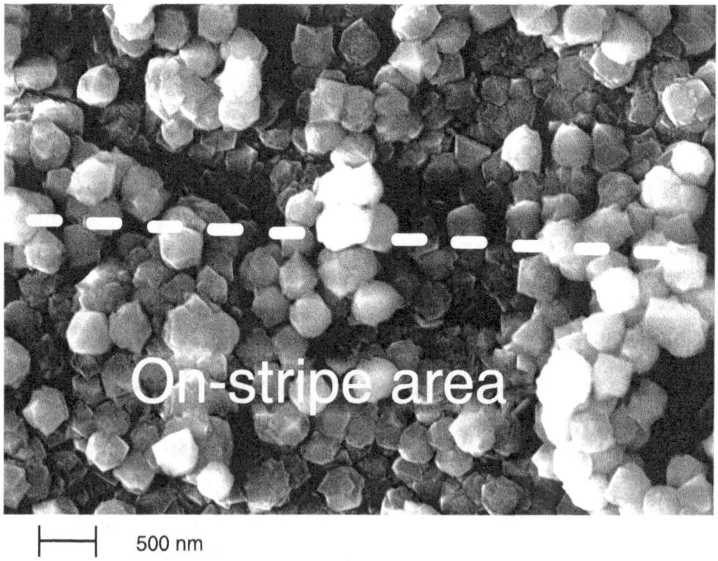

9.26 SEM morphology of 'high UDD' seeded sample after growth.

compact and fully closed, except of linear gaps (1 μm in width) formed in a repeating array. Third, formation of the fine-grained film with isolated grains sitting on top was not observed. As the nucleation was done by the 'UDD drop technique', some areas exhibited a three-dimensional growth and a self-standing

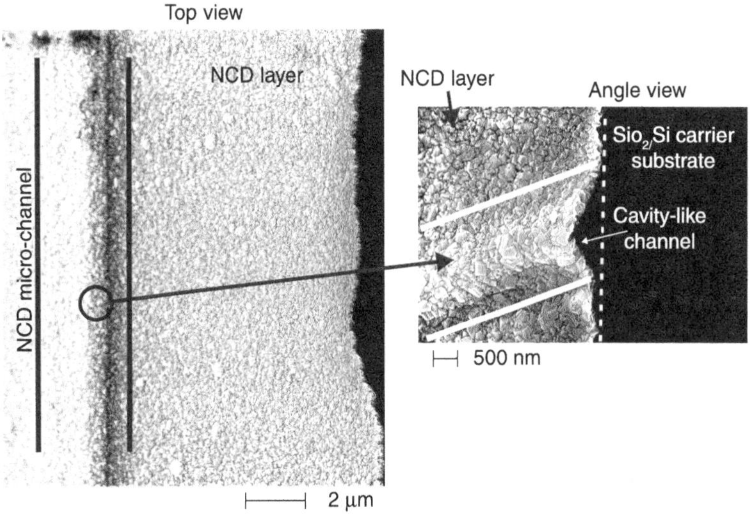

9.27 Top and cross-sectional views (angle 30°) of continuous NCD film formed in a cavity-like channel.

cavity-like channel is observed (Fig. 9.27) (Kromka *et al.*, 2009b). The cavity is about 600 nm in width and up to 400 nm in height.

These results confirm that 3D growth of diamond structures implementing the primary polymer is an interesting feature. We observed that the highest 3D structuring was achieved for sample seeded by the 'UDD drop technique', that is a liquid drop of UDD (6.7 wt.%) was spin-coated on the substrate. On the other hand, samples nucleated by ultrasonic seeding (the treatment described in previous chapters) exhibited the highest damage of the primary polymer edges due to the mechanical abrasion of polymer by diamond nanoparticles, while formation of combined 3D shapes exhibiting a porous-like structure was observed.

A common feature of high temperature growths was almost complete loss of the primary polymer pattern. We propose that in high temperature processes the primary polymer is etched away very fast and thus plays a minor role for the NCD growth.

9.6.2 Polymer/ultra-dispersed diamond (UDD) heterostructures

Diamond structuring is an important technological issue. The chemical inertness and mechanical hardness of a diamond make conventional structuring methods challenging, time consuming and thus less favourable. The direct growth of diamond structures combined with polymer transformation therefore represents a promising alternative solution. This direct growth, also known as selective area deposition (SAD), is generally achieved by applying the treatment of a seeding (i.e. nucleation) layer before the diamond growth (Fu *et al.*, 2003; Bongrain *et al.*,

2009). The SAD growth of diamond structures has been achieved using several treatment techniques such as the removal of the diamond nuclei (seeds) from defined areas (Hirabayashi *et al.*, 1988; Liu *et al.*, 2002), bias enhanced diamond nucleation process on pre-defined areas (Chen *et al.*, 1997; Sakamoto *et al.*, 1998), the direct 'printing' of diamond seeds onto the selected area by ink-jet printing (Fox *et al.*, 2000) or wet chemical etching of SiO_2 on selected areas by buffer oxide etchant (Kromka *et al.*, 2009d).

Common limitations of the above mentioned treatments are either aggressive wet chemistries or the need for a specific type of substrate material. A technological approach suitable for SAD growth with minimal damage to the substrate surface utilizing polymer/UDD/polymer structures has been shown as the optimal treatment technique for patterned diamond growth.

To study thin polymer/UDD heterostructures, we first tested the efficiency of removing diamond seeds using reactive ion etching through a photolithographic mask (Babchenko *et al.*, 2010). Ultrasonically seeded substrates were photolithographically processed using an OFPR polymer. Polymer structures with stripes and gaps 100 μm wide were prepared using the photolithography process. A dry etching process using CF_4/O_2 RF plasma was then used to remove seeds from the areas not protected by the polymer. The density of 'parasitic' (residual) diamond crystals on the unwashed area was up to 8×10^6 cm^{-2}, which may not provide a high enough selectivity. The main disadvantage of this strategy is the low resistance of the used polymer to the plasma treatment and thus the lower efficiency in removing the diamond seeds from the photolithographically defined regions.

Higher selectivity was achieved by implementing two OFPR layers, that is Si/SiO_2 wafers which were first covered by OFPR polymer seeded with diamond nanoparticles by ultrasound agitation, and packed by a second OFPR layer. Such polymer/UDD/polymer sandwich films exhibited nicely patterned structures after optical lithography. The detected density of the parasitic crystals was, however, as high as 5×10^7 cm^{-2}. This was attributed to UDD sedimentation on the wafer after polymer dissolution. From a technological point of view we observed that turning the sample upside down in a solvent partially decreased the density of remaining diamond seeds.

We continued our efforts by combining the first technique (i.e. removing the seed by RIE) and the second one (i.e. polymer/UDD/polymer films). The result was that the density of residual diamond crystals decreased to values as low as 10^5 cm^{-2}. Such a combination makes the process more complex as it employs two gentle treatments. The main advantage of this technique is its suitability for mechanically and chemically sensitive substrates (plastic substrates, ultrathin metal films, etc.).

It should be noted that all tested strategies resulted in the direct growth of diamond structures as confirmed by Raman and SEM measurements. The obtained results clearly confirmed that the main differences in achieving a high enough selective area deposition lie in the proper patterning of the seeding layer and its processing before the CVD growth. It should be also noted that the SAD growth proceeds in a 3D way, that is both upwards and laterally from the seeding patterns (Babchenko *et al.*, 2012).

9.6.3 Polymer composite nanofibres

Successful use of polymer composites opened the way for the use of organic nanofibres for diamond growth. Electrostatic spinning (ES) is a useful method of producing non-woven layers of submicron fibres (Li and Xia, 2004). Common ES techniques based on the use of a syringe (Li and Xia, 2004) produce nanofibre layers in low quantities. Needle-less electrospinning (Jirsak, 2005) allows the industrial-scale production of nanofibres with high productivity, scalability and quality of nanofibres. This is a versatile method for the production of thin fibres (diameter of 50 nm and more) from polymer solutions. The feasibility of using nanodiamond–polymer composite fibres manufactured by standard ES methods for diamond growth was shown by Behler *et al.* where fusing around 200°C was used for production of film coatings with high diamond content (Behler *et al.*, 2009).

In our case, the solutions of PVA and UDD were electrospun using a roller electrospinner on a polypropylene spunbond supporting web with an areal weight of 18 g/m^2. The average nanofibre diameter was 100 nm. The weight concentration of UDD in the PVA solution was prepared at five equally distributed concentrations between 0.001725 wt.% up to 0.023 wt.%. The concentration of PVA was 14 wt.%.

Silicon samples were used as substrates and cleaned by our standard methods. After removing the spunbond supporting web the composite nanofibre textiles were transferred onto Si substrates. CVD deposition was then performed in a microwave plasma-enhanced CVD reactor using the standard process parameters of a total power of 2500 W, total gas pressure 50 mbar, 1% of CH_4 diluted in H_2, the substrate temperature $T_s \approx 820°C$ and deposition time $t = 1$ h.

The surface morphology of diamond fibres grown on Si substrates patterned by the primary polymer structure is shown in Fig. 9.28. This SEM image shows growth using the polymer composite nanofibres with the highest concentration of UDD (i.e. 0.023 wt.%). Decreasing the concentration of UDD in the polymer matrix resulted in a shortening of the diamond fibres and lower density of the grown diamond web structure. This is due to the UDD particles which play a dominant role as seeds for diamond growth concentrated within the polymer fibres. Nevertheless, the effect of complex 3D geometry is pronounced. The highly curved surface of the polymer fibres generates a capillary pressure difference across the interface given by the Young–Laplace equation (Chen *et al.*, 2006). Assuming surface tension in the order of 10^{-1} J/m^2 and fibre radius of approximately 50 nm, the pressure difference is 10^6 Pa. We propose that, because of this effect, nucleation along the fibres with even the lowest concentration of UDD is preferred against spontaneous nucleation on a clean Si surface.

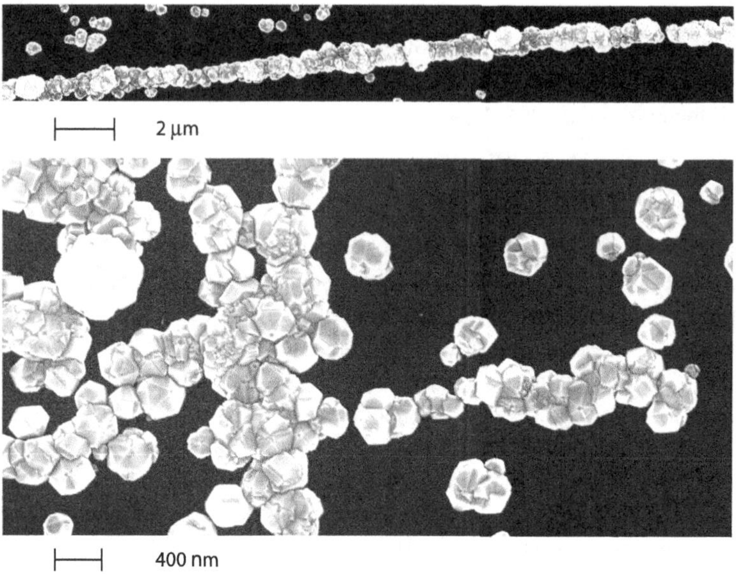

9.28 SEM morphology of the structures grown at the highest concentration of UDD nanoparticles in polymer matrix.

A diamond layer on a polymer composite nanofibre structure was also created in which the surface morphology was patterned by the fingerprint on the primary polymer. Surface coverage after 1 h growth of NCD film was higher than 90%. The tendency to form a diamond film decreased with the decreasing concentration of UDD in the polymer matrix as a result of the decreasing influence of the diamond seeds against the surface tension effect for the nucleation mechanism of diamond grain growth. The average diameter of crystals in all experiments was approximately 250 nm. The decrease in concentration of UDD in the polymer matrix results in a decreasing nucleation density from 1.2×10^{9} cm^{-2} down to 1.9×10^{8} cm^{-2}. The lowest nucleation density was achieved for only 0.001725 wt.% of UDD in the polymer matrix, which is a value three to four orders of magnitude higher than that achieved using spontaneous nucleation (Yang and Je, 1996; Prelas *et al.*, 1998). We suppose that such a high value is not only caused by the UDD seeds, but also by the complex 3D structure. A representative Raman measurement exhibited a dominant diamond peak of the formed fibrous layer and two broad D- and G-bands.

9.6.4 Fundamental processes during the early stages of chemical vapour deposition (CVD) growth

CVD growth from a polymer composite is a complex process. Previously it was shown that some fragments of a polymer can play an important role in CVD growth

(Jingsheng *et al.*, 1999). Direct polymer transformations into carbon materials were achieved without addition of UDD particles to polymer. In these studies, a complex composition of carbon materials containing, among others, nanodiamond crystals can be found both with (Sedov *et al.*, 2012) and without (Nur *et al.*, 2012) further growth by plasma process. The sequence of carbon reactions can be initialized to transform a limited number of carbon atoms into the sp^3-bonded form, which are then further stabilized by atomic hydrogen coming from plasma. The growth of continuous diamond films can be achieved only on the substrates where the nucleation or seeding densities are initially high enough. Using a polymer layer, the seeding density was enhanced up to as much as 10^{11} cm^{-2} (Jingsheng *et al.*, 1999). The increased nucleation density was assigned to the sp^3-bonded carbon coming from the polymer and to the local transport of carbon from polymer to diamond particles. They suggested that sp^3-bonded carbon with dangling bonds could be formed during CVD growth at certain temperatures (Sun *et al.*, 1996). It was proposed that atomic hydrogen coming from plasma plays an important role in stabilizing the dangling bonds of the sp^3-bonded amorphous carbon matrix and that this matrix can be converted to the crystalline diamond phase. It is notable that the presence of atomic hydrogen is not always a crucial issue. Bianconi *et al.* have shown that using a thermal treatment without the presence of atomic hydrogen can convert polymer into a sp^3-bonded carbon matrix, or even into diamond crystals (Sun *et al.*, 1997c; Bianconi *et al.*, 2004).

In our studies, where the patterned primary polymer stripes were used, we propose that the primary polymer acted as the carbon source and enhanced the diamond nucleation leading to homogenous CVD growth. In our experiments, the PVA polymer played a dominant role as the carrier for spin-coating of the diamond powder on flat substrates and allowed a good dispersion of UDD. Using low temperature deposition and a low amount of PVA resulted in the optimal process conditions for a homogenous NCD growth. The fully closed layer was found only over the primary polymer stripes. This bears a resemblance to the NNP process (see works by Rotter, 1999 and Sumant *et al.*, 2007), where the formation of an amorphous-carbon (a-C) layer before the CVD diamond growth was a crucial issue. Furthermore, the diamond layer formed on the polymer exhibited a tendency towards the growth of 3D-like structures. In such cases, equilibrium between the CVD growth and consumption and/or etching of the primary polymer stripes in plasma can be optimized to achieve the growth of self-standing cavities.

In addition, using a polymer layer seems to be effective for the SAD of diamond structures. Combining standard optical lithography with dry plasma etching (CF_4/O_2) of *photoresist-seeding layer-photoresist* multilayers resulted in a high degree of SAD selectivity with a residual density as low as spontaneous nucleation (~10^5 cm^{-2}). The main advantages of using a *multilayer* structure are its efficiency, simplicity and the minimal damage to the substrate surface.

Finally, novel nanofibre–UDD composites offer a new way of seeding three-dimensional, mechanically unstable and large area substrates. The diamond growth was primarily initialized via UDD particles. Yet we assume that the highly curved surfaces of nanofibres help to overcome the energy barrier required for diamond nucleation. This technique represents a bottom-up strategy for nanocrystalline diamond growth of complex shapes, or even porous films.

9.7 Spontaneous nucleation

As previously mentioned, the most commonly used nucleation techniques are bias enhanced nucleation, ultrasonic seeding with diamond powder and transformation of polymers into diamond films, but we have yet to cover finding optimized process conditions for diamond growth on substrates without any pretreatment. This condition can be classified as spontaneous or self-nucleation process.

Spontaneous nucleation is a very slow process in comparison with other nucleation methods. But it can offer a fundamental insight into a better understanding of diamond nucleation. It can also potentially find applications such as the overcoating of substrates with complex geometries.

Let us briefly summarize process conditions that can enhance the diamond nucleation. Figure 9.29 schematically shows possible ways for enhancing the formation of diamond nuclei in the spontaneous nucleation processes. The main requirement is achieving not only high nucleation densities, but also reproducibility and homogeneity over large areas.

For this study, we used two different plasma systems: focused microwave plasma with ellipsoidal cavity (Kromka *et al.*, 2008b) and pulsed linear-antenna

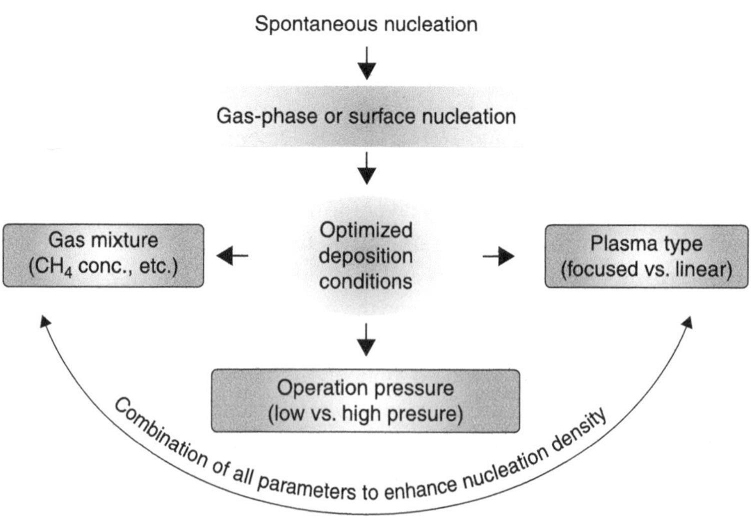

9.29 Schematic diagram of process conditions influencing spontaneous nucleation of diamond (self-nucleation).

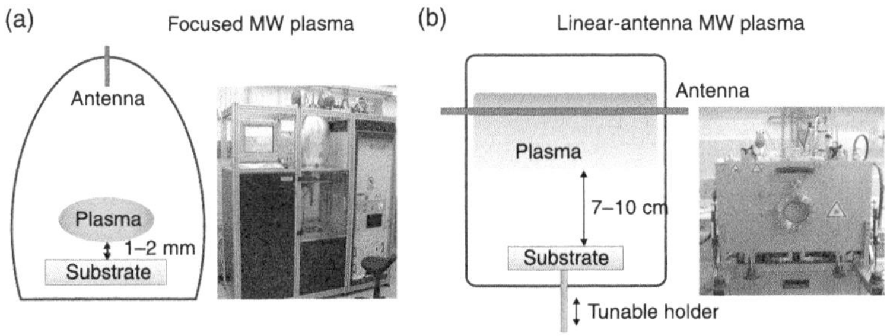

9.30 Schematic view of chemical vapour deposition systems in focused (a) and pulsed linear-antenna (b) microwave arrangement.

microwave plasma (Fig. 9.30). The experiments were conducted on silicon substrates. Focused plasma represents the standard ball-type system, where plasma is localized closely to the substrate surface at a distance of 1–2 mm. In the employed focused plasma system, stable plasma is ignited in the pressure range 20–200 mbar. Because of the high pressure, the substrate is heated by hot plasma which limits the lowest possible temperature of the process. The substrate temperature varies between 370°C and 1100°C, and the deposition diameter is limited to 5–7 cm.

Linear-antenna plasma represents a complementary system to focused plasma. Microwave plasma is ignited at a low pressure range (0.01–10 mbar) and the substrate is localized at a larger distance (7–10 cm) from the hottest plasma region (Kromka *et al.*, 2012). Thus, the substrate is not directly heated by plasma and its temperature can be as low as 100°C (Tsugawa *et al.*, 2010).

An additional advantage of this system is plasma stability with much broader range of gas mixtures, for example methane concentration >20% in hydrogen-rich plasma.

9.7.1 Influence of CH_4 in focused plasma

It is well known that increasing CH_4 concentration in CH_4/H_2 gas mixture results in an increased amount of sp^2 carbon phases during the diamond CVD growth. As previously discussed, a higher amount of sp^2 phases also can be energetically favourable for enhancing secondary re-nucleation in some cases, for example it can enhance spontaneous nucleation on non-treated substrates. The study was carried out for methane concentration from 0.5% to 10% in an H_2 atmosphere in standard growth conditions (i.e. a microwave power of 2500 W, a total gas pressure of 50 mbar, a temperature of 700°C and a growth time of 1 h). We observed that an increase in CH_4 increased the nucleation density from 10^6 cm^{-2} (0.5% CH_4) to 10^8 cm^{-2} (10% CH_4). This is partially caused by a lower concentration of hydrogen atoms, that is by the less efficient etching of sp^2 carbon phases being formed during the growth process. In addition, supersaturation due to the high level of methane leads to the formation of an amorphous carbon interlayer used as a diamond nucleation promoter (Mitsuda *et al.*, 1993, Feng *et al.*, 1996). SEM images of samples using the focused plasma CVD process at 0.5% and 10% are shown in Fig. 9.31(a,b).

9.7.2 Influence of plasma type

Figure 9.31(c,d) shows the surface morphology of samples grown using two different systems. A direct comparison of these systems is difficult, however, as a result of fundamental plasma principles (standing versus surface wave plasma). To minimize this limitation, we used standard deposition conditions of high-quality microcrystalline diamond characteristic for each system. Growth conditions in a focused plasma system were as follows: microwave power of 2500 W, total gas pressure of 50 mbar, temperature of ~700°C, process time 1 h and gas composition 1% of CH_4 in H_2. The experiment for linear-antenna plasma was completed under the following process conditions: pulsed microwave power of 2×2500 W, total gas pressure 0.2 mbar, temperature of ~700°C and process time 15 h. The distance of the substrate from the antennas was 8 cm and the gas composition was set to 2.5% of CH_4 in H_2. P-type Si wafers were used as substrates.

The sample deposited by the focused plasma revealed small diamond clusters (40–80 nm) and their density was slightly higher than 10^6 cm^{-2} (Fig. 9.31(c)). This

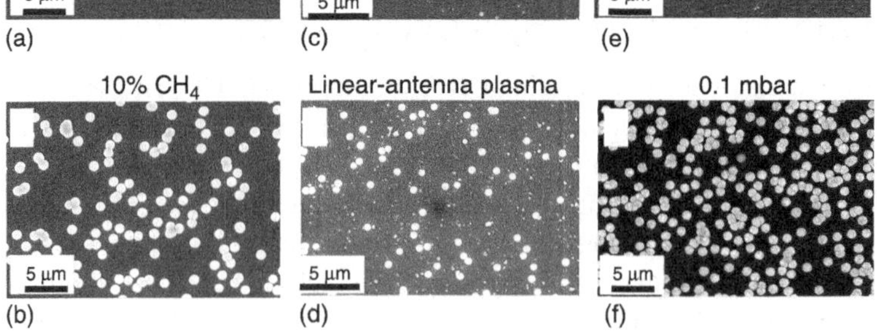

9.31 SEM images of samples deposited at different process conditions. (a,b) samples grown by focused plasma at 0.5% and 10% methane. (c,d) Samples grown by focused and linear-antenna plasma. (e,f) Samples grown by linear-antenna plasma at 2 and 0.1 mbar. Silicon substrates were wet-cleaned and no pretreatment method was applied.

corresponded well with previous results, where a higher spontaneous nucleation was achieved for a higher methane concentration. Similar process conditions with respect to methane concentration and substrate temperature resulted in a higher spontaneous nucleation density of 2×10^7 cm^{-2} achieved by linear-antenna plasma (Fig. 9.31(d)). Moreover, this sample consisted of small diamond crystals ($\phi\approx100$ nm) and large clustered features ($\phi\approx500$ nm). We attribute this to a time-dependent re-nucleation process. In the re-nucleation process small diamond clusters were formed on the substrate during the deposition. Some of these clusters are etched by plasma or spontaneously decomposed. Some clusters are stable and increase their size with deposition time.

The lower density for spontaneous nucleation in focused plasma is attributed to a more aggressive etching of carbon/diamond species by atomic hydrogen as a result of 1) the closer distance to the substrate; and 2) the higher concentration of atomic hydrogen. Also, it should be mentioned that both types of plasma differ in electron temperature, which can be as high as 10 eV in the focused plasma or lower than 3 eV in the linear-antenna plasma (Tsugawa *et al.*, 2011, Sugai *et al.*, 2000). Tsugawa *et al.* proposed that the gas-phase nucleation is a key process in the linear-antenna plasma (Tsugawa *et al.*, 2011).

9.7.3 Influence of pressure, CH_4 and CO_2 in linear-antenna plasma

Our previous studies have shown that diamond crystallographic character is strongly influenced by the total pressure (Kromka *et al.*, 2012). Based on these results we also investigated the influence of pressure on spontaneous nucleation. Except for pressure, experimental conditions were kept the same as in the previous experiments. SEM images of the samples grown by linear-antenna plasma at 2 and 0.1 mbar are shown in Fig. 9.31(e,f). At a pressure of 2 mbar, very small (<100 nm) diamond clusters are observed and their density is ~10^7 cm^{-2}. Lowering the pressure down to 0.1 mbar increases the nucleation density to 10^8 cm^{-2}. We also carried out an experiment at even lower pressure of 0.07 mbar, but the plasma was not stable and only a few large diamond clusters were observed (SEM images not showed here). We proposed that the effect of pressure on the diamond's spontaneous nucleation and growth can be explained by a change in the plasma density and distribution in the deposition chamber. In other words, lower pressure results in an increased mean free path and therefore enlarges the plasma volume close to the substrate.

Complementary to the focused plasma, we also investigated the influence of gas composition on spontaneous nucleation, particularly the effect of CO_2 and CH_4 concentration. We found that *oxygen-rich gas chemistry* (i.e. the addition of CO_2 to CH_4/H_2) resulted in the preferential etching of small clusters and only larger diamond clusters were detected. Even a small amount of CO_2 (5%) inhibited the formation of smaller diamond clusters. This can be explained by an etching effect of oxygen to unstable carbon species. The nucleation densities achieved in the oxygen-rich gas mixture were in the range of 10^7–10^8 cm^{-2}.

The influence of methane concentration was studied too. Samples grown by linear-antenna plasma from the gas mixture of 5% of CH_4 and 10% of CO_2 diluted in hydrogen exhibited the highest nucleation density of ~10^9 cm^{-2}. Work is in progress to identify the main origin of this observation.

The re-nucleation process is important for nanocrystalline- or ultrananocrystalline diamond film formation with very low surface roughness. The experiments on spontaneous nucleation indicated promising ways to define the balance between diamond growth and the re-nucleation regime and thus, methods for controlling grain size or even multilayered diamond growth (nano- and micro-sized stack layers).

9.8 Biological and tissue engineering applications

In the previous sections we have explored the varied methods for controlling nucleation and the growth of diverse diamond films and nanostructures. In combination with the unique properties of the diamond (Nebel *et al.*, 2007) such as the control of surface atoms or the stable grafting of organic molecules, this is an extremely useful feature for a range of applications, in particular for bio-sensor, prosthetics and tissue engineering.

The interaction of cells with as-grown and nanostructured diamond surfaces indicates that the diamond surface morphology can be tailored in a controlled way with respect to bio-technological and bio-medical requirements. A wide range of diamond surface morphologies have been found which are acceptable for cell growth. This corresponds with experiments on diamond films in which hierarchically modified substrate roughness was employed (Kalbacova *et al.*, 2009). The results showed an enhanced osteoblast adhesion as well as an increased differentiation (raised alkaline phosphatase activity and mineral deposition) on NCD surfaces (most significantly on RMS 20 nm) compared with tissue culture polystyrene. This is attributed mainly to the specific surface topography as well as to the biocompatible properties of the diamond. The controlled (topographically structured) diamond coating of various substrates may therefore offer a faster colonization by specific cells as well as longer-term stability. Nanostructured diamond surfaces can also modify the adhesion of human osteoblast-like cells (Babchenko *et al.*, 2009). Osteoblasts cultivated on relatively short and broad nano-cones form well pronounced, large focal adhesions with intensive vinculin staining indicating a larger surface available for adhesion and thus stronger adhesion contacts between the cell and the diamond. On the other hand, cells cultivated on relatively high and thin nanorods form very thin and fine focal adhesions indicating weaker adhesion.

Similarly, patterning of the nucleation layer prior to the diamond growth is a powerful procedure for fabricating three-dimensional nanocrystalline diamond microstructures that are of electronic-grade quality. They exhibit nanocrystalline morphology and yet have good electronic quality in terms of a clear transistor characteristics for field-effect transistor configurations employing the surface conductivity of the hydrogen-terminated diamond (Kozak *et al.*, 2010). As solution-gated field effect transistors (FETs) they also exhibit sensitivity to pH of electrolyte solution as well as to protein adsorption. They can therefore be employed in electrochemical and (bio) electronic applications. Compared with the common diamond post-growth patterning, for example by the dry etching process, this procedure is simple, inexpensive and fully compatible with the semiconductor industry.

When we compared hydrogen- and oxygen-terminated microstructures, cells preferably self-assembled on the oxygen-terminated surface regions (Rezek *et al.*, 2009). The growth of cells over the hydrogen-terminated areas, mostly at high cell concentrations, is presumably enabled by their linkage to the O-diamond layers because individual cells exhibit poor adhesion to H-diamond and reduced metabolic activity (Kalbacova *et al.*, 2008).

The described technologies, results and conclusions are significant and offer promising prospective applications for diamonds in biosensors, bioelectronics, microelectronics and other fields.

9.9 Acknowledgements

In the Czech Republic, this work was supported by the Academy of Sciences of the Czech Republic by J. E. Purkyne Fellowship, and by the P08/12/G108 grant (GACR Excellence Centre).

We would like to gratefully appreciate Karel Hruska and Jitka Libertinova for SEM, Josef Zemek for XPS, Cestmir Konak for DLS and Zdenek Remes for optical measurements, Milan Vanecek for valuable discussions, Jiri Potmesil and Ondrej Rezek for technical assistance and Zdenka Polackova for chemical treatments.

The HF CVD experiments were performed at the Department of Microelectronics, Faculty of EE & IT, Slovak University of Technology (FEI STU), Bratislava, the Slovak Republic. We would like to acknowledge the kind assistances of Miroslav Michalka and Alexander Satka for SEM measurements, Ivan Cerven for XRD measurements, Jan Janik, Viera Dubravcova, Marian Vesely and Stefan Bederka for valuable discussions, Tibor Danis and Frantisek Balon for BEN experiments and Jozef Kral for technical assistance.

There were also small contributions from undergraduate and PhD. students.

This work was carried out in the frame of the LNSM infrastructure.

9.10 References

Arnault, J., 2003. Highly oriented diamond films on heterosubstrates: Current state of the art and remaining challenges. *Surf. Rev. Lett.* 10, 127–146.

Avrami, M., 1939. Kinetics of Phase Change. I General Theory. *Journal of Chemical Physics* 7, 1103.

Babchenko, O., Izak, T., Ukraintsev, E., *et al.*, 2010. Toward surface-friendly treatment of seeding layer and selected-area diamond growth. *Physica Status Solidi (b)* 247, 3026–3029.

Babchenko, O., Kromka, A., Hruska, K., *et al.*, 2009. Fabrication of nano-structured diamond films for SAOS-2 cell cultivation. *Physica Status Solidi (a)* 206, 2033–2037.

Babchenko, O., Remes, Z., Izak, T., *et al.*, 2011. Deposition of nanocrystalline diamond films on temperature sensitive substrates for infrared reflectance spectroscopy. *Physica Status Solidi (b)* 248, 2736–2739.

Babchenko, O., Verveniotis, E., Hruska, K., *et al.*, 2012. Direct growth of sub-micron diamond structures. *Vacuum* 86, 693–695.

Behler, K.D., Stravato, A., Mochalin, V., *et al.*, 2009. Nanodiamond-Polymer Composite Fibers and Coatings. *ACS Nano* 3, 363–369.

Bianconi, P.A., Joray, S.J., Aldrich, B.L., *et al.*, 2004. Diamond and Diamond-Like Carbon from a Preceramic Polymer. *Journal of the American Chemical Society* 126, 3191–3202.

Bienk, E.J., and Eskildsen, S.S., 1993. The effect of surface preparation on the nucleation of diamond on silicon. *Diamond and Related Materials* 2, 432–437.

Bongrain, A., Scorsone, E., Rousseau, L., *et al.*, 2009. Selective nucleation in silicon moulds for diamond MEMS fabrication. *Journal of Micromechanics and Microengineering* 19, 074015.

Broz, A., Baresova, V., Kromka, A., *et al.*, 2009. Strong influence of hierarchically structured diamond nanotopography on adhesion of human osteoblasts and mesenchymal cells. *Physica Status Solidi (a)* 206, 2038–2041.

Bühlmann, S., Blank, E., Haubner, R., and Lux, B., 1999. Characterization of ballas diamond depositions. *Diamond and Related Materials* 8, 194–201.

Buijnsters, J.G., Vázquez, L., and ter Meulen, J.J., 2009. Substrate pre-treatment by ultrasonication with diamond powder mixtures for nucleation enhancement in diamond film growth. *Diamond and Related Materials* 18, 1239–1246.

Castro, M., Domnguez-Adame, F., Sánchez, A., and Rodrguez, T., 1999. Model for crystallization kinetics: Deviations from Kolmogorov–Johnson–Mehl–Avrami kinetics. *Applied Physics Letters* 75, 2205.

Chavanne, A., Arnault, J.-C., Barjon, J., and Arabski, J., 2011. Bias-enhanced nucleation of diamond on iridium: A comprehensive study of the first stages by sequential surface analysis. *Surface Science* 605, 564–569.

Chen, T., Chiu, M.-S., and Weng, C.-N., 2006. Derivation of the generalized Young-Laplace equation of curved interfaces in nanoscaled solids. *Journal of Applied Physics* 100, 074308.

Chen, Y.-H., Hu, C.-T., and Lin, I.-N., 1997. Selected-area Deposition of Diamond Films on Silicon Nitride-coated Silicon Substrates Using Negatively Biased Microwave Plasma Enhanced Chemical Vapor Deposition Technique. *Japanese Journal of Applied Physics* 36, 6900–6904.

Cui, J., and Fang, R., 1996. Evidence of the role of positive bias in diamond growth by hot filament chemical vapor deposition. *Applied Physics Letters* 69, 3507.

Daenen, M., Zhang, L., Erni, R., *et al.*, 2009. Diamond Nucleation by Carbon Transport from Buried Nanodiamond TiO2 Sol-Gel Composites. *Advanced Materials* 21, 670–673.

Das, D., and Singh, R.N., 2007. A review of nucleation, growth and low temperature synthesis of diamond thin films. *International Materials Reviews* 52, 29–64.

Demo, P., Kožíšek, Z., and Šášik, R., 1999. Analytical approach to time lag in binary nucleation. *Physical Review E* 59, 5124–5127.

Demo, P., Sveshnikov, A.M., and Kožíšek, Z., 2000. Comment on 'Propagator of the Fokker-Planck equation with a linear force—Lie-algebraic approach' by C. F. Lo. *Europhysics Letters (EPL)* 50, 278–279.

Feldman, A., 1995. *Applications of diamond films and related materials: third international conference: proceedings of the Applied Diamond Conference 1995: National Institute of Standards and Technology*, Gaithersburg, MD, August 21–24, 1995. The Institute; U.S. G.P.O.: For sale by the Supt. of Docs., Gaithersburg, MD; Washington, DC.

Feng, Z., Komvopoulos, K., Bogy, D.B., *et al.*, 1996. Effect of pretreatment process parameters on diamond nucleation on unscratched silicon substrates coated with amorphous carbon films. *Journal of Applied Physics* 79, 485.

Fox, N.A., Youh, M.J., Steeds, J.W., and Wang, W.N., 2000. Patterned diamond particle films. *Journal of Applied Physics* 87, 8187.

Fu, Y., Du, H., and Miao, J., 2003. Patterning of diamond microstructures on Si substrate by bulk and surface micromachining. *Journal of Materials Processing Technology* 132, 73–81.

Girard, H.A., Scorsone, E., Saada, S., *et al.*, 2012. Electrostatic grafting of diamond nanoparticles towards 3D diamond nanostructures. *Diamond and Related Materials* 23, 83–87.

Hassan, I.U., Rego, C.A., Ali, N., *et al.*, 1999. An investigation of the structural properties of diamond films deposited by pulsed bias enhanced hot filament CVD. *Thin Solid Films* 355–356, 134–138.

Hees, J., Kriele, A., and Williams, O.A., 2011. Electrostatic self-assembly of diamond nanoparticles. *Chemical Physics Letters* 509, 12–15.

Higa, A., Hatta, A., Ito, T., *et al.*, 1996. Effect of CO_2 Addition on Diamond Growth by DC Arc Plasma Jet Chemical Vapour Deposition. *Japanese Journal of Applied Physics* 35, 216–220.

Hirabayashi, K., Taniguchi, Y., Takamatsu, O., *et al.*, 1988. Selective deposition of diamond crystals by chemical vapor deposition using a tungsten-filament method. *Applied Physics Letters* 53, 1815.

Hsieh, C.-T., Lin, Y.-T., Lin, J.-Y., and Wei, J.-L., 2009. Synthesis of carbon nanotubes over Ni- and Co-supported $CaCO_3$ catalysts using catalytic chemical vapor deposition. *Materials Chemistry and Physics* 114, 702–708.

Hsu, C.-H., Cloutier, S.G., Palefsky, S., and Xu, J., 2010. Synthesis of Diamond Nanowires Using Atmospheric-Pressure Chemical Vapor Deposition. *Nano Letters* 10, 3272–3276.

Jiang, X., Schiffmann, K., and Klages, C.-P., 1994. Nucleation and initial growth phase of diamond thin films on (100) silicon. *Physical Review B* 50, 8402–8410.

Jingsheng, C., Xuejun, W., Zhihao, Z., and Fengyuan, Y., 1999. Nucleation and growth of diamond on silicon substrate coated with polymer. *Thin Solid Films* 346, 120–124.

Jirsak, O., Sanetrnik, F., Lukas, D., Kotek, V., Martinova, L., and Chaloupek, J., 2005. Method of nanofibres production from a polymer solution using electrostatic spinning and a device for carrying out the method, U.S. Patent WO/2005/024101.

Kalbacova, M., Michalikova, L., Baresova, V., *et al.*, 2008. Adhesion of osteoblasts on chemically patterned nanocrystalline diamonds. *Physica status solidi (b)* 245, 2124–2127.

Kalbacova, M., Rezek, B., Baresova, V., *et al.*, 2009. Nanoscale topography of nanocrystalline diamonds promotes differentiation of osteoblasts. *Acta Biomaterialia* 5, 3076–3085.

Kang, J.L., Li, J.J., Du, X.W., *et al.*, 2008. Synthesis and growth mechanism of metal filled carbon nanostructures by CVD using Ni/Y catalyst supported on copper. *Journal of Alloys and Compounds* 456, 290–296.

Kozak, H., Kromka, A., Babchenko, O., and Rezek, B., 2010. Directly Grown Nanocrystalline Diamond Field-Effect Transistor Microstructures. *Sensor Letters* 8, 482–487.

Kožíšek, Z., and Demo, P., 1995. Transient nucleation in binary ideal solution. *The Journal of Chemical Physics* 102, 7595.

Kromka, A., 2001. *Growth of Diamond Thin Films by a Hybrid Hot Filament CVD Technique*. PhD thesis – Slovak Technical University, Bratislava, Slovak Republic.

Kromka, A., Babchenko, O., Izak, T., *et al.*, 2012. Linear antenna microwave plasma CVD deposition of diamond films over large areas. *Vacuum* 86, 776–779.

Kromka, A., Babchenko, O., Kozak, H., *et al.*, 2009b. Seeding of polymer substrates for nanocrystalline diamond film growth. *Diam. Relat. Mater.* 18, 734–739.

Kromka, A., Babchenko, O., Rezek, B., *et al.*, 2009d. Simplified procedure for patterned growth of nanocrystalline diamond micro-structures. *Thin Solid Films* 518, 343–347.

Kromka, A., Daniš, T., Balon, F., *et al.*, 2003a. Influence of nucleation parameters on growth of diamond thin films by hybrid hot filament CVD. *Diamond and Related Materials* 12, 356–360.

Kromka, A., Janik, J., Balon, F., *et al.*, 2003b. Comparison of diamond nucleation in DC and AC substrate bias mode. *Thin Solid Films* 433, 73–77.

Kromka, A., Janik, J., Satka, A., *et al.*, 2001a. Investigation of carburisation of tungsten-carbide formation by hot-filament CVD technique. *Acta Phys. Slovaca* 51, 359–368.

Kromka, A., Malcher, V., and Cerven, I., 2001b. Influence of long time nucleation on homogeneity of diamond films grown on silicon substrates. *Acta Phys. Slovaca* 51, 27–34.

Kromka, A., Potocký, S., Cermák, J., *et al.*, 2008b. Early stage of diamond growth at low temperature. *Diam. Relat. Mater.* 17, 1252–1255.

Kromka, A., Potocky, S., Rezek, B., *et al.*, 2009c. Role of polymers in CVD growth of nanocrystalline diamond films on foreign substrates. *Physica Status Solidi (b)* 246, 2654–2657.

Kromka, A., Rezek, B., Kalbacova, M., *et al.*, 2009a. Diamond Seeding and Growth of Hierarchically Structured Films for Tissue Engineering. *Advanced Engineering Materials* 11, B71–B76.

Kromka, A., Rezek, B., Remes, Z., *et al.*, 2008a. Formation of Continuous Nanocrystalline Diamond Layers on Glass and Silicon at Low Temperatures. *Chem. Vap. Deposition* 14, 181–186.

Kruger, A., Kataoka, F., Ozawa, M., *et al.*, 2005. Unusually tight aggregation in detonation nanodiamond: Identification and disintegration. *Carbon* 43, 1722–1730.

Lee, H.-J., Jeon, H., and Lee, W.-S., 2011. Ultrathin ultrananocrystalline diamond film synthesis by direct current plasma-assisted chemical vapor deposition. *Journal of Applied Physics* 110, 084305.

Lee, Y.H., Richard, P.D., Bachmann, K.J., and Glass, J.T., 1990. Bias-controlled chemical vapor deposition of diamond thin films. *Applied Physics Letters* 56, 620.

Li, D., and Xia, Y., 2004. Electrospinning of Nanofibers: Reinventing the Wheel? *Advanced Materials* 16, 1151–1170.

Li, X., Hayashi, Y., and Nishino, S., 1997. An improved method for large-area oriented nucleation of diamond during bias process via hot-filament chemical vapor deposition. *Thin Solid Films* 308–309, 163–167.

Liang, Z.Z., Jia, X., Zang, C.Y., *et al.*, 2005. The influences of N and H on diamond synthesized with Ni–Mn–Co catalyst by HPHT. *Diamond and Related Materials* 14, 243–247.

Lifshitz, Y., 2002. The Mechanism of Diamond Nucleation from Energetic Species. *Science* 297, 1531–1533.

Liu, H., and Dandy, D.S., 1995. *Diamond chemical vapor deposition nucleation and early growth stages*. Noyes Publications, Park Ridge, N.J.

Liu, H., Wang, C., Gao, C., *et al.*, 2002. New insights into selected-area deposition of diamond films by means of selective seeding. *Journal of Physics: Condensed Matter* 14, 10973–10977.

Lu, Y.-G., Verbeeck, J., Turner, S., *et al.*, 2012. Analytical TEM study of CVD diamond growth on TiO2 sol–gel layers. *Diamond and Related Materials* 23, 93–99.

Mitsuda, Y., Moriyasu, T., and Masuko, N., 1993. Effect of high supersaturation at the initial stage on diamond nucleation phenomena. *Diamond and Related Materials* 2, 333–336.

Moulder, J.F., Chastain, J., and King, R.C., 1995. *Handbook of x-ray photoelectron spectroscopy: a reference book of standard spectra for identification and interpretation of XPS data*. Physical Electronics, Eden Prairie, Minn.

Muller, J., Antoni, F., Fogarassy, E., and Le Normand, F., 1998. HFCVD diamond nucleation and growth on DLC carbon films obtained by laser ablation. *Carbon* 36, 565–568.

Nebel, C.E., Shin, D., Rezek, B., *et al.*, 2007. Diamond and biology. *Journal of The Royal Society Interface* 4, 439–461.

Nur, Y., Duygulu, Ş., Pitcher, M.W., and Toppare, L., 2012. The electrochemical synthesis of poly(methylcarbyne) for diamond film coatings. *Journal of Applied Polymer Science* 124, 3626–3632.

Ōsawa, E., 2008. Monodisperse single nanodiamond particulates. *Pure and Applied Chemistry* 80, 1365–1379.

Perng, K., Liu, K.-S., and Lin, I.-N., 2002. Study on bias-enhanced nucleation of diamonds by simulating the time dependence of bias current. *Journal of Applied Physics* 91, 3934.

Potocký, Š., Kromka, A., Babchenko, O., Rezek, B., Martinova, L., Pokorny, P., 2013. Diamond structures growth from polymer composite, *Advanced Science, Engineering and Medicine*, accepted for publications.

Prelas, M.A., Popovici, G., and Bigelow, L.K., 1998. *Handbook of Industrial Diamonds and Diamond Films*. Marcel Dekker Inc, New York.

Ray, S.C., Fanchini, G., Tagliaferro, A., *et al.*, 2003. Amorphous carbon films prepared by the 'dip' technique: Deposition and film characterization. *J. Appl. Phys.* 94, 870.

Rezek, B., Michalíková, L., Ukraintsev, E., *et al.*, 2009. Micro-Pattern Guided Adhesion of Osteoblasts on Diamond Surfaces. *Sensors* 9, 3549–3562.

Robertson, J., Gerber, J., Sattel, S., *et al.*, 1995. Mechanism of bias-enhanced nucleation of diamond on Si. *Applied Physics Letters* 66, 3287.

Rotter, S., 1999. in: *Proceedings of the Applied Diamond Conference/Frontier Carbon Technologies—ADC/FCT 99*, Edited by M. Yoshikawa, Y. Koga, Y. Tzeng, C.-P. Klages, and K. Miyoshi, (MYU K.K., Tokyo, 1999). p. 25.

Sakamoto, Y., Takaya, M., Sugimura, H., *et al.*, 1998. Fabrication of a micro-patterned diamond film by site-selective plasma chemical vapor deposition. *Thin Solid Films* 334, 161–164.

Sawabe, A., and Inuzuka, T., 1985. Growth of diamond thin films by electron assisted chemical vapor deposition. *Applied Physics Letters* 46, 146.

Schreck, M., Thürer, K.-H., and Stritzker, B., 1997. Limitations of the process window for the bias enhanced nucleation of heteroepitaxial diamond films on silicon in the time domain. *Journal of Applied Physics* 81, 3092.

Scorsone, E., Saada, S., Arnault, J.C., and Bergonzo, P., 2009. Enhanced control of diamond nanoparticle seeding using a polymer matrix. *Journal of Applied Physics* 106, 014908.

Sedov, V.S., Ral'chenko, V.G., Khomich, A.A., *et al.*, 2012. Stimulation of the diamond nucleation on silicon substrates with a layer of a polymeric precursor in deposition of diamond films by microwave plasma. *Journal of Superhard Materials* 34, 37–43.

Spitsyn, B.V., Bouilov, L.L., and Derjaguin, B.V., 1981. Vapor growth of diamond on diamond and other surfaces. *Journal of Crystal Growth* 52, 219–226.

Stoner, B., Ma, G.-H., Wolter, S., and Glass, J., 1992. Characterization of bias-enhanced nucleation of diamond on silicon by invacuo surface analysis and transmission electron microscopy. *Physical Review B* 45, 11067–11084.

Sugai, H., Ghanashev, I., and Mizuno, K., 2000. Transition of electron heating mode in a planar microwave discharge at low pressures. *Applied Physics Let*ters 77, 3523.

Sumant, A.V., Gilbert, P.U.P.A., Grierson, D.S., *et al.*, 2007. Surface composition, bonding, and morphology in the nucleation and growth of ultra-thin, high quality nanocrystalline diamond films. *Diamond and Related Materials* 16, 718–724.

Sun, Z., Shi, X., Tay, B., *et al.*, 1997b. Low pressure polymer precursor for synthesis of diamond at low temperature. *Journal of Materials Science Letters* 16, 933–935.

Sun, Z., Shi, X., Tay, B.., *et al.*, 1997c. Growth of flake-like diamond crystal using polymer precursor. *Thin Solid Films* 308–309, 159–162.

Sun, Z., Shi, X., Tay, B.K., *et al.*, 1997a. Low pressure polymer precursor process for synthesis of hard glassy carbon and diamond films. *Diamond and Related Materials* 6, 230–234.

Sun, Z., Sun, Y., Yang, Q., *et al.*, 1996. IR spectral investigation of the pyrolysis of polymer precursor to diamond-like carbon. *Surface and Coatings Technology* 79, 108–112.

Titantah, J.T., and Lamoen, D., 2005. sp3/sp2 characterization of carbon materials from first-principles calculations: X-ray photoelectron versus high energy electron energy-loss spectroscopy techniques. *Carbon* 43, 1311–1316.

Tsugawa, K., Ishihara, M., Kim, J., *et al.*, 2010. Nanocrystalline diamond film growth on plastic substrates at temperatures below 100°C from low-temperature plasma. *Physical Review B* 82.

Tsugawa, K., Kawaki, S., Ishihara, M., *et al.*, 2011. Nanocrystalline diamond growth in a surface-wave plasma. *Diamond and Related Materials* 20, 833–838.

Varga, M., Ižák, T., Kromka, A., *et al.*, 2011. Study of diamond film nucleation by ultrasonic seeding in different solutions. *Central European Journal of Physics* 10, 218–224.

Vehkamäki, H., 2006. Classical nucleation theory in multicomponent systems. Springer, Berlin; New York.

Vojs, M., Veselý, M., Redhammer, R., *et al.*, 2005. Double bias HF CVD multilayer diamond films on WC–Co cutting tools. *Diamond and Related Materials* 14, 613–616.

Wang, W., Gao, J., Liao, K., and Ji, R., 1992. Diamond-Film Synthesis Using Heating-Assisted Oxygen-Acetylene Flame. *Physica Status Solidi (a)* 132, K31–K34.

Wang, W.N., Fox, N.A., May, P.W., *et al.*, 1996. Laser Raman Studies of Polycrystalline and Amorphic Diamond Films. *Physica Status Solidi (a)* 154, 255–268.

Wang, X., Chen, J., Zheng, Z., *et al.*, 1997. Synthesis of diamond from polymer seeded with nanometer-sized diamond particles. *Journal of Crystal Growth* 181, 308–313.

Williams, O.A., Douhéret, O., Daenen, M., *et al.*, 2007. Enhanced diamond nucleation on monodispersed nanocrystalline diamond. *Chemical Physics Letters* 445, 255–258.

Williams, O.A., Hees, J., Dieker, C., *et al.*, 2010. Size-Dependent Reactivity of Diamond Nanoparticles. *ACS Nano* 4, 4824–4830.
Yang, W.S., and Je, J.H., 1996. Effects of Secondary Pretreatments of Substrate on the Nucleation of Diamond Film. *Journal of Materials Research* 11, 1787–1794.
Yoshikawa, M., Fukunaga, O., Saito, S., Japan New Diamond Forum (JNDF), 1990. *Science and technology of new diamond: proceedings of the 1st international conference of new diamond science and technology*, Tokyo, Japan, October 24–26, 1988. KTK Scientific Publishers: Terra Scientific Pub. Co., Tokyo.
Yugo, S., Kanai, T., Kimura, T., and Muto, T., 1991. Generation of diamond nuclei by electric field in plasma chemical vapor deposition. *Applied Physics Letters* 58, 1036.
Zemek, J., Houdkova, J., Lesiak, B., *et al.*, 2006. Electron spectroscopy of nanocrystalline diamond surfaces. *J. Optoelectron. Adv. Mater.* 8, 2133–2138.
Zhang, M., Yan, H., and Peng, F., 2008. Analysis of the Phenomena of Diamond Synthesis by Seeding with Diamond. *J. Mater. Sci. Technol.* 24, 809–812.
Zhou, X., Lai, H., Peng, H., *et al.*, 2000. Heteroepitaxial nucleation of diamond on Si(100) via double bias-assisted hot filament chemical vapor deposition. *Diamond and Related Materials* 9, 134–139.
Zhou, X.T., Li, Q., Meng, F.Y., *et al.*, 2002. Manipulation of the equilibrium between diamond growth and re-nucleation to form a nanodiamond/amorphous carbon composite. Applied Physics Letters 80, 3307.

10
Diamond materials for microfluidic devices

A. KARCZEMSKA, Lodz University of Technology, Poland

DOI: 10.1533/9780857093516.2.256

Abstract: This chapter discusses the possibilities and advantages offered by the use of diamond materials in the fabrication of microfluidic devices. The correct choice of material with optimal properties is crucial in the design of modern microfluidic devices. The different applications of diamond materials in this field are reviewed, along with a discussion of recent development and future trends.

Key words: diamond, diamond-like carbon (DLC), nanocrystalline diamond (NCD), chemical vapour deposition (CVD), microfluidic devices.

10.1 Introduction

The start of the twentieth century saw a number of highly significant developments in the field of physics, including quantum mechanics, the theory of relativity and particle physics. Scientific discoveries and new technologies later in the century led to a technological revolution, with the introduction of television, computers and fast cars; the Moon landings; and developments in medicine and biotechnology, such as the understanding of the structure of DNA. These discoveries and developments, along with extensive research into new and innovative materials, have led to significant improvements in many areas of people's lives.

One twentieth-century development that is key to the topic discussed in this chapter is miniaturization. In 1959 Richard Feynman, the famous physicist and Nobel Prize winner, gave a speech entitled 'There's Plenty of Room at the Bottom', which inspired the later development of the field of nanotechnology. His words proved to be prophetic:

> I would like to describe a field in which little has been done, but in which an enormous amount can be done in principle. This field is not quite the same as the others in that it will not tell us much of fundamental physics (in the sense of, "what are the strange particles?") but it is more like solid-state physics in the sense that it might tell us much of great interest about the strange phenomena that occur in the complex situations. Furthermore a point that is most important is that it would have an enormous number of technical applications (Feynman, 1959).

Since then, rapid technological developments in the area of miniaturization have taken place, particularly the miniaturization of electronic devices. Microelectronics, and more recently nanoelectronics, have changed our lives in numerous ways: the latter has become one of the most promising areas of research over the last decade. At the end of the 1970s, miniaturization technology extended to microelectromechanical systems (MEMS). Microfluidics, a branch of science and technology that processes or manipulates small amounts of fluids (10^{-9} to 10^{-18} kg) using channels with dimensions of tens to hundreds of micrometers (Whitesides, 2006), is one of the most dynamic branches of MEMS research. The aim of work in this field is to miniaturize the biochemical laboratory to a 'lab-on-a-chip' size; it offers new options for novel analysis techniques (Tian, 2008). In the history of microfluidics, the first silicon-based analysis systems were fabricated in the end of 1970s, but it was not until the work of Manz and others in the early 1990s that the full potential of microfluidic devices was realised (Manz, 1990, 1992) and the term microTotal Analysis Systems (μTAS) was introduced. The studies carried out in that period demonstrated the miniaturization of gas and liquid chromatography columns but also began to miniaturize electrophoretic techniques. A new era in separation sciences can be said to have begun when Manz *et al.* (1992) introduced the first capillary electrophoresis (CE) system on-chip. Microchip electrophoresis allows the separation of DNA and proteins in a very short time (as little as a few seconds), with only a small volume of analytes required while still allowing high reproducibility. Subsequent years saw the development of new concepts and applications of microfluidic devices, such that two decades later it is difficult to describe them all. Most applications of microfluidic devices can be split into those relying on pressure and those relying on electrokinetically driven mechanisms of fluid transport. The samples and different reagents can be diluted, separated, mixed and controlled using mixers, micropumps, microvalves, systems of microcapillaries and different types of electronic devices such as biosensors and detectors, which may be included inthe chip.

Microfluidic systems offer a number of advantages, including enhanced heat transfer; improved laminar flow (low Reynolds number $Re<1$); lower consumption of reagents and samples; faster separations; and improved efficiency (Sommer, 2008). They also display a high degree of integration, portability and excellent performance. Although a great deal of work has already been carried out, studies are ongoing and more research in the field is still required. The apparatus currently in use is automated, and has become much smaller and quicker in recent years, but many problems remain to be solved. The main aim of current studies in the area is the development of modern cheap microfluidic and nanofluidic devices that are still quicker and cheaper (Tian, 2008, Hesketh, 2008).

Extensive developments and discoveries in the fields of biology and biotechnology can be expected in the twenty-first century. The understanding of the human genome and proteome will provide information about ourselves that we cannot even anticipate currently. These developments allow us, and will continue to allow us, to access a wealth of information that will have widespread applications for the future. Different kinds of microfluidic devices will soon allow diagnostic techniques in hospitals and homes to be revolutionized, and will lead to the development of new tools for biochemical laboratories, environmental monitoring, pharmaceutical analysis, clinical diagnostics and food production, among many other applications. Research into new materials for these applications will also help to achieve new goals and go right to the limits of this technique. One such material is diamond.

10.2 Materials for the manufacture of microfluidic devices

Polymers, glass or silicon are most frequently used for manufacturing microfluidic devices (Lysko, 2012). Historically, many technologies used in the fabrication of microfluidic devices were adapted from the semiconductor industry (such as photolithography and wet etching), so early microfluidic chips were often manufactured in silicon (Zhang, 2006). However, there are other materials that possess better optical and biological properties for such applications, so similar technologies began to be used with silica glass, Pyrex and quartz, and some combined silicon/glass devices have also been manufactured. Today, however, there is growing interest in the use of moulded fabrication techniques. Such techniques allow the inexpensive, simple and rapid production of microfluidic devices using polymer materials. Polydimethylosiloxane (PDMS) is particularly widely used in this area, because of the low costs involved and the simplicity of manufacturing PDMS microfluidic devices. PDMS also has quite good optical and electrical properties, but a very low thermal conductivity coefficient.

The correct choice of the optimal material and fabrication technique is a very important issue in the design and manufacture of microfluidic devices: it can affect the performance of the final device, and there is still much work to be done in this area. A number of different properties should be taken into consideration when selecting the optimal material: the most general of these are shown in Table 10.1 for a range of materials that are most frequently used in microfluidic devices. A range of microfabrication methods are available, including photolithography, laser micromachining, injection moulding and hot embossing. A variety of surface modification techniques are also used to modify the surface of the material, such as plasma treatment, surface functionalization by binding biological molecules, or the application of different kinds of coatings. This allows certain surface properties to be changed, such as electric charge, wettability and surface energy.

Diamond possesses unique properties that allow it to be applied in many fields of science and technology (Sussmann, 1998): it has good optical properties, which means it has a broad transmission spectrum; is very hard and rigid; shows the highest known thermal conductivity and a low thermal expansion coefficient; is chemically inert, and therefore not affected by alkaline or acid reagents; and is bioactive (Mitura, 2006). Diamond also can be an insulator or a semiconductor. Some monocrystalline diamond properties are shown in Table 10.2.

Table 10.1 Example properties of materials commonly used for manufacturing of microfluidic devices

Property	PDMS	Glass	Si (monocrystalline)	SiO_2
Thermal conductivity (W/m·K)	0.18	1.1	157	1.4
>70% optical transmittance (nm)	400–700	>350	>700	>350
Maximum processing temperature (K)	~420	~820	1688	1973
Dielectric strength (×10^6V/cm)	2.1	5~10	3	2~3
Contact angle for water (°)	~110	20~35	110	~30

Source: Zhang, 2006.

Table 10.2 Diamond properties

Property	Value
Density	3.52 g/cm^3
Vickers hardness	10 000 kg/mm^2
Young's modulus	1050 GPa
Coefficient of friction	0.1
Refractive index	2.417
Bandgap	5.45 eV
Resistivity	10^{13}–10^{16} Ω·cm
Specific heat at 20°C	0.502 J/gK
Thermal conductivity	2200 W/mK

Source: Yoder, 1993; Kidalov, 2009.

In recent years, advances in diamond materials technology, especially different chemical vapour deposition (CVD) techniques, have allowed the manufacture of both CVD polycrystalline diamond plates of different grades with large surface areas, and different kinds of diamond-like coatings and powders. Depending on the grade of the polycrystalline material and its composition (sp^3 to sp^2 content), carbon materials can possess a wide range of properties. Changes in these properties can occur because of reductions in crystal size, the presence of defects and grain boundaries, increases in sp^2 bonds in the material and changes in material composition (i.e. presence of impurities). For instance, the thermal conductivity coefficient can range from 0.1 W/mK for diamond-like carbon amorphous coatings (DLC) to almost ~3000–5300 W/mK for graphene (Ghosh, 2012). The thermal conductivity coefficients for different diamond materials (monocrystalline diamond, polycrystalline CVD diamond with different crystal grades, nanocrystalline diamond, and DLC) and different materials used for manufacturing microfluidic devices (PDMS, glass, silicon) are compared in the graph in Fig. 10.1. The thermal conductivity of monocrystalline diamond is about

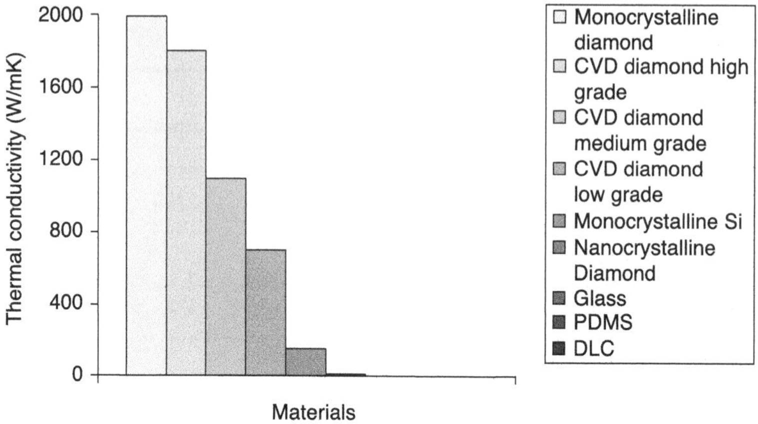

10.1 Comparison of thermal conductivity properties for different diamond materials and materials most often used for manufacturing microfluidic devices (PDMS, glass, Si) (Karczemska, 2002; Kidalov, 2009; Diamond Materials, 2008).

2200 W/mK, whereas isotopically pure diamond ^{12}C or ^{13}C has thermal conductivity of around 50% higher. Diamond is therefore useful as a heat sink material.

It is likely that different diamond and diamond-like materials, as well as other allotropic forms of carbon, still have further undiscovered properties, which may offer other new application possibilities (Karczemska, 2010a, Karczemska, 2010b). For instance, polytypes of diamond other than 'conventional' cubic diamond have been discovered in meteorites: some of these are shown in Fig. 10.2. Hexagonal diamond, known as lonsdaleite, was initially discovered in a meteorite and was subsequently manufactured in a laboratory. Many other polytypes have been discovered, such as 2H, 6H, 8H, 10H and 21R. However, meteoritic polytypes of diamond are found in small quantities and always with other phases. In the future it is likely that an increased understanding of the properties of these diamonds, along with further developments in large-scale manufacturing technologies, will allow new diamond materials to be designed, and large high quality diamond monocrystals to be obtained.

Diamond materials offer great potential for microfluidic devices because of their unique biological, chemical, mechanical and optical properties: the combination of electrical insulating capability and high thermal conductivity is particularly advantageous. For electrokinetically driven microfluidic devices, materials with a high coefficient of thermal conductivity are especially useful because Joule heating occurs as the electric field is applied. Electrophoretic microchips manufactured from materials with high thermal conductivity could be faster, because higher electric fields can be applied. The velocities of analysed biomolecules are dependent on the mass/charge proportion and the electric field:

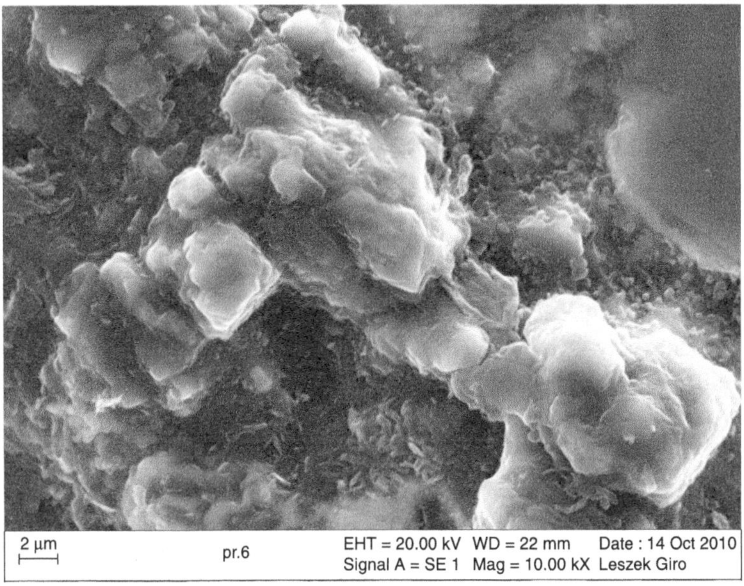

10.2 SEM image of diamonds in meteorite – ureilite DaG 868.

higher electric fields mean shorter separation times, but also increased Joule heat generation, which is undesirable. The use of diamond (instead of plastics or glass) as the material for manufacturing electrophoretic microchips, allows much better heat dissipation from the microchannels. The other properties of diamond also make it a very interesting material for some extreme applications.

10.3 Diamond microfluidic devices

A variety of different diamond materials such as CVD polycrystalline diamond, nanocrystalline diamond coatings (NCD) and DLC coatings have been used in the manufacture of different elements of microfluidic devices. The methods and results have been reported in a number of studies, a selection of which are discussed below.

10.3.1 Studies into the use of diamond in microfluidic devices

Björkman *et al.* (2001) presented the first diamond microchips for chromatography. Columns 40 mm long, 100 µm wide and 40 or 70 µm high were fabricated using a silicon-based microengineering technology, using firstly silicon microstructuring and then diamond replication. The diamond surface inside the capillaries was modified, changing from hydrophobic to hydrophilic. Channels in the 40 mm long straight columns were filled with continuous polymer beds and the separations were performed in less than 30 seconds.

A diamond micro-reaction system for chemical reactions was described by Adamschik *et al.* (2001). Micro-reactors are essential parts of biochemical synthesis and analysis systems. The microdevice presented in this study consists of reaction chambers with a removable bottom and micro-dosage elements which allow the ejection and mixture of two fluids. CVD diamond films were used at specific locations, specifically at the microheater elements, the reaction chamber surface and the nozzle plate. The use of diamond meant that the system was chemically inert, and the study was also able to describe the application of this system for the DNA synthesis cycle.

Guillaudeu *et al.* (2003) demonstrated narrow freestanding polycrystalline diamond (poly-C) microfluidic channels (microcapillaries) 100 μm long, 2 μm wide and 10 μm high. This type of channel can carry any chemical because of the non-reactivity of diamond. The authors reported that the specific properties of diamond make it suitable for use in micro-chemical laboratories (i.e. lab-on-a-chip).

Müller *et al.* (2004, 2005) also used CVD diamond to manufacture surface microfluidic elements for lab-on-a-chip systems. They described a new approach using surface channels and chambers fabricated from diamond to provide a covered fluidic system. High aspect ratio microchannels with a large cross-section were obtained by using electroplated copper as a sacrificial layer, which was overgrown with CVD diamond (and the copper layer was etched out after the diamond deposition). This technique can be used to fabricate microfluidic devices. An integrated micro-membrane pump with thermal actuation was also discussed in the same studies. The unique properties of diamond and the possibility of changing the properties of diamond materials (such as modifying the electrical conductivity by incorporating additional element atoms into the diamond crystal structure) allows diamond to be used in both passive and active elements.

In Khanna *et al.* (2006), NCD is presented as an attractive material for lab-on-a-chip devices. Khanna *et al.* (2009) also demonstrated the use of NCD microspikes for microfluidic lab-on-a-chip. NCD microspikes in the microfluidic chamber increased the efficiency of the mechanical cell lysis. NCD has attractive properties for cell lysis applications because it is biologically inert, robust, and easy to fabricate. Moreover, it is possible to create microspikes with an extremely sharp nanocrystalline tip, which are able to survive multiple experiments without damage.

Forsberg *et al.* (2011) also described applications of nanocrystalline diamond for microfluidic devices. The array of boron-doped nanocrystalline diamond microband electrodes were used in a PDMS-based microfluidic system by placing them in the PDMS microchannel. The electrodes demonstrated very good stability and well-defined electrochemical responses. The electrodes can be cleaned and reused, can work for several hundred hours and are better than the more commonly used gold electrodes.

In Chen's (2007) review paper, boron-doped diamond and carbon nanotubes were investigated and found to be highly suitable for electrochemical sensing in conventional CE as well as in microchip electrophoresis. The attractive properties of these carbon materials make them very promising materials for applications in a variety of microfluidic analysis systems. Diamond is an electrical insulator but it becomes a conductor when doped by other elements such as boron. Boron-doped diamond electrodes exhibit very good properties, such as favourable signal to background characteristics, low noise, stable background currents, wide potential window and low adsorption of organic compounds.

Massi *et al.* (2003) studied the use of the plasma etching process in DLC films for the construction of microfluidic channels. The technique of DC magnetron sputtering was used to deposit DLC films onto p-type silicon wafers. One major advantage of DLC mentioned in this paper is that its properties can be easily changed by controlling the sp^3/sp^2 ratio.

In Saha *et al.* (2010), the surface properties of Si micromoulds used in the replication process during the manufacture of microfluidic polymethlyl methacrylate (PMMA) were investigated. DLC coatings were selected because of their excellent tribological and mechanical properties, and were applied as the coatings on Si moulds used for a micro-hot-embossing process. DLC coatings helped to minimize the coefficient of friction, which is very important during the demoulding process as the surface-to-volume ratio of a microdevice is very high. The surface adhesion and coefficient of friction were reduced by the application of N:DLC:Ni coatings: this allowed improved replications, and resulted in coated micromoulds and longer lifetimes (3–18 times longer) in the hot-embossing process.

PMMA microchannels with a micropillar array structure and modified channel surfaces with DLC coatings are presented in Mukhopadhyay *et al.* (2011). This study investigated the effects of surface modifications such as changes in surface energy and surface chemistry. The PMMA surfaces were coated with hydrogenated amorphous carbon (a-C:H) and with Si-doped a-C:H using the plasma-enhanced chemical vapour deposition (PECVD) technique. Investigations were carried out into the surface energy (static contact angle), the surface chemistry, the surface roughness and the fluidic measurements, and it was found that this type of surface engineering can be used in a variety of applications, including in microfluidics.

Fu *et al.* (2012) demonstrated surface acoustic wave devices (SAW) fabricated on zinc oxide deposited on the ultra-smooth nanocrystalline diamond (UNCD) coating. Finally, Kumar *et al.* (NSF NIRT Grant) also showed the application of nanocrystalline diamond thin films for a microfluidic lab-on-a-chip.

The devices manufactured in all the studies discussed above were reproducible and functional, showing that diamond surface microfluidic technology can be used to fabricate all types of diamond microfluidic devices.

10.3.2 Techniques and problems in diamond microfluidic device fabrication

Electrophoresis is a method of separating large molecules (such as DNA fragments, peptides or proteins) from a mixture of similar molecules. An electric current is passed through a medium (gel) containing the mixture of molecules. Agarose and acrylamide gels are the mediums most commonly used for the electrophoresis of proteins and nucleic acids. The various molecules travel through the medium at different rates depending on their electrical charge and size. The separation of the molecules is based on these differences: smaller fragments typically travel further through the medium in which the separation is carried out.

Joule heating is a major problem in CE processes. The capillary tube, filled by an electrophoretic medium, behaves as a cylindrical ohmic conductor when the electric field is applied. The conductance of an electric current through an electrolyte solution results in the generation of heat due to frictional collisions between mobile ions and medium (buffer or gel) molecules. As high field strengths are employed in CE, this so-called Joule heating can be significant (Grossman and Colburn, 1992, Beckman Instruments 1994, Chankvetache, 1997), and, combined with temperature gradients, can cause a number of problems with respect to reproducibility, band broadening and migration properties. Non-uniform column temperatures across the diameter or length of the column can decrease efficiency and resolution. Cylindrical capillaries are not as effective in heat dissipation because the channel surface/channel volume ratio is minimal. Rectangular channels with a large aspect ratio can provide much better temperature stabilization (Ermakov, 1998). Such channel geometries are typical of microfabricated devices.

The combination of very good properties, such as the highest thermal conductivity, transparency to UV light and high breakdown voltage, makes wide bandgap materials the most promising candidates for use in future microfluidic devices.

10.3.3 Recent developments in diamond microengineering

The microengineering of diamond has until recently not been possible due to its extreme hardness. However, the development of CVD diamond has opened up new possibilities in this area, and several new techniques to shape diamond have been developed, such as the replication of diamond in a mould, laser ablation and plasma etching. It must be stressed, however, that CVD diamond plates and technologies to shape diamond are currently too expensive for use in commercial applications.

Karczemska *et al.* (2010, 2011) and Fijalkowski (2012) described the technology of fabrication of diamond microfluidic devices with microstructures of a high aspect ratio of depth to width. The polycrystalline diamond thick layers were deposited on the silicon moulds using the microwave plasma chemical vapor deposition (MPCVD) reactor system DF – 100. A CH_4/H_2 gas mixture was used under the following conditions: microwave power 3.6 kW; methane content 2%; total flow rate 800 sccm; pressure 87 Tr; substrate temperature 820°C. Silicon mould nucleaction was provided by a bath with detonation nanodiamond dissolved in ethanol. After about 2 weeks of diamond deposition, the silicon mould was chemically etched off and the diamond chips were finished with the laser, specifically by wafer edge cutting and upper surface polishing. The first silicon mould and microfluidic chip obtained using this method is shown in Fig. 10.3(a) and (b), whereas Fig. 10.4 shows the diamond microfluidic device with four channels. Microchannels with a high aspect ratio of depth to width (shown in Fig. 10.5 and 10.6) and multichannels (Fig. 10.7) have also been fabricated.

PDMS, as mentioned above, is the material widely used for manufacturing microfluidic devices. Its main advantages are that it is a very cheap and easy to

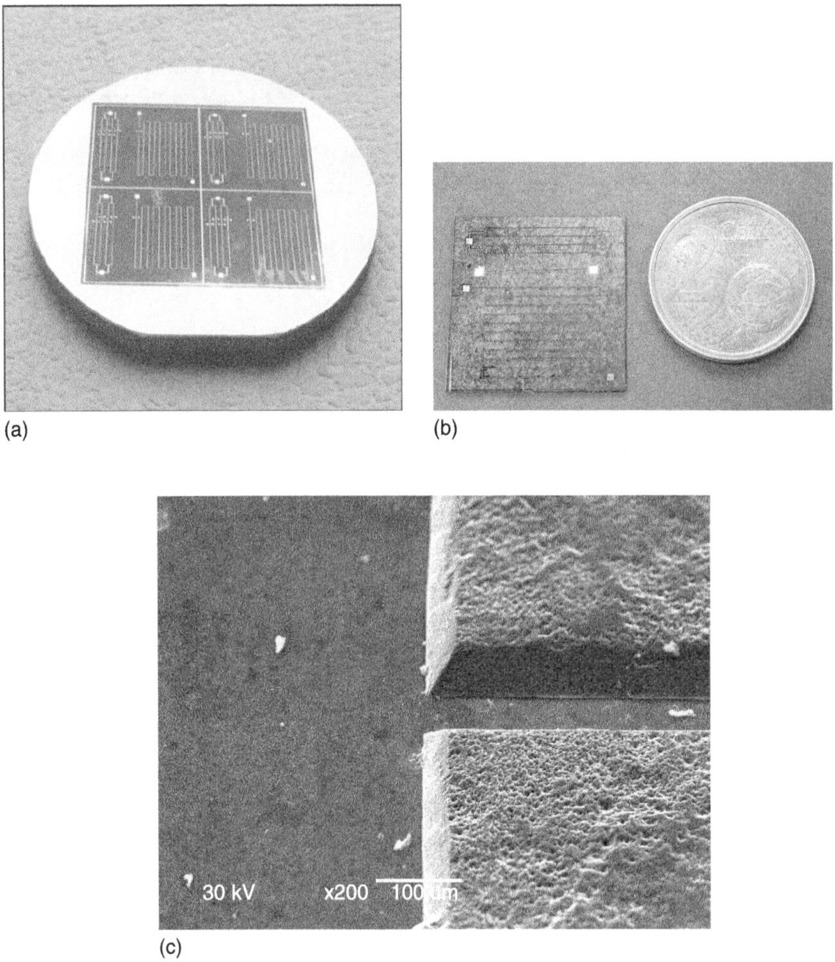

10.3 (a) The first silicon mould. (b) Microfluidic channels on the surface of the CVD polycrystalline diamond plate. (c) SEM image of the microfluidic channels manufactured in diamond with transfer moulding technique (replica method).

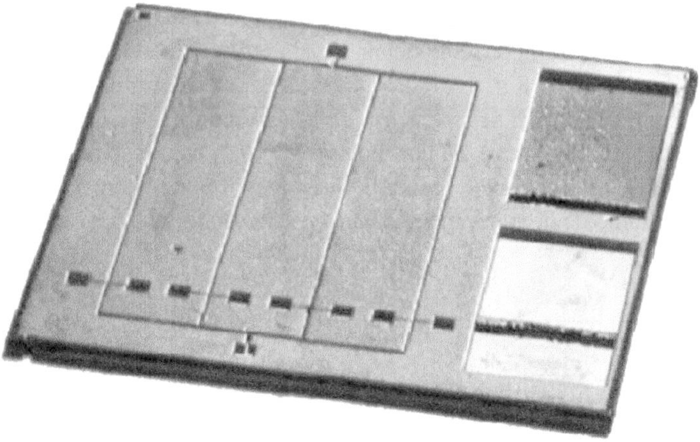

10.4 Four channel diamond microfluidic device manufactured with transfer moulding technique.

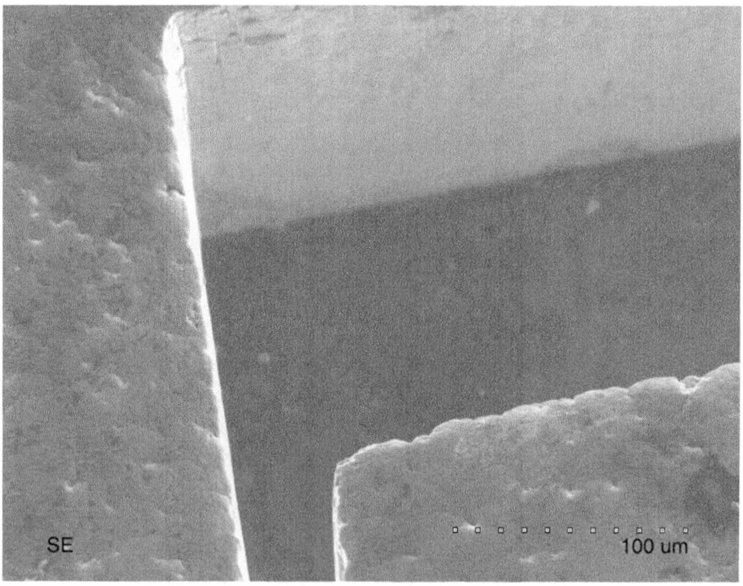

10.5 SEM image of the microstructure in diamond.

shape material. Modifications of PDMS surface by deposition of different kinds of carbon coatings can change the surface properties of this material in a wide range and are under investigation in the project 'Micro- and nano- systems for chemistry and biomedical diagnostics – MNS-DIAG'. The properties such as

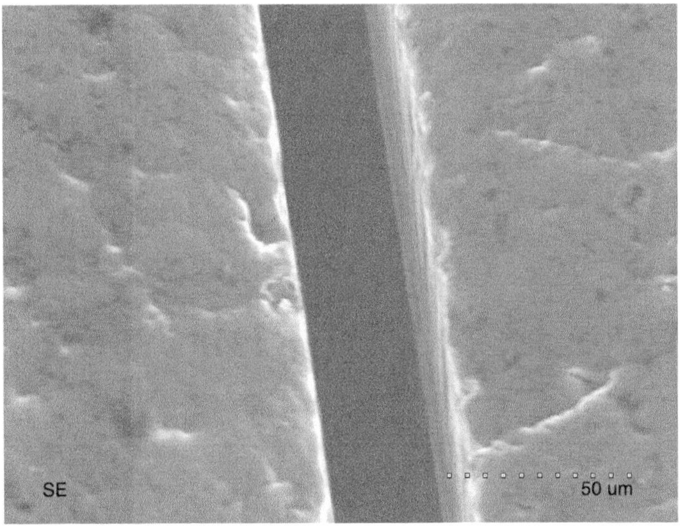

10.6 SEM image of the microchannel in diamond.

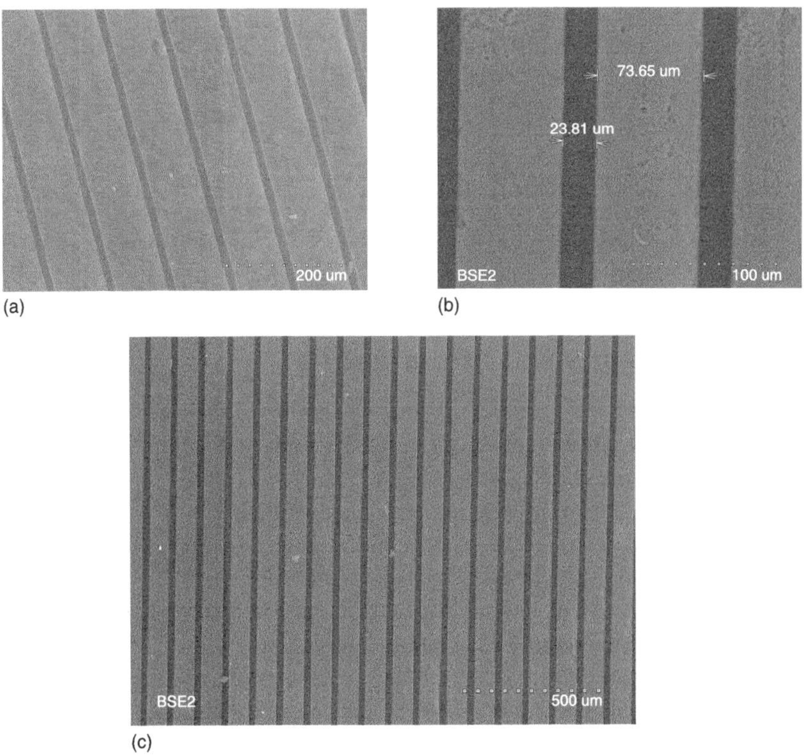

10.7 (a–c) SEM images of the multiple microfluidic channels in diamond.

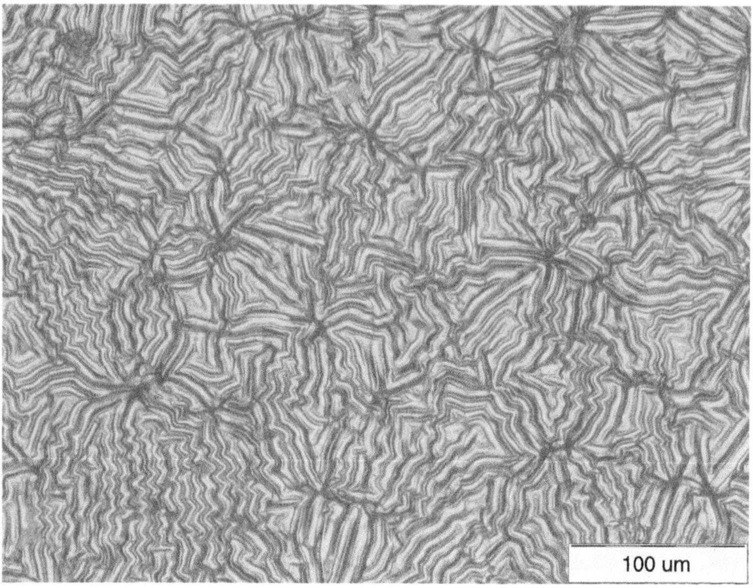

10.8 Optical microscope image of PDMS surface modified with diamond-like carbon coating.

hydrophobicity, surface energy, surface chemistry, roughness and interaction with biological molecules can be modified. This can allow manufacture of specific material for specific application (Kaczorowski 2010, Lysko 2012). Finally, Fig. 10.8 presents a PDMS surface modified with a DLC coating.

10.4 Conclusions and future trends

Diamond materials have great potential for a variety of applications in the field of microfluidic devices. The aim of research in this area is to develop technology to manufacture large polycrystalline diamond plates, and also to manufacture monocrystalline diamonds in large quantities and at low cost. The synthesis of large plates of polycrystalline CVD diamond is now possible but remains too expensive.

Another goal is the development of new diamond and diamond-like materials with extreme properties (perhaps including diamond polytypes). There is also a need to develop technologies for the manufacture of micro- and nanostructures in diamond. The use of diamond in microfluidic devices can be considered analogous to the use of silicon in electronics and computers. Silicon technology was initially very expensive and exclusive, but today silicon technology is readily available at low cost.

These few examples of diamond applications are only the first step towards making diamond a suitable material for microfluidic devices. It could be especially interesting for extreme applications where the other materials cannot be used, such as in harsh environments or in situations where effective heat conductivity is required. Novel applications of microfluidic devices are dependent on the creativity and ideas of designers. There may even be potential in the future for diamond nanofluidic devices to be introduced.

10.5 Acknowledgments

Supported by the project 'Micro- and nano- systems for chemistry and biomedical diagnostics – MNS-DIAG' co-financed by the European Union via the European Regional Development Fund and the Polish state budget in the framework of the Operational Programme Innovative Economy 2007–2013, contract No. UDAPOIG.01.03.01-00-014/08.

10.6 References

Adamschik M, Hinz M, Maier C, *et al.*, 'Diamond micro system for bio-chemistry', *Diamond and Related Materials*, 2001, 10, 722–730.

Björkman H, Rangsten P, Hollman P, and Hjort K, 'Diamond replicas from microstructured silicon masters', *Sensors and Actuators*, 1999, 73, 24–29.

Björkman H., Ericson C., Hjertén S., and Hjort K., 'Diamond microchips for fast chromatography of proteins', *Sensors and Actuators B*, 2001, 79, 71–77.

Chankvetache B, '*Capillary Electrophoresis in chiral analysis*', 1997 John Wiley & Sons Ltd. England.

Chen G., 'Carbon nanotube and diamond as electrochemical detectors in microchip and conventional capillary electrophoresis', *Talanta*, 2007, 74, 326–332.

Ermakov S V, Jacobson S C, and Ramsey J M, 'Computer Simulations of Electrokinetic transport in Microfabricated Channel Structures', *Anal. Chem.*, 1998, 70, 4494–4504.

Feynman R, 1959 *'There's Plenty of Room at the Bottom'*, Miniaturization, Horace D. Gilbert Ed. Van Nostrand Reinhold.

Fijalkowski M, *'Diamond Electrophoretic Microchip cooled by the Peltier Device'*, PhD thesis, Lodz University of Technology, Poland, 2012.

Forsberg P, Jorge E O, Nyholm L, *et al.*, 'Fabrication of boron doped diamond microband electrodes for electrochemical detection in a microfluidic channel', *Diamond & Related Materials*, 2011, 20, 1121–1124.

Fu Y Q, Garcia-Gancedo L, Pang H F, *et al.*, 'Microfluidics based on ZnO/nanocrystalline diamond surface acoustic wave devices', *Biomicrofluidics* 2012, 6, 024105.

Grossman P D, and Colburn J C, *'Capillary Electrophoresis – Theory and Practice'*, Copyright Academic Press, Inc. 1992, USA.

Ghosh S, and Balandin A A, *'Graphene: Thermal and Thermoelectric Properties'*, in. *'Graphene Synthesis and Applications'* Ed. By Wonbong Choi Jo-Won Lee, Taylor & Francis Group 2012.

Guillaudeu S, Zhu X, and Aslam D M, 'Fabrication of 2-μm wide poly-crystalline diamond channels using silicon molds for micro-fluidic applications', *Diamond and Related Materials* 2003, 12, 65–69.

Hassard J, US Patent 6752914 – *Capillary Electrophoresis device* (2004).
Hesketh PJ, *BioNanoFluidic MEMS*, Springer 2008.
Kaczorowski W, Batory D, Karczemska A, *et al.*, *Diamond-like Coatings as Supports for Cell Culturing* abstract in 5th Wide Bandgap Materials – progress in synthesis and applications and 7th Diamond & Related Films jointly with 2nd International Workshop on Science and Applications of Nanoscale Diamond, 28 June–2 July, Zakopane 2010, Poland.
Karczemska A, and Sokolowska A, 'Materials for DNA sequencing chip', *Journal of Wide Bandgap Materials*, 2002, Vol.9, No.4, 243.
Karczemska A, *New Generation DNA Sequencing Chip – Selection of Material*, PhD thesis Warsaw University of Technology, 2002
Karczemska A, Witkowski D, Ralchenko V, *et al.*, *Diamond microfluidic devices manufactured with replica method*, Proc. of the Vth International Conference MEMSTECH 2009, Polyana, Ukraine 2009.
Karczemska AT, Diamonds in meteorites – Raman mapping and cathodoluminescence studies, *Journal of Achievements in Materials and Manufacturing Engineering*, 2010a, 43, 94–107.
Karczemska AT, 'Meteoritic matter and materials manufacturing', *Archives of Materials Science and Engineering*, 2010b, 45, 114–119.
Karczemska A T, Witkowski D, Ralchenko V, *et al.*, 'Diamond electrophoretic microchips – Joule heating effects', *Materials Science and Engineering B*, 2011, 176, 326–330.
Karczemska A, Ralchenko V, Bolshakov A, *et al.*, 'Application of Diamond for Microfluidic Devices'; in *Implant Expert* edited by Zbigniew Nawrat, ISBN 978-83-62023-72-1 Zabrze 2011, 107–116.
Khanna P, Villagra A, Kim S, *et al.*, 'Use of nanocrystalline diamond for microfluidic lab-on-a-chip', *Diamond & Related Materials* 2006, 15, 2073–2077.
Khanna P, Ramachandran N, Yang J, *et al.*, 'Nanocrystalline diamond microspikes increase the efficiency of ultrasonic cell lysis in a microfluidic lab-on-a-chip', *Diamond & Related Materials*, 2009, 18, 606–610.
Kidalov S V, and Shakhov F M, 'Thermal conductivity of diamond composites', *Materials*, 2009, 2, 2467–2495.
Kohn E, Adamschik M, Schmid P, *et al.*, 'Diamond electro-mechanical micro devices – technology and performance', *Diamond & Related Materials*, 2001, 10, 1684–1691.
Kumar A, Bhansali S, Oleynik I I, and Weller T M, *'Nanocrystalline Diamond Thin Films for MEMS and Biomedical Devices'*, NSF NIRT Grant 0404137.
Lysko J M, Witkowski D, Obidowski D, and Karczemska A, 'Numerical Simulations of Diamond Microfluidic Device for the Biomolecules Electrophoretic Separations' *Computer Methods in Material Science*, 9, 1 (2009) 97.
Lysko J M, Pijanowska D G, Baraniecka A, *et al.*, 2012 'Microfluidic devices for biomedical applications', *Electrical Review*, ISSN 0033-2097, R. 88 NR 3a/2012.
Manz A, Graber N, and Widmer H M, 'Miniaturised total chemical analysis systems: a novel concept for chemical sensing', *Sensors and Actuators B*, 1990, 1, 244–248.
Manz A, Harrison D, Verpoorte E, *et al.* 'Planar chips technology for miniaturization and integration of separation techniques into monitoring systems: Capillary electrophoresis on a chip', *Chromatogr*. A593 (1992) 253.
Massi M *et al.*; 'Plasma etching of DLC films for microfluidic channels', *Microelectronics Journal* 2003, 34, 635–638.
Mitura S, Mitura K, Niedzielski P, *et al.*, 'Nanocrystalline diamond, its synthesis, properties and applications', *Journal of Achievements in Materials and Manufacturing Engineering*, 2006, 16(1–2), 9–16.

Mukhopadhyay S, Roy S S, D'Sa R A *et al.*, 'Nanoscale surface modifications to control capillary flow characteristics in PMMA microfluidic devices', *Nanoscale Research Letters*, 2011, 6, 411–422.

Müller R, Schmid P, Munding A, *et al.*; 'Elements for surface microfluidics in diamond'; *Diamond and Related Materials* 2004, 13, 780–784.

Müller R, Gronmaier R, Janischowsky K, *et al.*, 'An "all-diamond" inkjet realized in sacrificial layer technology', *Diamond & Related Materials*, 2005, 14, 504–508.

Narayan R J, Boehm R D, and Sumant A V, 'Medical applications of diamond particles & surfaces', *Materials Today*, 2011, 14(4), 154–163.

Ralchenko V G, and Pimenov S M, 'Laser Processing of Diamond Films', Diamond Films and Technology, 1997, 7(1), MYU Tokyo.

Ralchenko V, *'Nano- and Microstructural Features in CVD Diamond Growth'*, NATO ASI School 'Nanostructured Carbon for Advanced Applications', Erice, Italy, 19–31 July 2000.

Ralchenko V, Vlasov I, Frolov V, *et al.*, 'CVD diamond films on surfaces with intricate shape' ed. A.A. Voevodin *et al.*, *Nanostructured Thin Films and Nanodispersion Strengthened Coatings*, Kluver, 2004, 209–220.

Ralchenko V, Schirone L, Sotgiu G, *et al.*, *Proc. 6th Int. Symp. on Diamond Materials*, The Electrochem. Soc., Pennington, USA, vol. 99–32 (2000) 72.

Saha B *et al.*; 'Improvement in lifetime and replication quality of Si micromold using N:DLC:Ni coatings for microfluidic devices'; *Sensors and Actuators B* 2010, 150, 174–182.

Sussmann R S, Brandon J R, Coe S E, *et al.*, 'CVD diamond: a new engineering material for thermal, dielectric and optical applications', *Industrial Diamond Review* 3/98, 1998.

Tian W-Ch, and Finehout E, *'Microfluidics for Biological Applications'*, Springer 2008.

Whitesides G M, 'The origin and the future of microfluidics', *Nature* 442/27 July 2006.

Witkowski D, Obidowski D, Lysko J, and Karczemska A, '3D Simulations of Microfluidic Devices', *Cieplne Maszyny Przepływowe – Turbomachinery*, 133 (2008) 359.

Wu D, Qin J, and Lin B, 'Electrophoretic separations on microfluidic chips', *Journal of Chromatography A*, 2008, 1184 (1–2), 542–559.

Yoder M N, *'Diamond Properties and Applications'*; in 'Diamond Films and Coatings' Edited by R.F. Davies; Noyes Publications 1993; ISBN 0-8155-1323-2.

Zhang X, and Haswell S J, 'Materials Matter in Microfluidic Devices', *MRS Bulletin* 31, February 2006.

'*Diamond Microfluidic Devices for Genomics and Proteomics*', EU project ERA-NET MNT/98/2006, 2007–2010.

'*The CVD diamond booklet*'; Diamond Materials 2008 available at: www.diamond-materials.com/download

'*Introduction to Capillary Electrophoresis*'; 1994 Beckman Instruments, Inc.

Index